2012
YEAR BOOK OF
CRITICAL CARE
MEDICINE®

The 2012 Year Book Series

Year Book of Anesthesiology and Pain Management™: Drs Chestnut, Abram, Black, Gravlee, Lien, Mathru, and Roizen

Year Book of Cardiology®: Drs Gersh, Cheitlin, Elliott, Gold, Graham, and Thourani

Year Book of Critical Care Medicine®: Drs Dries, Zanotti-Cavazzoni, Latenser, Martinez, Rincon, and Zwank

Year Book of Dermatology and Dermatologic Surgery™: Dr Del Rosso

Year Book of Diagnostic Radiology®: Drs Elster, Abbara, Oestreich, Offiah, Rosado de Christenson, Stephens, and Strickland

Year Book of Emergency Medicine®: Drs Hamilton, Bruno, Handly, Minczak, Mullin, Quintana, and Ramoska

Year Book of Endocrinology®: Drs Schott, Apovian, Clarke, Eugster, Ludlam, Meikle, Oetgen, Ovalle, Schteingart, and Toth

Year Book of Hand and Upper Limb Surgery®: Drs Yao, Adams, Isaacs, Lee, and Rizzo

Year Book of Medicine®: Drs Barker, Garrick, Gersh, Khardori, LeRoith, Panush, Talley, and Thigpen

Year Book of Neonatal and Perinatal Medicine®: Drs Fanaroff, Benitz, Donn, Neu, Papile, Polin, and Van Marter

Year Book of Neurology and Neurosurgery®: Drs Klimo, Minagar, Gandhi, House, Kevill, Liu, Mazia, Panagariya, Ragel, Riesenburger, Robottom, Schwendimann, Shafazand, Uhm, and Yang

Year Book of Obstetrics, Gynecology, and Women's Health®: Drs Dungan and Shulman

Year Book of Oncology®: Drs Arceci, Bauer, Chiorean, Gordon, Lawton, Murphy, Thigpen, and Tsao

Year Book of Ophthalmology®: Drs Rapuano, Cohen, Flanders, Hammersmith, Milman, Myers, Nagra, Nelson, Penne, Pyfer, Sergott, Shields, Talekar, and Vander

Year Book of Orthopedics®: Drs Morrey, Huddleston, Rose, Swiontkowski, and Trigg

Year Book of Otolaryngology-Head and Neck Surgery®: Drs Sindwani, Balough, Franco, Gapany, and Mitchell

Year Book of Pathology and Laboratory Medicine®: Drs Raab and Bissell

Year Book of Pediatrics®: Dr Stockman

Year Book of Plastic and Aesthetic Surgery™: Drs Miller, Gosman, Gurtner, Gutowski, Ruberg, Salisbury, and Smith

Year Book of Psychiatry and Applied Mental Health®: Drs Talbott, Ballenger, Buckley, Frances, Krupnick, and Mack

Year Book of Pulmonary Disease®: Drs Barker, Jones, Maurer, Spradley, Tanoue, and Willsie

Year Book of Sports Medicine®: Drs Shephard, Cantu, Feldman, Galea, Jankowski, Janssen, Lebrun, and Nieman

Year Book of Surgery®: Drs Copeland, Behrns, Daly, Eberlein, Fahey, Huber, Klodell, Mozingo, and Pruett

Year Book of Urology®: Drs Andriole and Coplen

Year Book of Vascular Surgery®: Drs Moneta, Gillespie, Starnes, and Watkins

2012 The Year Book of CRITICAL CARE MEDICINE®

Editors-in-Chief

David J. Dries, MSE, MD

John F. Perry, Jr. Chair of Trauma Surgery, Professor of Anesthesiology, Adjunct Professor of Clinical Emergency Medicine, University of Minnesota; Assistant Medical Director for Surgical Care, HealthPartners Medical Group, Minneapolis, Minnesota; Director of Critical Care Services and Director of Academic Programs, Department of Surgery, Regions Hospital, St. Paul, Minnesota

Sergio L. Zanotti-Cavazzoni, MD

Assistant Professor of Medicine, Cooper Medical School of Rowan University; Adjunct Professor, Robert Wood Johnson Medical School, University of Medicine and Dentistry of New Jersey; Program Director, Critical Care Medicine Fellowship, Division of Critical Care Medicine, Cooper University Hospital, Camden, New Jersey

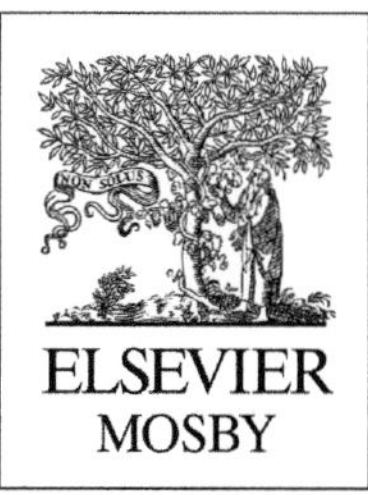

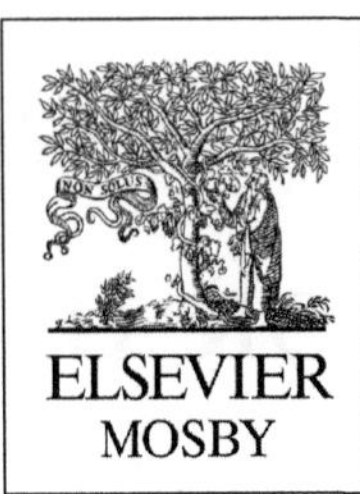

Vice President, Continuity: Kimberly Murphy
Developmental Editor: Patrick Manley
Production Supervisor, Electronic Year Books: Donna M. Skelton
Electronic Article Manager: Mike Sheets
Illustrations and Permissions Coordinator: Dawn Vohsen

2012 EDITION

Printed and bound by CPI Group (UK) Ltd, Croydon, CR0 4YY
Transferred to Digital Print 2012

Composition by TNQ Books and Journals Pvt Ltd, India

Editorial Office:
Elsevier
Suite 1800
1600 John F. Kennedy Blvd.
Philadelphia, PA 19103-2899

International Standard Serial Number: 0734-3299
International Standard Book Number: 978-0-323-08875-6

Associate Editors

Barbara A. Latenser, MD
Professor of Surgery, Division of Acute Care Surgery, Department of Surgery, University of Iowa, Iowa City, Iowa

Elizabeth A. Martinez, MD, MHS
Associate Professor of Anesthesia, Critical Care and Pain Medicine, Massachusetts General Hospital, Harvard University, Boston, Massachusetts

Fred Rincon, MD, MSc, FACP
Assistant Professor of Neurology and Neurological Surgery, Department of Neurological Surgery, Thomas Jefferson University and Jefferson College of Medicine; Staff Neurointensivist, Division of Critical Care and Neurotrauma, Jefferson Hospital for Neurosciences, Philadelphia, Pennsylvania

Michael D. Zwank, MD, RDMS, FACEP
Assistant Professor, Department of Emergency Medicine, University of Minnesota Medical School, Minneapolis, Minnesota; Staff Physician, Emergency Department, Regions Hospital, St. Paul, Minnesota

Guest Editors

Guest Editor for Quality Improvement

Gary B. Collins, MD, MBA

Department Head, Surgery; Associate Medical Director, Quality & Safety, Regions Hospital, St. Paul, Minnesota

Guest Editor for Transfusion in the Critically Ill

David R. Gerber, DO

Associate Professor of Medicine, Cooper Medical School of Rowan University; Adjunct Professor, Robert Wood Johnson Medical School, University of Medicine and Dentistry of New Jersey; Associate Director, Medical/Surgical Intensive Care Unit, Cooper University Hospital, Camden, New Jersey

Guest Editor for Infection

Anand Kumar, MD

Associate Professor of Medicine, Cooper Medical School of Rowan University; Adjunct Professor, Robert Wood Johnson Medical School, University of Medicine and Dentistry of New Jersey; Division of Critical Care Medicine and Division of Infectious Diseases, Cooper University Hospital, Camden, New Jersey; Associate Professor of Medicine, Sections of Critical Care Medicine and Infectious Disease, University of Manitoba, Winnipeg, Canada

Guest Editor for Ethics

Vijay K. Rajput, MD

Associate Professor of Medicine and Assistant Dean for Curriculum, Cooper Medical School of Rowan University; Adjunct Professor, Robert Wood Johnson Medical School, University of Medicine and Dentistry of New Jersey; Program Director, Internal Medicine Residency, Cooper University Hospital, Camden, New Jersey; Associate Fellow, Center for Bioethics, University of Pennsylvania, Philadelphia, Pennsylvania

Guest Editor for Cardiology

Steven W. Werns, MD

Professor of Medicine, Cooper Medical School of Rowan University; Adjunct Professor, Robert Wood Johnson Medical School, University of Medicine and Dentistry of New Jersey; Director, Invasive Cardiovascular Services, Cooper University Hospital, Camden, New Jersey

Contributing Editors

Robert A. Balk, MD

J. Bailey Carter, MD, Professor of Medicine, Rush Medical College; Director, Division of Pulmonary and Critical Care Medicine, Rush University Medical Center, Chicago, Illinois

Saugat Dey, MBBS

Clinical Observer and Research Volunteer, Neurological Surgery, Thomas Jefferson University, Philadelphia, Pennsylvania

Duane Funk, MD

Assistant Professor of Anesthesia, University of Manitoba; Department of Anesthesia and Section of Critical Care Medicine, Winnipeg Health Sciences Center, Winnipeg, Manitoba, Canada

Sayantani Ghosh, MBBS

Clinical Observer and Research Volunteer, Neurological Surgery, Thomas Jefferson University, Philadelphia, Pennsylvania

Zoulficar Kobeissi, MD

Assistant Professor of Clinical Medicine, Weill-Cornell School of Medicine, New York, New York; Intensivist, Division of Critical Care Medicine, The Methodist Hospital, Houston, Texas

Jocelyn Mitchell-Williams, MD, PhD

Associate Dean for Multicultural and Community Affairs, Cooper Medical School of Rowan University; Adjunct Professor, Robert Wood Johnson Medical School, University of Medicine and Dentistry of New Jersey; Department of Obstetrics and Gynecology, Cooper University Hospital, Camden, New Jersey

Nitin Puri, MD

Medical Intensivist, Inova Fairfax Hospital, Falls Church, Virginia

Collaborative Reviewers

Marcus Blouw, MD
Postdoctoral Fellow, Department of Medicine, Section of Critical Care, University of Manitoba, Winnipeg, Canada

Mariane Charron, MD
Postdoctoral Fellow, Department of Medicine, Division of Critical Care Medicine, Cooper University Hospital, Camden, New Jersey

Emily Damuth, MD
Postdoctoral Fellow, Department of Medicine, Division of Critical Care Medicine, Cooper University Hospital, Camden, New Jersey

Ben Goodgame, MD
Postdoctoral Fellow, Department of Medicine, Division of Critical Care Medicine, Cooper University Hospital, Camden, New Jersey

Shravan Kethireddy, MD
Postdoctoral Fellow, Department of Medicine, Section of Critical Care, University of Manitoba, Winnipeg, Canada

Munira Mehta, MD
Postdoctoral Fellow, Department of Medicine, Division of Critical Care Medicine, Cooper University Hospital, Camden, New Jersey

Utkal Patel, MD
Postdoctoral Fellow, Department of Medicine, Division of Critical Care Medicine, Cooper University Hospital, Camden, New Jersey

Vivek Punjabi, MD
Postdoctoral Fellow, Department of Medicine, Division of Critical Care Medicine, Cooper University Hospital, Camden, New Jersey

Ulug M. Unligil, MD
Postdoctoral Fellow, Department of Medicine, Section of Critical Care, University of Manitoba, Winnipeg, Canada

Travante Cartwright, MD
Resident, Department of Medicine, Division of Internal Medicine, Cooper University Hospital, Camden, New Jersey

Robert C. Perez, MD
Resident, Department of Surgery, Cooper University Hospital, Camden, New Jersey

Krysta Contino, BS
Medical Student, Robert Wood Johnson Medical School, University of Medicine and Dentistry of New Jersey, Camden, New Jersey

Lydia Irwin, BS
Medical Student, Robert Wood Johnson Medical School, University of Medicine and Dentistry of New Jersey, Camden, New Jersey

Christie Mannino, BS
Medical Student, Robert Wood Johnson Medical School, University of Medicine and Dentistry of New Jersey, Camden, New Jersey

William M. Rafelson, MBA
Medical Student, Robert Wood Johnson Medical School, University of Medicine and Dentistry of New Jersey, Camden, New Jersey

Table of Contents

Journals Represented

Journals represented in this YEAR BOOK are listed below.

Academic Emergency Medicine
Acta Anaesthesiologica Scandinavica
American Journal of Cardiology
American Journal of Clinical Pathology
American Journal of Emergency Medicine
American Journal of Otolaryngology
American Journal of Respiratory and Critical Care Medicine
American Journal of Surgery
American Surgeon
Anaesthesia
Anaesthesia and Intensive Care
Anesthesiology
Annals of Emergency Medicine
Annals of Plastic Surgery
Annals of Surgery
Annals of Thoracic Surgery
Archives of Internal Medicine
Archives of Surgery
British Journal of Surgery
Burns
Canadian Journal of Anaesthesia
Chest
Circulation
Circulation Cardiovascular Quality and Outcomes
Clinical Infectious Diseases
Critical Care Medicine
Current Opinion in Anaesthesiology
European Journal of Vascular and Endovascular Surgery
Heart
Infection
Injury
Intensive Care Medicine
Journal of Bone and Joint Surgery (American)
Journal of Burn Care & Research
Journal of Emergency Medicine
Journal of Neurosurgery
Journal of Orthopaedic Trauma
Journal of Pediatrics
Journal of Surgical Research
Journal of the American College of Surgeons
Journal of the American Medical Association
Journal of the American Society of Nephrology
Journal of Thoracic and Cardiovascular Surgery
Journal of Trauma
Journal of Ultrasound in Medicine
Journal of Vascular and Interventional Radiology
Lancet

Neurosurgery
New England Journal of Medicine
Obstetrics & Gynecology
Pharmacotherapy
Plastic and Reconstructive Surgery
Prehospital Emergency Care
Science
Spine
Stroke
Thrombosis Research
Transfusion
Transplantation
World Journal of Surgery

Standard Abbreviations

The following terms are abbreviated in this edition: acquired immunodeficiency syndrome (AIDS), cardiopulmonary resuscitation (CPR), central nervous system (CNS), cerebrospinal fluid (CSF), computed tomography (CT), deoxyribonucleic acid (DNA), electrocardiography (ECG), health maintenance organization (HMO), human immunodeficiency virus (HIV), intensive care unit (ICU), intramuscular (IM), intravenous (IV), magnetic resonance (MR) imaging (MRI), and ribonucleic acid (RNA).

Note

The Year Book of Critical Care Medicine® is a literature survey service providing abstracts of articles published in the professional literature. Every effort is made to assure the accuracy of the information presented in these pages. Neither the editors nor the publisher of the Year Book of Critical Care Medicine® can be responsible for errors in the original materials. The editors' comments are their own opinions. Mention of specific products within this publication does not constitute endorsement.

To facilitate the use of the Year Book of Critical Care Medicine® as a reference tool, all illustrations and tables included in this publication are now identified as they appear in the original article. This change is meant to help the reader recognize that any illustration or table appearing in the Year Book of Critical Care Medicine® may be only one of many in the original article. For this reason, figure and table numbers will often appear to be out of sequence within the Year Book of Critical Care Medicine®.

Preface

Welcome to the YEAR BOOK OF CRITICAL CARE MEDICINE for 2012!

A new editorial team wishes to acknowledge the invaluable input and example set by our predecessors. Dr R. Phillip Dellinger and Dr Joseph E. Parrillo continue to be international thought leaders in our field. This partnership has made the YEAR BOOK OF CRITICAL CARE MEDICINE a reality.

This edition introduces new lead editors: Dr David J. Dries in Surgery from Regions Hospital and the University of Minnesota and Dr. Sergio L. Zanotti-Cavazzoni from the Cooper Medical School of Rowan University and Cooper University Hospital. We will do our best to live up to the standard of our predecessors.

The other senior members of the editorial team are a diverse associate editor group. Dr Barbara Latenser of the University of Iowa provides her insight into burn care. Dr Fred Rincon of Thomas Jefferson University Hospitals adds his passion and expertise in neurologic critical care. Dr Elizabeth Martinez from Massachusetts General Hospital is leading our reviews in critical care anesthesiology while Dr Michael Zwank of the University of Minnesota and Regions Hospital reviews emergency medicine management for critical illness.

The editors and associate editors continue to receive invaluable input from a group of national authorities serving as guest editors for this edition. For the input of all, we are most grateful.

In addition to the print volume for the YEAR BOOK OF CRITICAL CARE MEDICINE, we are giving additional emphasis to development of the online portion of this reference with earlier availability to key articles identified by the editors. Dr Dries and Dr Zanotti-Cavazzoni will lead this project with specific input from associate and guest editors as necessary. Thus, more of our reviews will be available online in real time and in our annual bound collection.

Most important are the individuals facilitating our editorial process. Ms. Toni Piper at Cooper University Hospital remains an editorial resource for the YEAR BOOK OF CRITICAL CARE MEDICINE. She is joined by Mrs Sherry Willett at Regions Hospital in St Paul, Minnesota. Finally, the editorial team and offices at Cooper University Medical Center and Regions Hospital acknowledge the invaluable support of Mr Patrick Manley and the editorial team at Elsevier.

We hope you enjoy this issue of the YEAR BOOK OF CRITICAL CARE MEDICINE.

Respectfully,

David J. Dries, MSE, MD
Sergio Zanotti-Cavazzoni, MD

1 Airways/Lungs

Airway

Trauma patients can be safely extubated in the emergency department

Weingart SD, Menaker J, Truong H, et al (Mount Sinai School of Medicine, NY; Shock Trauma Ctr, Baltimore, MD)

J Emerg Med 40:235-239, 2011

Background.—Many trauma patients are intubated for conditions that fully resolve during their emergency department (ED) stay. Often, these patients remain intubated until after they leave the ED.

Objective.—The objective of this study was to examine the prognosis of patients extubated in the ED.

Methods.—Data from the records of adult trauma patients who were intubated and then extubated in the ED at a single trauma referral center were prospectively collected for a quality initiative. Two trained abstractors retrospectively recorded these data as well as additional information from the trauma registry and patient charts. The primary outcome was the need for unplanned reintubation during hospitalization. Additional outcomes were disposition and complications from the extubation.

Results.—There were 50 eligible patients identified and included in the study. Reasons for the intubation included combative behavior or decreased mental status before computed axial tomography (CT) scan in 24 patients (48%), sedation before the performance of a painful procedure in 18 patients (36%), and seizures before CT scan in 3 patients (6%). None of the patients (0%; 95% confidence interval 0–6%) required unplanned reintubation. Eight (16%) of the patients were able to be discharged from the ED before admission.

Conclusions.—Although our findings must be verified in larger, controlled studies, it may be safe to extubate patients in the ED, if the condition necessitating intubation has fully resolved. This practice may reduce admission rates and limit the need for intensive care unit beds for the patients who are admitted (Fig 1).

▶ As critical care resources become increasingly limited and emergency department stays lengthened, we must be willing to extubate patients without obvious problems after initial workup is complete. A protocol for doing this, which evaluates both readiness to extubate and respiratory muscle capacity, is included.[1,2]

ED Extubation Protocol

Inclusion

- Resolution of clinical issue requiring intubation
- Sat > 95% on FiO2 ≤ 40%, PEEP ≤ 5 cm H_2O
- RR < 30, SBP > 100, HR < 130
- Patient not known to be a difficult intubation

Preparation

- Turn off sedatives
- Leave opioids on at a low dose (e.g., fentanyl 50 μg/h)
- Allow patient to regain full mental status
- If patient shows signs of discomfort, consider administering more pain medication.
- Patient should be able to understand and respond to commands

Testing for Readiness

- Ask patient to raise arm and leave in air for 15 seconds
- Ask patient to raise their head off the bed
- Ask patient to cough, they should be able to generate a strong cough
- Place Patient on Pressure Support at a setting of 5 cm H_2O. Sit patient up to at least 45°. Observe for 15-30 minutes. If Sat < 90%, HR > 140, SBP > 200, severe anxiety, or decreased LOC–discontinue extubation attempt.

Procedure

- Have a nebulizer filled with normal saline attached to a mask
- Sit pt up to at least 45°
- Suction ET tube with bronchial suction catheter
- Suction oropharynx with Yankeur suction
- Deflate the ET tube cuff
- Have the patient cough, pull the tube during the cough
- Suction the oropharynx again
- Encourage the patient to keep coughing up any secretions
- Place the nebulizer mask on the patient at 4–6 LPM

After Extubation

- Patient should receive close monitoring for at least 60 minutes
- If patient develops respiratory distress, NIV will often be sufficient to avoid reintubation.

FIGURE 1.—Protocol for ED extubation. When first starting to perform ED extubation, all patients should be admitted to the hospital for further observation. Sat = oxygen saturation; PEEP = positive end-expiratory pressure; RR = respiratory rate; SBP = systolic blood pressure; HR = heart rate; LOC = level of consciousness; ET = endotracheal; LPM = liters per minute; NIV = non-invasive ventilation. (Reprinted from Weingart SD, Menaker J, Truong H, et al. Trauma patients can be safely extubated in the emergency department. *J Emerg Med.* 2011;40:235-239, Copyright 2011, with permission from Elsevier.)

I note that the authors recommend 1 hour of observation for these patients after extubation. Given the increasing length of emergency department stays, this should not be a problem.

Intubation is frequently appropriate to facilitate expeditious workup, which will frequently allow exclusion of potential injuries. Admission of these patients to the intensive care unit to simply go through a weaning protocol is a waste of resources.

D. J. Dries, MSE, MD

References

1. Ely EW, Bennett PA, Bowton DL, Murphy SM, Florance AM, Haponik EF. Large scale implementation of a respiratory therapist-driven protocol for ventilator weaning. *Am J Respir Crit Care Med.* 1999;159:439-446.
2. Dries DJ, McGonigal MD, Malian MS, Bor BJ, Sullivan C. Protocol-driven ventilator weaning reduces use of mechanical ventilation, rate of early reintubation, and ventilator-associated pneumonia. *J Trauma.* 2004;56:943-952.

Usefulness and Safety of Open Tracheostomy by a Paramedian Approach for Cervical Infection: Esophageal and Tracheal Injury and Necrotizing Fasciitis

Moriwaki Y, Sugiyama M, Iwashita M, et al (Yokohama City Univ Med Ctr, Japan)

Am Surg 76:1251-1254, 2010

Tracheostomy is hardly performed in patients with cervical infection close to the site of the tracheostomy. This study aimed to present and clarify the usefulness and safety of open tracheostomy performed by the paramedian approach technique. The procedure is as follows. A 2.5-cm paramedian incision is made for the tracheostomy on the opposite side of infectious focus; the anterior neck muscles are dissected and split; the trachea is fenestrated by a reverse U-shaped incision; and the fenestral flap of the trachea is fixed to the skin. We used this technique in five patients. There were no complications such as bleeding, desaturation, and displacement of the tube; and there were no postoperative complications such as severe contamination or infection of the tracheostomy site from the nearby cervical wound, difficulty in securing the tracheostomy tube and connecting device to the ventilator, difficulties in daily management and care, or dislocation of the tracheostomy tube. All wounds resulting from the tracheostomy were kept separate from and not contaminated by the nearby dirty wounds. Open tracheostomy by the paramedian approach technique is useful and

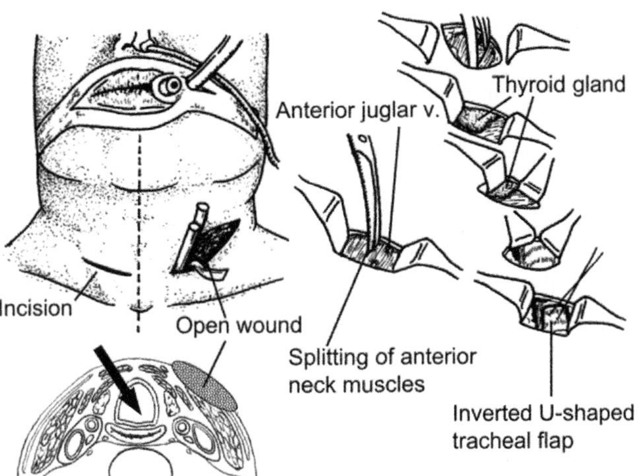

FIGURE 1.—The schema of the technique: a 2.5-cm transverse paramedian incision on the opposite side against to the dirty wound; dissecting, splitting, and cutting if necessary of the anterior neck muscles; ligation of the anterior jugular vein if necessary; disclosure of the cervical tracheal surface; and reverse U-shaped incision of the trachea. (Reprinted from Moriwaki Y, Sugiyama M, Iwashita M, et al. Usefulness and safety of open tracheostomy by a paramedian approach for cervical infection: esophageal and tracheal injury and necrotizing fascitis. *Am Surg*. 2010;76:1251-1254, Copyright 2010, with permission from Elsevier.)

safe for patients with severe cervical infection requiring open drainage and long ventilatory management (Fig 1).

▶ This is an interesting extension of a common open procedure that may be appropriate in patients with localized central soft tissue injury or an operative procedure in which the midline should be avoided.[1] Obviously, the infection, if infection is to be avoided, must be superficial. A deep infection could easily involve the paratracheal tissues, even if its cutaneous manifestation is lateral to the midline.

The authors describe only open procedures. They do believe that this approach can be used with a percutaneous technique as well and suggest this in the article. I was encouraged to see that the authors develop an inferior tracheal flap as part of the open procedures which, in my opinion, helps to protect the mediastinum and inferior structures.

Finally, the authors demonstrate durability of this approach and suggest that no medial tissue breakdown occurs. I believe that it is pragmatic to image the neck prior to placing a tracheostomy via a paramedian approach.

D. J. Dries, MSE, MD

Reference

1. Rana S, Pendem S, Pogodzinski MS, Hubmayr RD, Gajic O. Tracheostomy in critically ill patients. *Mayo Clin Proc.* 2005;80:1632-1638.

Emergency surgical airway in life-threatening acute airway emergencies – why are we so reluctant to do it?

Greenland KB, Acott C, Segal R, et al (The Univ of Queensland, Brisbane, Australia; Royal Adelaide Hosp, South Australia, Australia; Royal Melbourne Hosp, Victoria, Australia; et al)

Anaesth Intensive Care 39:578-584, 2011

'Can't intubate, can't oxygenate' scenarios are rare but are often poorly managed, with potentially disastrous consequences. In our opinion, all doctors should be able to create a surgical airway if necessary. More practically, at least all anaesthetists should have this ability. There should be a change in culture to one that encourages and facilitates the performance of a life-saving emergency surgical airway when required. In this regard, an understanding of the human factors that influence the decision to perform an emergency surgical airway is as important as technical skill. Standardisation of difficult airway equipment in areas where anaesthesia is performed is a step toward ensuring that an emergency surgical airway will be performed appropriately. Information on the incidence and clinical management of 'can't intubate, can't oxygenate' scenarios should be compiled through various sources, including national coronial inquest databases and anaesthetic critical incident reporting systems. A systematic approach to teaching and maintaining human factors in airway crisis management

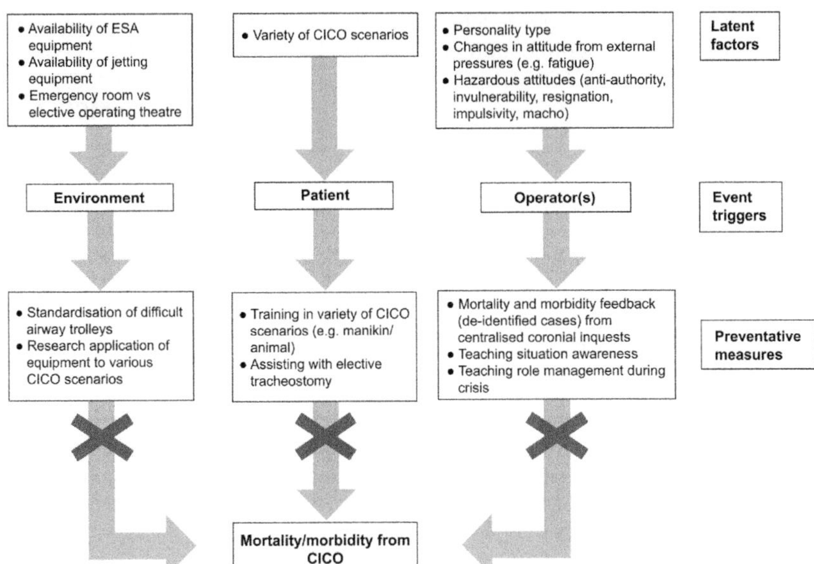

FIGURE 1.—Factors influencing the occurrence of 'can't intubate, can't oxygenate' scenarios. (Modified from Professor David Gaba's original figure[12], with kind permission). ESA=emergency surgical airway, CICO='can't intubate, can't oxygenate'. *Editor's Note*: Please refer to original journal article for full references. (Reprinted from Greenland KB, Acott C, Segal R, et al. Emergency surgical airway in life-threatening acute airway emergencies – why are we so reluctant to do it? *Anaesth Intensive Care*. 2011;39:578-584, with permission of the Australian Society of Anaesthetists.)

and emergency surgical airway skills to anaesthetic trainees and specialists should be developed: in our opinion participation should be mandatory. Importantly, the view that performing an emergency surgical airway is an admission of anaesthetist failure should be strongly countered (Fig 1).

▶ This presentation begins with case summaries of 4 patients dying after various oral surgical procedures. Patients were successfully extubated but later had airway obstruction that could not be addressed with reintubation. Frequently, a practitioner with surgical airway skills was not present. These authors argue for a broader approach to the emergency surgical airway among anesthesiologists who inevitably will be called upon to address this problem.[1,2]

In addition to careful evaluation of the patient, an appropriate environment with necessary equipment and training that includes the use of surgical airway techniques should be considered. These authors appropriately identify the human factors considerations, which are now receiving great attention in avoidance of wrong site surgery and other intraoperative problems.[3] The attached flow chart details some of the interventions and changes in intellectual approach that may be helpful in reducing mortality and morbidity from cerebral ischaemia of cardiac origin (Fig 1).

Perhaps the essential observations are the need for improved human factors management, broader training of the anesthesiologist, and a multidisciplinary airway team approach using general surgeons with head and neck specialists. Along with resource identification and improved training, a centralized reporting system with feedback and evaluation of near misses should be used.

D. J. Dries, MSE, MD

References

1. Heard AM, Green RJ, Eakins P. The formulation and introduction of a 'can't intubate, can't ventilate' algorithm into clinical practice. *Anaesthesia.* 2009;64:601-608.
2. Henderson JJ, Popat MT, Latto IP, Pearce AC. Difficult Airway Society guidelines for management of the unanticipated difficult intubation. *Anaesthesia.* 2004;59:675-694.
3. Cuschieri A. Nature of human error: implications for surgical practice. *Ann Surg.* 2006;244:642-648.

Temperature distribution in the upper airway after inhalation injury

Rong Y-H, Liu W, Wang C, et al (Beijing Jishuitan Hosp, PR China; Union Hosp Affiliated to Fujian Med Univ, PR China)

Burns 37:1187-1191, 2011

Objective.—The aim of the study was to establish an animal model of laryngeal burn and to investigate the temperature distribution of heated air in the upper airway.

Methods.—The animal model was established by inhalation of dry heated air at 80, 160 and 320°C in 18 healthy, male, adult hybrid dogs. Time for inducing injury was set at 20 min. The distribution of temperatures after heated-air inhalation was examined at different locations including the epiglottis, laryngeal vestibule, vocal folds and trachea.

Results.—The temperatures of the heated air decreased to 47.1, 118.4 and 193.8°C at the laryngeal vestibule and to 39.3, 56.6 and 137.9°C at the lower margin of vocal folds in the 80, 160 and 320°C groups, respectively.

Conclusion.—Due to its special anatomy and functions, the larynx has different responses to dry heated air at different temperatures. The air temperature decreases markedly when the air arrives at the larynx. By contrast, the larynx has a low capacity for blocking high-temperature air and retaining heat. As a result, high-temperature air often causes more severe injury to the larynx and the lower airway (Fig 1).

▶ The thermal injury to the respiratory tract in cases of inhalation injury is usually limited to the upper respiratory tract, mainly the trachea, and is due to 2 factors. There is heat conduction along the tracheal surface and convection from fluid flow of incoming air along the boundary of the tracheal lumen surface. Because the burn concentration is a function of temperature, the extent of the burn rises as temperature increases with inspiration and remains constant as temperature decreases during expiration. The 2 largest variations of fire are the temperature that the fire reaches depending on the material burnt (air, gasoline, chemical vapors, wood, or other insulation and building materials) and the duration of the exposure. However, the thermal changes within the tracheal

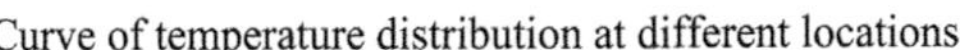

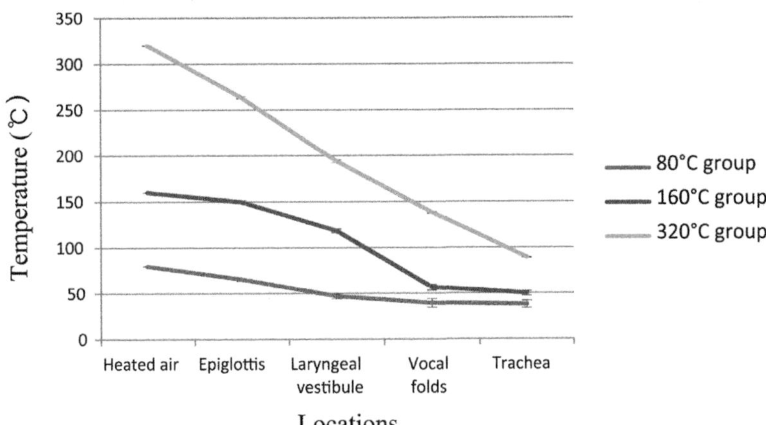

FIGURE 1.—Curve of temperature distribution at different locations in the three groups. (Reprinted from Rong Y-H, Liu W, Wang C, et al. Temperature distribution in the upper airway after inhalation injury. *Burns*. 2011;37:1187-1191, Copyright 2011, with permission from International Society for Burn Injuries.)

tissue do not depend merely on the inlet air temperature. The tissue is supplied by blood vessels, which play a role in heat exchange, and is also constantly carrying out metabolism. Thus, other factors taken into consideration when considering thermal injury include the metabolic rate of tissue, blood perfusion, and various arterial and metabolic effects.

The authors set out to develop an animal model of airway burns, looking at the effect of different air temperatures throughout the upper airway. The maximum temperature a human can incur before tissue damage is 45°C. In this study, the authors use temperatures of 80, 160, and 320°C. What they discovered is a simple but elegant demonstration of the effect of different air temperatures on various locations within the upper airways. Air temperatures do not diminish at the same rate over different locations in the upper airway (see Fig 1, curve of temperature distribution at different locations in the 3 groups). A better understanding of the interplay between transient temperature and injury distribution over the trachea may help to direct treatment of inhalation injury in the future.

B. A. Latenser, MD, FACS

Use of Sonography for Rapid Identification of Esophageal and Tracheal Intubations in Adult Patients

Muslu B, Sert H, Kaya A, et al (Fatih Univ, Ankara, Turkey)
J Ultrasound Med 30:671-676, 2011

Objectives.—The aim of this study was to investigate the usefulness of sonography for verifying tracheal tube placement within 3 seconds in adult surgical patients.

Methods.—This was a blinded prospective randomized study. The anesthesiologist placed the tracheal tube randomly in the trachea (n = 75) or in the esophagus (n = 75) with direct laryngoscopy. A sonographer identified all tracheal and esophageal intubations. The transducer was placed transversely on the neck just superior to the suprasternal notch. The position of the tracheal tube was determined by the sonographer within 3 seconds of tracheal tube placement in the trachea or in the esophagus.

Results.—We successfully identified 150 correct tracheal tube placements in tracheas and esophagi, resulting in sensitivity of 100% (95% confidence interval, 84%–100%) and specificity of 100% (95% confidence interval, 84%–100%).

Conclusions.—This investigation shows that sonography for confirming tracheal intubation is a fast and effective technique.

▶ Bedside ultrasound is increasingly ubiquitous in many medical specialties. This is a randomized controlled trial examining the reliability of bedside ultrasound in detecting tracheal and esophageal intubations. The ultrasounds were performed with a linear probe examining the tracheal and paratracheal neck in a transverse plane (Figs 2 and 3 in the original article). One hundred fifty patients were included, which fares well compared with similar ultrasound studies that examine novel techniques. Limitations to the study included generally young patients with normal body habitus and normal anatomy and a single experienced sonographer performing all ultrasounds. Within that context, the results were perfect. All intubations were correctly identified as esophageal or tracheal. The results do support the technique as a reasonable option for those performing intubations. Although this will not likely replace any of the more widely accepted methods of endotracheal tube placement confirmation, such as end-tidal CO_2 detectors, it can be considered as an adjunct. Its usefulness may be more pronounced in more resource-limited settings. As with any ultrasound application, the reliability of the ultrasound lies within the experience of the user.

M. D. Zwank, MD

Mechanical Ventilation/Weaning

Increase in Early Mechanical Ventilation of Burn Patients: An Effect of Current Emergency Trauma Management?

MacKie DP, van Dehn F, Knape P, et al (Red Cross Hosp, Beverwijk, The Netherlands; et al)

J Trauma 70:611-615, 2011

Background.—Data relating to patients admitted with extensive burn injuries in the Netherlands have revealed a marked increase in patients whose initial care included mechanical ventilation (MV). The increase was abrupt, dating from 1997, and has been sustained since. The aim of this study is to quantify this observation and to discuss possible causes.

Methods.—The study included 258 consecutive patients with burns >30% total body surface area admitted to the Beverwijk burns center. Patients were divided into two groups based on admission date: group 1 from 1987 to 1996 (n = 135) and group 2 from 1997 to 2006 (n = 123). Data were analyzed using χ^2 or analysis of variance.

Results.—There were no differences between groups in demographics, facial burns, inhalation injury, and % total body surface area. However, the number of patients subjected to MV at admission increased from 38% to 76% (group 1 vs. 2; $p < 0.001$). In 57% of patients who were intubated based on the suspicion of inhalation injury, this condition could not be confirmed ($p < 0.05$ vs. 9% [1987–1996]).

Conclusions.—This study has confirmed that a higher proportion of patients were treated with MV since 1997, whereas the severity of burn injury remained unchanged throughout the study period. In the absence of a clinical explanation, we surmise that there has been a change within Dutch casualty departments in the initial management of major burn injury. The change coincides with the implementation of the Advanced Life Trauma Support training course as the accepted standard of trauma care in Dutch hospitals.

▶ This small study is an important work. Using the Beverwijk Burns Center database from 1987 to 2006, the authors looked at airway management before and after the introduction of Advanced Trauma Life Support (ATLS) in the Netherlands. They describe what they call "ventilator creep" to describe the increase in mechanical ventilation (MV) in recent years. Although the impact of this increase in MV was not studied, one can certainly speculate about some of the effects of being intubated: increased fluid requirements, being in an intensive care unit, increase in health care costs, and the hazards of intubation in a prehospital setting: vocal cord injury, increased risk of respiratory infection/aspiration, and unnecessary medication, such as succinylcholine.

I suspect these data are reflective of practices in other high-income countries where ATLS has been taught and is practiced. I believe one of the main issues is the teaching that facial burns = inhalation injury = endotracheal tube. Education of emergency care providers will allow them to understand that although 85% of patients with inhalation injuries have facial burns, 85% of patients with facial burns do not have an inhalation injury. Other factors, such as being in an enclosed space, carbonaceous sputum, history of unconsciousness, and stridor, are much more concerning for inhalation injury. Let's educate our colleagues and reverse this dangerous trend.

B. A. Latenser, MD, FACS

Other

Timing is Everything: Delayed Intubation is Associated with Increased Mortality in Initially Stable Trauma Patients

Miraflor E, Chuang K, Miranda MA, et al (UCSF-East Bay, Oakland)

J Surg Res 170:286-290, 2011

Background.—The indications for immediate intubation in trauma are not controversial, but some patients who initially appear stable later deteriorate and require intubation. We postulated that initially stable, moderately injured trauma patients who experienced delayed intubation have higher mortality than those intubated earlier.

Methods.—Medical records of trauma patients intubated within 3 h of arrival in the emergency department at our university-based trauma center were reviewed. Moderately injured patients were defined as an ISS < 20. Early intubation was defined as patients intubated from 10–24 min of arrival. Delayed intubation was defined as patients intubated ≥25 min after arrival. Patients requiring immediate intubation, within 10 min of arrival, were excluded.

Results.—From February 2006 to December 2007, 279 trauma patients were intubated in the emergency department. In moderately injured patients, mortality was higher with delayed intubation than with early intubation, 11.8% *versus* 1.8% ($P = 0.045$). Patients with delayed intubations had greater frequency of rib fractures than their early intubation counterparts, 23.5% *versus* 3.6% ($P = 0.004$). Patients in the delayed intubation group had lower rates of cervical gunshot wounds than the early intubation group, 0% *versus* 10.7% ($P = 0.048$) and a trend toward fewer of skull fractures 2.9% *versus* 16.1%, ($P = 0.054$).

Conclusions.—These findings suggest that delayed intubation is associated with increased mortality in moderately injured patients who are initially stable but later require intubation and can be predicted by the presence of rib fractures (Figs 2-4).

▶ The authors identify a group of patients at increased risk for late complications, including the need for an artificial airway. Rib fractures appear to be the most important indicator (Fig 3). The difference in morality between early and late intubation is striking (Fig 2).

I find the title in this paper to be somewhat deceptive. The authors describe a relationship between delayed intubation and adverse outcome. What they do not provide us with is a mechanism. In fact, there is no difference in length of stay or ventilator days in patients treated with early versus late intubation. Insertion of the airway may not be the critical intervention. Perhaps some of these patients could be adequately served with noninvasive ventilation.[1,2] Clearly, we must be cautious in the patient group with multiple rib fractures, providing aggressive respiratory monitoring and airway and ventilator support as necessary.

I was interested to see that neurologic decompensation did not strongly affect the incidence of early versus late intubation (Fig 4). This observation

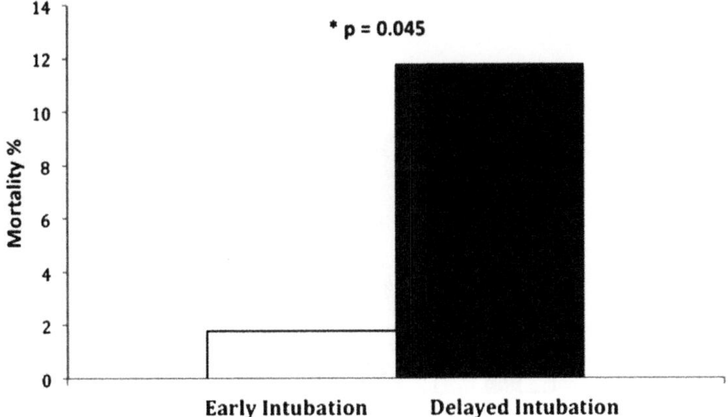

FIGURE 2.—Mortality in moderately injured patients by timing of intubation. Moderately injured patients (ISS < 20) intubated late had a higher mortality, 11.8%, than those intubated early, 1.8% ($P = 0.045$). The mortality risk reduction with earlier intubation was 85%. (Reprinted from Miraflor E, Chuang K, Miranda MA, et al. Timing is everything: delayed intubation is associated with increased mortality in initially stable trauma patients. *J Surg Res*. 2011;170:286-290, with permission from Elsevier.)

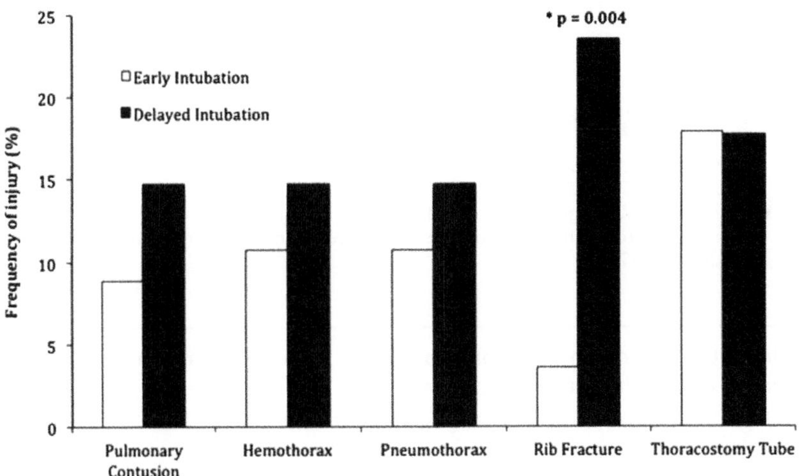

FIGURE 3.—Frequency of pulmonary contusion, hemothorax, pneumothorax, rib fracture, and thoracostomy tube by timing of intubation in moderately injured patients (ISS < 20). Patients in the delayed intubation group had a greater frequency of rib fractures, 23.5% versus 3.6% ($P = 0.004$). (Reprinted from Miraflor E, Chuang K, Miranda MA, et al. Timing is everything: delayed intubation is associated with increased mortality in initially stable trauma patients. *J Surg Res*. 2011;170:286-290, with permission from Elsevier.)

differs from the observations of respiratory management in trauma from other sites.[3]

D. J. Dries, MSE, MD

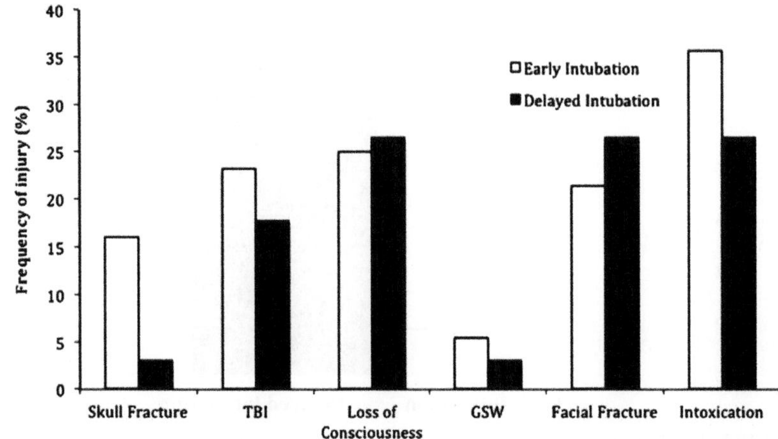

FIGURE 4.—Frequency of skull fracture, traumatic brain injury (TBI), loss of consciousness, gunshot wounds to the head (GSW), facial fractures, and intoxication by timing of intubation in moderately injured patients (ISS < 20). Patients requiring delayed intubation did not have a greater frequency of neurologic injury or intoxication. (Reprinted from Miraflor E, Chuang K, Miranda MA, et al. Timing is everything: delayed intubation is associated with increased mortality in initially stable trauma patients. *J Surg Res*. 2011;170:286-290, with permission from Elsevier.)

References

1. Hillberg RE, Johnson DC. Noninvasive ventilation. *N Engl J Med*. 1997;337: 1746-1752.
2. Garpestad E, Brennan J, Hill NS. Noninvasive ventilation for critical care. *Chest*. 2007;132:711-720.
3. Brown CV, Daigle JB, Foulkrod KH, et al. Risk factors associated with early reintubation in trauma patients: a prospective observational study. *J Trauma*. 2011;71:37-42.

A Novel CT Volume Index Score Correlates with Outcomes in Polytrauma Patients with Pulmonary Contusion

Strumwasser A, Chu E, Yeung L, et al (Univ of California, San Francisco-East Bay, Oakland)

J Surg Res 170:280-285, 2011

Background.—Exact quantification of pulmonary contusion by computed tomography (CT) may help trauma surgeons identify high-risk populations. We hypothesized that the size of pulmonary contusions, measured accurately, will predict outcomes. Our specific aims were to (1) precisely quantify pulmonary contusion size using pixel analysis, (2) correlate contusion size with outcomes, and (3) determine the threshold contusion size portending complications.

Methods.—Thoracic CTs of 106 consecutive polytrauma patients with pulmonary contusion were evaluated at a university-based urban trauma

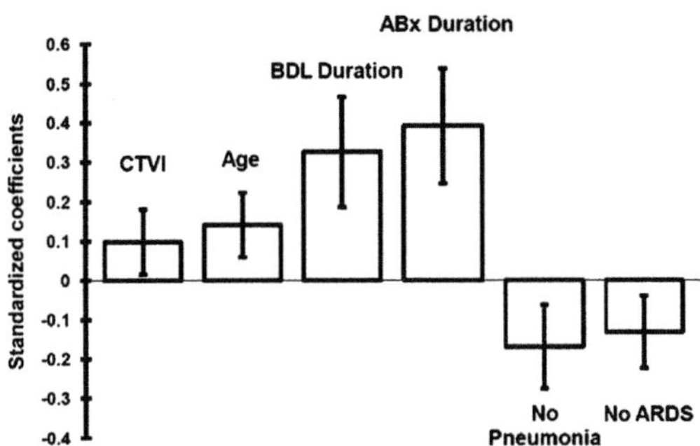

FIGURE 2.—Multivariate model (ICU LOS) standardized coefficients including pneumonia and ARDS (95% confidence intervals). On histogram analysis, CTVI is contributory to a multivariate model predicting ICU LOS, however, it is less in magnitude than age and length of antibiotic and bronchodilator support, as is evidenced by a smaller coefficient of contribution to the model. In addition, the absence of pneumonia and/or ARDS is associated with shorter ICU LOS. BDL = duration of bronchodilator therapy; Abx = duration of antibiotic therapy. (Reprinted from Strumwasser A, Chu E, Yeung L, et al. A novel CT volume index score correlates with outcomes in polytrauma patients with pulmonary contusion. *J Surg Res.* 2011;170:280-285, with permission from Elsevier.)

center. A novel CT volume index (CTVI) score was calculated based on the ratio of affected lung to total lung [slices of lung on CT × affected pixel region/lung pixel region × 0.45 (left side) + slices of lung on CT × affected pixel region/lung pixel region × 0.55 (right side)]. Multivariate analysis correlated CTVI and patient predictors' impact on outcomes.

Results.—Of 106 polytrauma patients (mean ISS = 28 ± 1.2, AIS chest = 3.5 ± 0.1), 39 developed complications (acute respiratory distress syndrome [ARDS], pneumonia, and/or death). Mean CTVI was significantly higher in the group with complications (0.28 ± 0.03 *versus* 17 ± 0.02, $P = 0.01$). By multivariate analysis, CTVI predicted longer ICU LOS ($R^2 = 0.84, P < 0.01$). A receiver operating curve (ROC) analysis identified a CTVI threshold score of 0.2 (AUC 0.67, $P < 0.01$) for developing pneumonia, ARDS or death. Patients with CTVI scores of 0.2 or more had longer hospitalization, longer ICU LOS, more ventilator days, and developed pneumonia ($P < 0.01$).

Conclusions.—Higher CTVI scores predicted prolonged ICU LOS across all sizes of pulmonary contusion. Pulmonary contusion volumes greater than 20% of total lung volume specifically identify patients at risk for developing complications (Fig 2).

▶ Similar to another study reported a number of years ago from the Memphis group, these authors demonstrate a correlation between the volume of lung involved with pulmonary contusion and a variety of outcomes, including resource consumption and mortality.[1] The authors appropriately performed additional multivariate analyses, demonstrating that pharmacotherapy (antibiotics and bronchodilators) and age also contribute to outcomes. The relative contribution of factors included in the multivariate model is indicated in Fig 2.

Multivariate models do not lend themselves readily to bedside utilization. However, it is important to take away the value of quantification for size of pulmonary contusions if decisions regarding patient disposition need to be made.

D. J. Dries, MSE, MD

Reference

1. Miller PR, Croce MA, Bee TK, et al. ARDS after pulmonary contusion: accurate measurement of contusion volume identifies high-risk patients. *J Trauma.* 2001; 51:223-230.

Pulmonary function, exercise capacity and physical activity participation in adults following burn

Willis CE, Grisbrook TL, Elliott CM, et al (Univ of Western Australia, Perth; et al)
Burns 37:1326-1333, 2011

Purpose.—To determine the relationship between pulmonary function, aerobic exercise capacity and physical activity participation in adults following burn.

Methods.—Eight burn injured males aged 20–55 years (%TBSA 33.3 ± 18.7, 5.1 years ± 1.8 post injury), and 30 healthy adult controls participated. Pulmonary function was assessed during rest via spirometry. A graded exercise test measuring peak oxygen consumption (VO_{2peak}) and oxygen saturation (S_pO_2) was conducted, and physical activity was assessed via the Older Adult Exercise Status Inventory (OA-EI).

Results.—No significant correlation was observed between resting pulmonary function, aerobic capacity and physical activity participation for burn injured patients or controls. Two burn injured patients presented with obstructive ventilatory defects, and one displayed a restrictive ventilatory defect. Burn injured patients had a significantly lower VO_{2peak} ($p < 0.001$) and time to fatigue ($p = 0.026$), and a greater degree of oxygen desaturation ($p = 0.063$, Effect Size = 1.02) during a graded exercise test. Burn injured patients reported significantly less participation in leisure-related activity >9 METs ($p = 0.01$), and significantly greater participation in work-related activity ($p = 0.038$), than healthy controls.

Conclusion.—Compromised lung function, decreased aerobic capacity and reduced participation in leisure-related physical activity may still exist in some adults, even up to 5 years post injury. Limitations and long term outcomes of cardiopulmonary function and physical fitness need to be considered in the prescription of exercise rehabilitation programmes following burn.

▶ The authors have looked at the difference between postburn and never-burned adults in terms of cardiopulmonary function and physical fitness. Using a very small ($n = 8$) group of burn patients culled from their outpatient list, they compare these men to 30 never-burned men who were comparable in age and body mass index. It appears that the burn group comprised at least 1 smoker

(12.5% of the study population), and the control group comprised all never-smoked patients without past or present respiratory disease. Although not statistically significant, the burn population is 5 years older than the control group. The burn patients report significantly less participation in leisure activity (eg, physical fitness activities that I would presume include activities such as regular walking, running, bicycle riding, tennis, golf, or rock climbing) than those of the control group. If the burned patients do not participate in regular physical activity, their reduction in aerobic capacity may be more reflective of their lack of participation in leisure-related exercise due to lack of money or disabilities resulting from the burn and not an alteration in their pulmonary mechanics. Information about presence of inhalation injury at the time of admission, length of time on a ventilator, and the potential long-term sequelae of ventilators such as tracheomalacia, subglottic stenosis, or bronchiolitis is not presented. In summary, the data presented by these authors in this small, nonrandomized (and potentially biased) article does not convince me that the cardiopulmonary effects of a small (15% total body surface area [TBSA]) burn have such large effects years later. Only 1 patient had more than 40% TBSA burns, making analysis of the larger burn injury impossible. Before accepting these findings as gospel, a randomized case-controlled study should be performed. Patients with and without inhalation injury should be treated as separate entities, and knowledge of preburn physical activity status should be included in the analysis.

B. A. Latenser, MD, FACS

Two Days of Dexamethasone Versus 5 Days of Prednisone in the Treatment of Acute Asthma: A Randomized Controlled Trial

Kravitz J, Dominici P, Ufberg J, et al (St Barnabas Health System, Toms River, NJ; Albert Einstein Med Ctr, Philadelphia, PA; Temple Univ, Philadelphia, PA; et al)

Ann Emerg Med 58:200-204, 2011

Study Objective.—Dexamethasone has a longer half-life than prednisone and is well tolerated orally. We compare the time needed to return to normal activity and the frequency of relapse after acute exacerbation in adults receiving either 5 days of prednisone or 2 days of dexamethasone.

Methods.—We randomized adult emergency department patients (aged 18 to 45 years) with acute exacerbations of asthma (peak expiratory flow rate less than 80% of ideal) to receive either 50 mg of daily oral prednisone for 5 days or 16 mg of daily oral dexamethasone for 2 days. Outcomes were assessed by telephone follow-up.

Results.—Ninety-six prednisone and 104 dexamethasone subjects completed the study regimen and follow-up. More patients in the dexamethasone group reported a return to normal activities within 3 days compared with the prednisone group (90% versus 80%; difference 10%; 95% confidence interval 0% to 20%; P=.049). Relapse was similar between groups (13% versus 11%; difference 2%; 95% confidence interval −7% to 11%, P=.67).

Conclusion.—In acute exacerbations of asthma in adults, 2 days of oral dexamethasone is at least as effective as 5 days of oral prednisone in returning patients to their normal level of activity and preventing relapse.

▶ Asthma exacerbation is a very common diagnosis seen in the emergency department (ED). Although possibly lethal, it is a diagnosis that is generally easily treated, with most patients being discharged from the ED. However, one of the great challenges in treating this patient population is compliance with the treatment plan. This randomized controlled trial conducted at two urban emergency departments examined the efficacy of a 2-day course of oral dexamethasone versus a 5-day course of prednisone, which is often a standard treatment in the United States. Slightly more patients in the dexamethasone group reported returning to normal activity within 3 days (90% vs 80%; $P = .049$). There was similar use of rescue inhalers and similar relapse between the two groups (13% vs 11%). Not surprisingly, 22% of patients were lost to follow-up. Those that have frequently treated asthmatics will realize that compliance with a 2-day therapy will almost certainly exceed that of a 5-day therapy in this patient group. I would strongly recommend considering oral dexamethasone (16 mg) for 2 days when treating asthma exacerbation.

M. D. Zwank, MD

2 Cardiovascular

Cardiopulmonary Resuscitation/Other

Surgery in Adults With Congenital Heart Disease

Zomer AC, Verheugt CL, Vaartjes I, et al (Academic Med Ctr, Amsterdam, the Netherlands; VU Univ Med Ctr, Amsterdam, the Netherlands; Univ Med Ctr Utrecht, the Netherlands; et al)
Circulation 124:2195-2201, 2011

Background.—A significant proportion of patients with congenital heart disease require surgery in adulthood. We aimed to give an overview of the prevalence, distribution, and outcome of cardiovascular surgery for congenital heart disease. We specifically questioned whether the effects of surgical treatment on subsequent long-term survival depend on sex.

Methods and Results.—From the Dutch Congenital Corvitia (CONCOR) registry for adults with congenital heart disease, we identified 10 300 patients; their median age was 33.1 years. Logistic and Cox regression models were used to assess the association of surgery in adulthood with sex and with long-term survival. In total, 2015 patients (20%) underwent surgery for congenital heart disease in adulthood during a median follow-up period of 15.1 years; in 812 patients (40%), it was a reoperation. Overall, both first operations and reoperations in adulthood were performed significantly more often in men compared with women (adjusted odds ratio=1.4 [95% confidence interval, 1.2–1.6] and 1.2 [95% confidence interval, 1.0–1.4], respectively). Patients with their third and fourth or more surgery in adulthood had a 2- and 3-times-higher risk of death compared with patients never operated on (adjusted hazard ratio=1.9 [95% confidence interval, 1.0–3.6] and 2.7 [95% confidence interval, 1.1–6.3], respectively). Men with a reoperation in adulthood had a 2-times-higher risk of death than women (adjusted hazard ratio=1.9; 95% confidence interval, 1.0–3.5).

Conclusions.—Of predominantly young adults with congenital heart disease, one fifth required cardiovascular surgery during a 15-year period; in 40%, the surgery was a reoperation. Men with congenital heart disease have a higher chance of undergoing surgery in adulthood and have a consistently worse long-term survival after reoperations in adulthood compared with women (Fig, Table 4).

▶ The estimated number of adults with congenital heart disease is 1 million in the United States and 1.2 million in Europe. Given the improved early and

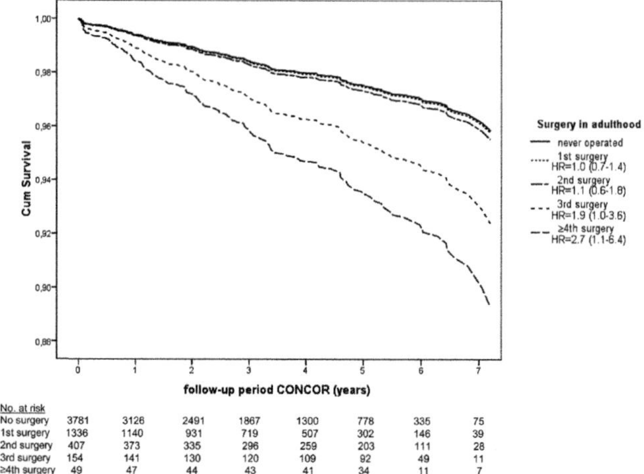

FIGURE.—Survival curves of adult patients who were never operated on (reference group), who had their first surgery in adulthood, and who had their second, third, fourth, or more surgery in adulthood. Hazard ratios (HR) (95% confidence interval) are for a median follow-up period of 3.8 years; they are shown after adjustment for age at inclusion, underlying defect, and multiple defects. CONCOR indicates Congenital Corvitia. (Reprinted from Zomer AC, Verheugt CL, Vaartjes I, et al. Surgery in adults with congenital heart disease. *Circulation*. 2011;124:2195-2201, with permission from American Heart Association, Inc.)

TABLE 4.—Sex Differences in Risk of Death in Patients Who Were Never Operated on, Who Had Their First Surgery in Adulthood, and Who Had Their Second or Third or More Surgery in Adulthood

Surgery in Adulthood	HR (95% CI)*
No surgery at all	1.84 (1.21–2.78)
First-time surgery	0.97 (0.60–1.59)
Reoperation	1.89 (1.02–3.50)
Second surgery	1.10 (0.47–2.55)
Third or more surgery†	3.78 (1.33–10.79)

*Hazard ratio (HR) (95% confidence interval [CI]) for a median follow-up period of 3.8 years, males vs females. HRs are shown after adjustment for age of inclusion, underlying defect, and multiple defects.

†Because of the small number in the category of ≥4 surgeries, this category could not be validly analyzed separately; therefore, it was combined with the category of 3 surgeries.

long-term management, many are surviving to adulthood, and a substantial number of them require additional cardiac operations.[1] This group of patients poses unique challenges to perioperative providers, and understanding their perioperative risks is important. The current article and the one that follows by Kim et al[2] evaluate outcomes in this unique patient population.

In the current study, Zomer and colleagues used the Dutch Congenital Corvitia (CONCOR) registry for adults with congenital heart disease. Of the 10 300 patients in the registry, 2015 (20%) underwent surgery for congenital heart disease in adulthood, 745 of these had their first surgery in adulthood, 213 of these had a subsequent operation as an adult, and 216 patients had an operation as a child and then subsequent operation as an adult. In this national registry, they showed that mortality risk increased with each reoperation (Fig) and that men are at higher risk than women (Table 4). The strength of this study is that it used a national registry with quality control checks to develop this risk model. While these findings may not be generalizable to non-Dutch patients because of the possibility of unique genetic variations or local differences in selection bias for surgical intervention, they are consistent with other literature sources.

The second study is from the United States and used data from the Pediatric Health Information System (PHIS) from January 2000 to 2008.[2] PHIS is an administrative database with comprehensive inpatient data from 42 not-for-profit children's hospitals. The authors evaluated the impact of clinical and admission (baseline) characteristics and adult and total (adult and pediatric) congenital heart surgery volume in each of the pediatric hospitals performing adult congenital cardiac surgery. Of the 97 563 total congenital heart surgery admissions between 2000 and 2008, 3061 were adults who underwent cardiac surgery. In their multivariate analysis, they identified age, gender, and surgical complexity (RACHS-1 score; Risk Adjustment for Congenital Heart Surgery-1) as important risk factors. They also identified that the annual adult congenital surgical volume was associated with outcomes. Those centers with ≥20 adult congenital cases had better outcomes, with an adjusted odds ratio of 0.4 (95% confidence interval, 0.2–0.7; $P = .003$). However, the total number of congenital heart surgeries, which includes both pediatric and adult procedures, was not associated with outcomes (Fig 4 in the original article). This study highlights that there may be a difference in experience and procedure technique in adult versus pediatric congenital heart procedures and that the overall experience, as represented by number of cases for both pediatric and adult patients with congenital heart disease, doesn't necessarily convey a reduced risk for the adults cared for in that hospital. This might imply that the techniques differ and thus they require different expertise. Alternatively, there may be other structures and processes of care that are in place at pediatric centers that perform ≥20 adult congenital heart procedures that impact the improved outcomes, such as the organization of the intensive care unit, the perfusionist team, or other ancillary practices.

Both studies identified a greater risk for men. In the Dutch study, they also note that men are more likely to undergo surgery and acknowledge that the women may be undertreated or that, conversely, perhaps the men are overtreated, and this increased rate of going to surgery is a potential unmeasured confounder. Increased knowledge about the risk factors for mortality and perhaps improved, standardized guidelines for surgical interventions may improve outcomes. In addition, identifying other contributors to differences in outcomes that could be implemented in lower-volume centers could be important.

E. A. Martinez, MD, MHS

References

1. van der Bom T, Zomer AC, Zwinderman AH, Meijboom FJ, Bouma BJ, Mulder BJ. The changing epidemiology of congenital heart disease. *Nat Rev Cardiol.* 2011;8: 50-60.
2. Kim YY, Gauvreau K, Bacha EA, Landzberg MJ, Benavidez OJ. Risk factors for death after adult congenital heart surgery in pediatric hospitals. *Circ Cardiovasc Qual Outcomes.* 2011;4:433-439.

Risk Factors for Death After Adult Congenital Heart Surgery in Pediatric Hospitals

Kim YY, Gauvreau K, Bacha EA, et al (Univ of Pennsylvania School of Medicine, Philadelphia; Harvard Med School, Boston, MA; Columbia Univ College of Physicians and Surgeons, NY)

Circ Cardiovasc Qual Outcomes 4:433-439, 2011

Background.—Despite the central role that pediatric hospitals play in the surgical treatment of congenital heart disease, little is known about outcomes of adult congenital cardiac surgical care in pediatric hospitals. Risk factors for inpatient death, including adult congenital heart (ACH) surgery volume, are poorly described.

Methods and Results.—We obtained inpatient data from 42 free-standing pediatric hospitals using the Pediatric Health Information System data base 2000 to 2008 and selected ACH surgery admissions (ages 18 to 49 years). We examined admission characteristics and hospital surgery volume. Of 97 563 total (pediatric and adult) congenital heart surgery admissions, 3061 (3.1%) were ACH surgery admissions. Median adult age was 22 years and 39% were between ages 25 to 49 years. Most frequent surgical procedures were pulmonary valve replacement, secundum atrial septal defect repair, and aortic valve replacement. Adult mortality rate was 2.2% at discharge. Multivariable analyses identified the following risk factors for death: age 25 to 34 years (adjusted odds ratio [AOR], 2.1; $P=0.009$), age 35 to 49 years (AOR, 3.2; $P=0.001$), male sex (AOR, 1.8; $P=0.04$), government-sponsored insurance (AOR, 1.8; $P=0.03$), and higher surgical risk categories 4+ (AOR, 21.5; $P=0.001$). After adjusting for case mix, pediatric hospitals with high ACH surgery volume had reduced odds for death (AOR, 0.4; $P=0.003$). There was no relationship between total congenital heart surgery volume and ACH inpatient mortality.

Conclusions.—Older adults, male sex, government-sponsored insurance, and greater surgical case complexity have the highest likelihood of in-hospital death when adult congenital surgery is performed in free-standing pediatric hospitals. After risk-adjustment, pediatric hospitals with high ACH surgery volume have the lowest inpatient mortality (Fig 4).

▶ The estimated number of adults with congenital heart disease is 1 million in the United States and 1.2 million in Europe. Given the improved early and long-term management, many are surviving to adulthood, and a substantial number of them require additional cardiac operations.[1] This group of patients poses unique challenges to perioperative providers, and understanding their perioperative risks is important. The current article and the preceding article by Zomer et al evaluate outcomes in this unique patient population.

In the first study, Zomer and colleagues[2] used the Dutch Congenital Corvitia (CONCOR) registry for adults with congenital heart disease. Of the 10 300 patients in the registry, 2015 (20%) underwent surgery for congenital heart disease in adulthood, 745 of these had their first surgery in adulthood, 213 of these had a subsequent operation as an adult, and 216 patients had an operation as a child

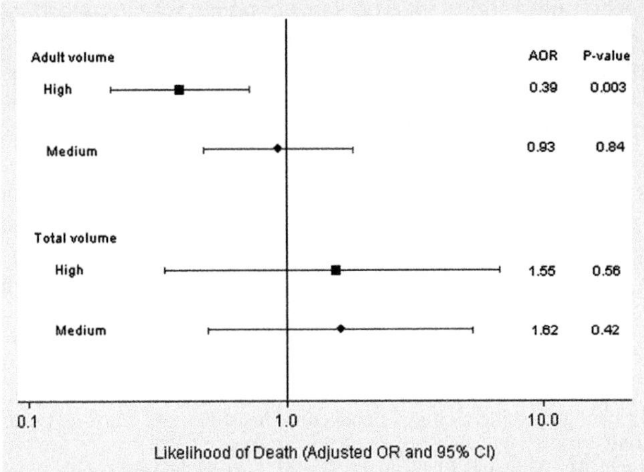

FIGURE 4.—Adjusted odds ratio (OR) for in-hospital mortality after ACH surgery in pediatric hospitals by surgery volume. Reference group is low surgery volume hospitals. High adult volume has significantly lower odds of death compared with low adult volume centers. Total (pediatric and adult) congenital heart surgery volume was not associated with in-hospital death. Error bars represent 95% CIs. (Reprinted from Kim YY, Gauvreau K, Bacha EA, et al. Risk factors for death after adult congenital heart surgery in pediatric hospitals. *Circ Cardiovasc Qual Outcomes*. 2011;4:433-439, with permission from American Heart Association, Inc.)

and then subsequent operation as an adult. In this national registry, they demonstrated that mortality risk increased with each reoperation (Fig 4 in the original article) and that men are at higher risk than women (Table 4 in the original article). The strength of this study is that it used a national registry, with quality control checks to develop this risk model. While these findings may not be generalizable to non-Dutch patients because of the possibility of unique genetic variations or local differences in selection bias for surgical intervention, they are consistent with other literature sources.

The current study is from the United States and used data from the Pediatric Health Information System (PHIS) from January 2000 to 2008. PHIS is an administrative database with comprehensive inpatient data from 42 not-for-profit children's hospitals. The authors evaluated the impact of clinical and admission (baseline) characteristics, and adult and total (adult and pediatric) congenital heart surgery volume in each of the pediatric hospitals performing adult congenital cardiac surgery. Of the 97 563 total congenital heart surgery admissions between 2000 and 2008, 3061 were adults who underwent cardiac surgery. In their multivariate analysis, they identified age, gender, and surgical complexity (RACHS-1 score; Risk Adjustment for Congenital Heart Surgery-1) as important risk factors. They also identified that the annual adult congenital surgical volume was associated with outcomes. Those centers with ≥20 adult congenital cases had better outcomes, with an adjusted odds ratio of 0.4 (95% confidence interval, 0.2–0.7; $P = .003$). However, the total number of congenital heart surgeries, which includes both pediatric and adult procedures, was not associated with outcomes (Fig 4). This study highlights that there may be a difference in experience and procedure technique in adult versus pediatric congenital heart procedures and that the overall experience, as represented by number of cases for both pediatric and adult patients with congenital heart disease, doesn't necessarily convey a reduced risk for the adults cared for in that hospital. This might imply that the techniques differ and thus they require different expertise. Alternatively, there may be other structures and processes of care that are in place at pediatric centers that perform ≥20 adult congenital heart procedures that impact the improved outcomes, such as the organization of the intensive care unit, the perfusionist team, or other ancillary practices.

E. A. Martinez, MD, MHS

References

1. van der Bom T, Zomer AC, Zwinderman AH, Meijboom FJ, Bouma BJ, Mulder BJ. The changing epidemiology of congenital heart disease. *Nat Rev Cardiol.* 2011;8: 50-60.
2. Zomer AC, Verheugt EL, Vaartjes I, et al. Surgery in adults with congenital heart disease. *Circulation.* 2011;24:2195-2201.

A 2-year survey of treatment of acute atrial fibrillation in an ED

Hirschl MM, Wollmann C, Globits S (Landesklinikum St Pölten, Austria, Europe)

Am J Emerg Med 29:534-540, 2011

Objective.—Pharmacologic cardioversion of atrial fibrillation (AF) is a reasonable mode of treatment if the arrhythmia is of recent onset. Results concerning the response rates of different drugs, respectively, in daily clinical practice and data with regard to the parameters associated with successful cardioversion are not very prevalent.

Methods.—Three-hundred seventy-six patients who were admitted to the emergency department with acute AF and a duration of shorter than 48 hours were enrolled into the AF registry.

Results.—The most effective drugs were flecainide and ibutilide (95% and 76%). Low response rates were observed with amiodarone (36%) and the individual use of digoxin or diltiazem (19% and 18%). Factors associated with a successful cardioversion were a lower blood pressure on admission ($P = .002$), a shorter time interval between the onset of AF and admission to the ED ($P = .003$), and adherence to treatment guidelines ($P < .0001$).

Conclusion.—The use of flecainide and ibutilide is associated with a much higher rate of cardioversion than other drugs we studied.

▶ The safety of cardioversion of recent-onset (<48 hours) atrial fibrillation has been well established, especially in recent literature. Most physicians and patients choose electrical cardioversion because it is quick and effective. However, there remains a role for chemical cardioversion in those that wish to avoid electricity for various reasons. This article presents a retrospective analysis of 376 patients treated with various drugs in an emergency department in Austria. Flecainide and ibutilide provided the best success rates by far (95% and 76%, respectively). Other response rates were amiodarone (57%), magnesium (51%), and the combination of diltiazem and digoxin (72%). One patient who received flecainide experienced torsades, and two patients who received ibulitide experienced ventricular tachycardia. Nobody died. Flecainide was also the quickest acting, with a mean response time of 117 minutes. If chemical conversion is the route you choose, flecainide is the best choice and is a class I recommendation by the American Heart Association.

M. D. Zwank, MD

Myocardial Infarction/Cardiogenic Shocks

Conservative Versus Liberal Red Cell Transfusion in Acute Myocardial Infarction (the CRIT Randomized Pilot Study)

Cooper HA, Rao SV, Greenberg MD, et al (Washington Hosp Ctr, DC; Durham VA Med Ctr, NC; Washington, DC VA Med Ctr)

Am J Cardiol 108:1108-1111, 2011

Red blood cell transfusion is common in patients with acute myocardial infarction (AMI). However, observational data suggest that this practice may be associated with worse clinical outcomes and data from clinical trials are lacking in this population. We conducted a prospective multicenter randomized pilot trial in which 45 patients with AMI and a hematocrit level ≤30% were randomized to a liberal (transfuse when hematocrit <30% to maintain 30% to 33%) or a conservative (transfuse when hematocrit <24% to maintain 24% to 27%) transfusion strategy. Baseline hematocrit was similar in those in the liberal and conservative arms (26.9% vs 27.5%, $p = 0.4$). Average daily hematocrits were 30.6% in the liberal arm and 27.9% in the conservative arm, a difference of 2.7% ($p < 0.001$). More patients in the liberal arm than in the conservative arm were transfused (100% vs 54%, $p < 0.001$) and the average number of units transfused per patient tended to be higher in the liberal arm than in the conservative arm (2.5 vs 1.6, $p = 0.07$). The primary clinical safety measurement of in-hospital death, recurrent MI, or new or worsening congestive heart failure occurred in 8 patients in the liberal arm and 3 in the conservative arm (38% vs 13%, $p = 0.046$). In conclusion, compared to a conservative transfusion strategy, treating anemic patients with AMI according to a liberal transfusion strategy results in more patients receiving transfusions and higher hematocrit levels. However, this may be associated with worse clinical outcomes. A large-scale definitive trial addressing this issue is urgently required.

▶ It has historically been accepted as a matter of conventional wisdom that patients with coronary artery disease (CAD), especially those with active ischemia, require transfusion to relatively high hemoglobin levels, typically in the range of 10 g/dL. Although there are good data to support the premise that patients with CAD and anemia have worse outcomes than similar patients without anemia, it does not necessarily follow that transfusion is beneficial to anemic patients with CAD. In the last 10 to 15 years, a significant body of data has accumulated that has cast doubt on these assumptions, beginning with data generated from the initial TRICC trial.[1] Since then, numerous studies, primarily retrospective in nature, have indicated that patients with active coronary ischemia not only do not require hemoglobins as high as historically presumed, but may have better outcomes if not transfused and allowed to run modestly lower hemoglobins when compared with similar patients undergoing packed red blood cell (PRBC) transfusion.[2] However, until recently, this concept has not been specifically evaluated prospectively. These investigators report their results of a pilot study comparing a restrictive transfusion strategy (keeping hematocrit between 24% and 27%) and a liberal strategy (hematocrit between 30% and 33%) in patients with acute myocardial infarction (AMI). In this small study (45 patients) of mixed ST- and non–ST-elevation myocardial infarction (MI) patients, the investigators identified higher rates of the combined endpoint of death or recurrent MI or new or worse heart failure both in hospital and at 30 days after the liberal transfusion; the liberal transfusion group also has significantly more in-hospital new or worsening heart failure. No other parameters (death, recurrent MI, new or worsening heart failure), either alone or in combination, showed any significant differences, either in hospital or at 30 days. Nevertheless, this is the first prospective study to specifically show an adverse outcome impact of PRBC transfusion in the setting of AMI. These findings, while clearly preliminary, are consistent with the extensive body of data that precedes it. The ability of stored PRBC is less efficient in delivering oxygen to tissues than clinicians often appreciate, and carries a host of acute and less-acute complications, including inflammatory effects, immunosuppression, and the potential of fluid overload. There is an increasing body of literature accumulating that indicates that the deficiencies in the utility of stored PRBC, coupled with their detrimental effects, often result in adverse outcomes more often than beneficial ones. Although these are clearly preliminary data, they should support a conservative approach to the use of PRBC transfusion in patients with coronary ischemia and provide an impetus to ongoing prospective research in this area.

D. R. Gerber, DO, FCCP

References

1. Hebert PC, Yetisir E, Martin C, et al; Transfusion Requirements in Critical Care Investigators for the Canadian Critical Care Trials Group. Is a low transfusion threshold safe in critically ill patients with cardiovascular diseases? *Crit Care Med.* 2001;29:227-234.
2. Gerber DR. Transfusion of packed red blood cells in patients with ischemic heart disease. *Crit Care Med.* 2008;36:1068-1074.

Intra-aortic Balloon Counterpulsation and Infarct Size in Patients With Acute Anterior Myocardial Infarction Without Shock: The CRISP AMI Randomized Trial

Patel MR, Smalling RW, Thiele H, et al (Duke Univ Med Ctr, Durham, NC; Univ of Texas, Houston; Univ of Leipzig Heart Ctr, Germany; et al)

JAMA 306:1329-1337, 2011

Context.—Intra-aortic balloon counterpulsation (IABC) is an adjunct to revascularization in patients with cardiogenic shock and reduces infarct size when placed prior to reperfusion in animal models.

Objective.—To determine if routine IABC placement prior to reperfusion in patients with anterior ST-segment elevation myocardial infarction (STEMI) without shock reduces myocardial infarct size.

Design, Setting, and Patients.—An open, multicenter, randomized controlled trial, the Counterpulsation to Reduce Infarct Size Pre-PCI Acute Myocardial Infarction (CRISP AMI) included 337 patients with acute anterior STEMI but without cardiogenic shock at 30 sites in 9 countries from June 2009 through February 2011.

Intervention.—Initiation of IABC before primary percutaneous coronary intervention (PCI) and continuation for at least 12 hours (IABC plus PCI) vs primary PCI alone.

Main Outcome Measures.—Infarct size expressed as a percentage of left ventricular (LV) mass and measured by cardiac magnetic resonance imaging performed 3 to 5 days after PCI. Secondary end points included all-cause death at 6 months and vascular complications and major bleeding at 30 days. Multiple imputations were performed for missing infarct size data.

Results.—The median time from first contact to first coronary device was 77 minutes (interquartile range, 53 to 114 minutes) for the IABC plus PCI group vs 68 minutes (interquartile range, 40 to 100 minutes) for the PCI alone group (*P*=.04). The mean infarct size was not significantly different between the patients in the IABC plus PCI group and in the PCI alone group (42.1% [95% CI, 38.7% to 45.6%] vs 37.5% [95% CI, 34.3% to 40.8%], respectively; difference of 4.6% [95% CI, −0.2% to 9.4%], *P*=.06; imputed difference of 4.5% [95% CI, −0.3% to 9.3%], *P*=.07) and in patients with proximal left anterior descending Thrombolysis in Myocardial Infarction flow scores of 0 or 1 (46.7% [95% CI, 42.8% to 50.6%] vs 42.3% [95% CI, 38.6% to 45.9%], respectively; difference of 4.4% [95% CI, −1.0% to 9.7%], *P*=.11; imputed difference of 4.8% [95% CI, −0.6% to 10.1%], *P*=.08). At 30 days, there were no significant differences between the IABC plus PCI group and the PCI alone group for major vascular complications (n=7 [4.3%; 95% CI, 1.8% to 8.8%] vs n=2 [1.1%; 95% CI, 0.1% to 4.0%], respectively; *P*=.09) and major bleeding or transfusions (n=5 [3.1%; 95% CI, 1.0% to 7.1%] vs n=3 [1.7%; 95% CI, 0.4% to 4.9%]; *P*=.49). By 6 months, 3 patients (1.9%; 95% CI, 0.6% to 5.7%) in the IABC plus PCI group and 9 patients (5.2%; 95% CI, 2.7% to 9.7%) in the PCI alone group had died (*P*=.12).

Conclusion.—Among patients with acute anterior STEMI without shock, IABC plus primary PCI compared with PCI alone did not result in reduced infarct size.

Trial Registration.—clinicaltrials.gov Identifier: NCT00833612.

► The intra-aortic balloon pump (IABP) is utilized to provide hemodynamic support in a variety of critical care circumstances, especially in patients with hypotension or pulmonary edema caused by acute myocardial infarction (MI) complicated by cardiogenic shock or acute mitral regurgitation.[1] Afterload reduction and increased collateral blood flow are probably the major mechanisms that account for the benefit of the IABP in patients with acute MI.[2,3]

Based on the theoretical hemodynamic benefits of an IABP, both cardiologists and cardiac surgeons have advocated prophylactic insertion of an IABP to provide hemodynamic support in "high-risk" patients who require either percutaneous or surgical myocardial revascularization.[4-6] There has been a paucity of clinical trials, however, to justify widespread use of the IABP in patients with an acute MI not complicated by cardiogenic shock. Prophylactic use of the IABP was not associated with a decreased rate of reinfarction, enhanced myocardial recovery, or improved clinical outcomes among patients who received an IABP in a randomized trial of prophylactic insertion of an IABP in high-risk patients with acute MI who underwent primary angioplasty.[7]

The Counterpulsation to Reduce Infarct Size Pre-PCI Acute Myocardial Infarction (CRISP AMI) trial was a prospective, multicenter, randomized trial to determine if routine insertion of an IABP before primary percutaneous coronary intervention (PCI) reduces infarct size in patients with an acute anterior ST-segment elevation MI without cardiogenic shock. Unfortunately, insertion of an IABP was not associated with a reduction of infarct size as measured by cardiac magnetic resonance imaging 3 to 5 days after PCI. Therefore, the authors correctly concluded that an IABP should not be used routinely in high-risk anterior MI patients without cardiogenic shock.

S. W. Werns, MD

References

1. Stone GW, Ohman EM, Miller MF, et al. Contemporary utilization and outcomes of intra-aortic balloon counterpulsation in acute myocardial infarction: the benchmark registry. *J Am Coll Cardiol.* 2003;41:1940-1945.
2. Flynn MS, Kern MJ, Donohue TJ, Aguirre FV, Bach RG, Caracciolo EA. Alterations of coronary collateral blood flow velocity during intraaortic balloon pumping. *Am J Cardiol.* 1993;71:1451-1455.
3. Dekker AL, Reesink KD, van der Veen FH, et al. Intra-aortic balloon pumping in acute mitral regurgitation reduces aortic impedance and regurgitant fraction. *Shock.* 2003;19:334-338.
4. Kahn JK, Rutherford BD, McConahay DR, Johnson WL, Giorgi LV, Hartzler GO. Supported "high risk" coronary angioplasty using intraaortic balloon pump counterpulsation. *J Am Coll Cardiol.* 1990;15:1151-1155.
5. Brodie BR, Stuckey TD, Hansen C, Muncy D. Intra-aortic balloon counterpulsation before primary percutaneous transluminal coronary angioplasty reduces catheterization laboratory events in high-risk patients with acute myocardial infarction. *Am J Cardiol.* 1999;84:18-23.

6. Christenson JT, Badel P, Simonet F, Schmuziger M. Preoperative intraaortic balloon pump enhances cardiac performance and improves the outcome of redo CABG. *Ann Thorac Surg.* 1997;64:1237-1244.
7. Stone GW, Marsalese D, Brodie BR, et al. A prospective, randomized evaluation of prophylactic intraaortic balloon counterpulsation in high risk patients with acute myocardial infarction treated with primary angioplasty. *J Am Coll Cardiol.* 1997; 29:1459-1467.

Effect of Nesiritide in Patients with Acute Decompensated Heart Failure

O'Connor CM, Starling RC, Hernandez AF, et al (Univ of North Carolina Heart Failure Program, Chapel Hill; Cleveland Clinic, OH; et al)

N Engl J Med 365:32-43, 2011

Background.—Nesiritide is approved in the United States for early relief of dyspnea in patients with acute heart failure. Previous meta-analyses have raised questions regarding renal toxicity and the mortality associated with this agent.

Methods.—We randomly assigned 7141 patients who were hospitalized with acute heart failure to receive either nesiritide or placebo for 24 to 168 hours in addition to standard care. Coprimary end points were the change in dyspnea at 6 and 24 hours, as measured on a 7-point Likert scale, and the composite end point of rehospitalization for heart failure or death within 30 days.

Results.—Patients randomly assigned to nesiritide, as compared with those assigned to placebo, more frequently reported markedly or moderately improved dyspnea at 6 hours (44.5% vs. 42.1%, $P = 0.03$) and 24 hours (68.2% vs. 66.1%, $P = 0.007$), but the prespecified level for significance ($P \leq 0.005$ for both assessments or $P \leq 0.0025$ for either) was not met. The rate of rehospitalization for heart failure or death from any cause within 30 days was 9.4% in the nesiritide group versus 10.1% in the placebo group (absolute difference, −0.7 percentage points; 95% confidence interval [CI], −2.1 to 0.7; $P = 0.31$). There were no significant differences in rates of death from any cause at 30 days (3.6% with nesiritide vs. 4.0% with placebo; absolute difference, −0.4 percentage points; 95% CI, −1.3 to 0.5) or rates of worsening renal function, defined by more than a 25% decrease in the estimated glomerular filtration rate (31.4% vs. 29.5%; odds ratio, 1.09; 95% CI, 0.98 to 1.21; $P = 0.11$).

Conclusions.—Nesiritide was not associated with an increase or a decrease in the rate of death and rehospitalization and had a small, nonsignificant effect on dyspnea when used in combination with other therapies. It was not associated with a worsening of renal function, but it was associated with an increase in rates of hypotension. On the basis of these results, nesiritide cannot be recommended for routine use in the broad population of patients with acute heart failure. (Funded by Scios; ClinicalTrials.gov number, NCT00475852.)

▶ The saga of nesiritide, recombinant human brain natriuretic peptide, for treating patients with acute decompensated heart failure is well documented in 2 commentaries written by Eric Topol and published in the *New England Journal of Medicine* in July 2005 and July 2011, respectively.[1,2] Compared with placebo, intravenous nesiritide at a dose of 0.03 μg/kg/min for 6 hours reduced pulmonary capillary wedge pressure by nearly 10 mm Hg in patients hospitalized for acute decompensated heart failure.[3] A randomized, controlled trial that was conducted at Veterans Affairs Hospitals found similar hemodynamic and clinical effects of intravenous nesiritide and nitroglycerin in patients with acute decompensated heart failure.[4] Subsequent reports, however, raised concerns that nesiritide might increase the risk of death[5] and deterioration of renal function,[6] prompting Topol's 2005 commentary.[1]

The uncertainty regarding the efficacy and safety of nesiritide prompted the performance of a placebo-controlled clinical trial, known as the Acute Study of Clinical Effectiveness of Nesiritide in Decompensated Heart Failure (ASCEND-HF).[7] There were no significant differences in several outcomes, including the rates of improved dyspnea, death, or rehospitalization for heart failure within 30 days or worsening renal function. Hypotension occurred significantly more often among the patients who received nesiritide compared with the placebo group. The authors concluded that "nesiritide cannot be recommended in the broad population of patients with acute decompensated heart failure."[7] Their conclusion certainly seems justified by the data and should influence the next round of practice guidelines for the treatment of heart failure. It is possible that nesiritide will be downgraded to a class IIb recommendation from its current status as a class IIa recommendation.[8] Other options to relieve fluid overload include the combination of a loop diuretic with a second diuretic, eg, metolazone or spironolactone,[9] and the institution of venovenous ultrafiltration.[10]

S. W. Werns, MD

References

1. Topol EJ. Nesiritide - not verified. *N Engl J Med.* 2005;353:113-116.
2. Topol EJ. The lost decade of nesiritide. *N Engl J Med.* 2011;365:81-82.
3. Colucci WS, Elkayam U, Horton DP, et al. Intravenous nesiritide, a natriuretic peptide, in the treatment of decompensated congestive heart failure. *N Engl J Med.* 2000;343:246-253.
4. Publication committee for the VMAC Investigators (Vasodilatation in the Management of Acute CHF). Intravenous nesiritide vs nitroglycerin for treatment of decompensated congestive heart failure: a randomized controlled trial. *JAMA.* 2002;287:1531-1540.
5. Sackner-Bernstein JD, Kowalski M, Fox M, Aaronson K. Short-term risk of death after treatment with nesiritide for decompensated heart failure: a pooled analysis of randomized controlled trials. *JAMA.* 2005;293:1900-1905.
6. Sackner-Bernstein JD, Skopicki HA, Aaronson KD. Risk of worsening renal function with nesiritide in patients with acutely decompensated heart failure. *Circulation.* 2005;111:1487-1491.
7. O'Connor CM, Starling RC, Hernandez AF, et al. Effect of nesiritide in patients with acute decompensated heart failure. *N Engl J Med.* 2011;365:323-343.
8. Hunt SA, Abraham WT, Chin MH, et al. 2009 focused update incorporated into the ACC/AHA 2005 guidelines for the diagnosis and management of heart failure in adults a report of the American College of Cardiology Foundation/American Heart Association Task Force on Practice Guidelines Developed in Collaboration with the International Society for Heart and Lung Transplantation. *J Am Coll Cardiol.* 2009;53:e1-e90.

9. Channer KS, McLean KA, Lawson-Matthew P, Richardson M. Combination diuretic treatment in severe heart failure: a randomised controlled trial. *Br Heart J.* 1994;71:146-150.
10. Costanzo MR, Guglin ME, Saltzberg MT, et al. Ultrafiltration versus intravenous diuretics for patients hospitalized for acute decompensated heart failure. *J Am Coll Cardiol.* 2007;49:675-683.

Beneficial association of β-blocker therapy on recovery from severe acute heart failure treatment: Data from the Survival of Patients With Acute Heart Failure in Need of Intravenous Inotropic Support trial

Böhm M, Link A, Cai D, et al (Universitätsklinikum des Saarlandes, Homburg/Saar, Germany; Abbott Laboratories, Abbott Park, IL; et al)
Crit Care Med 39:940-944, 2011

Objectives.—Beta-blocker therapy is recommended for most patients with chronic heart failure, although such therapy may be discontinued or reduced during hospitalizations. The aim is to determine whether β-blocker use at study entry and/or at discharge has an impact on 31- and 180-day survival.

Design.—Survival of Patients With Acute Heart Failure in Need of Intravenous Inotropic Support study was designed as a randomized, double-blind, active-controlled, multi-center study.

Setting.—Multinational.

Patients.—A total of 1,327 critically ill patients hospitalized with low-output heart failure in need of inotropic therapy.

Intervention.—Levosimendan versus dobutamine.

Measurements.—All-cause mortality at 31 and 180 days in patients who survived initial hospitalization with/without β-blocker use at entry and/or at discharge.

Results.—Patients on β-blockers at entry and at discharge had significantly lower 31-day ($p < .0001$) and 180-day ($p < .0001$) mortality compared to patients without β-blockers use at both time points. The association was robust when adjusted for age and co-morbidities ($p = .006$ at 31 days; $p = .003$ at 180 days).

Conclusions.—Those results strongly suggest, in severe acutely decompensated heart failure patients, admitted on β-blockers, to continue on them at discharge.

▶ Bisoprolol,[1] sustained-release metoprolol,[2] and carvedilol[3] have been shown to reduce the risk of death in patients with chronic heart failure, and metoprolol and carvedilol also have been shown to improve functional class and reduce the need for hospitalization for worsening heart failure.[4,5] The Cardiac Insufficiency Bisoprolol Study II (CIBIS-II) was a double-blind, randomized, placebo-controlled trial that enrolled 2647 patients with New York Heart Association (NYHA) Class III or IV heart failure and a left ventricular ejection fraction (LVEF) ≤ 35%.[1] After a mean follow-up period of 1.3 years, all-cause mortality was significantly lower among patients who were randomized to the bisoprolol group (11.8% vs 17.3%; hazard ratio 0.66; 95% confidence interval [CI] 0.54–0.81; $P < .0001$). The Metoprolol CR/XL Randomised Intervention Trial in Congestive Heart Failure (MERIT-HF) was a double-blind, placebo-controlled, randomized trial that enrolled 3991 patients with NYHA class II, III, or IV heart failure and a LVEF ≤ 40%.[2] After a mean follow-up period of 1 year, all-cause mortality was significantly lower among patients who were randomized to metoprolol (7.2% vs 11.0%; relative risk 0.66; 95% CI 0.53–0.81; $P = .0062$). The Carvedilol Prospective Randomized Cumulative Survival (COPERNICUS) Study was a double-blind, placebo-controlled, randomized trial that enrolled 2290 patients with severe heart failure, that is, symptoms at rest or on minimal exertion, and a LVEF less than 25%.[3] After a mean follow-up period of 10.4 months, all-cause mortality was 11.4% in the carvedilol group compared with 18.5% in the placebo group (relative risk reduction 35%; 95% CI 19%–48%; $P = .0014$). A meta-analysis of 22 placebo-controlled trials that included 10 132 patients concluded that beta-blocker use reduced total mortality by 35% (odds ratio 0.65; 95% CI 0.53–0.80).[6]

When patients with chronic heart failure are hospitalized for acute decompensated heart failure, the clinician must decide whether to initiate a beta-blocker in patients not receiving them before admission and whether to continue or discontinue beta-blockers in patients who were receiving chronic beta-blocker therapy. Unfortunately, there are limited data regarding the safety of initiating beta-blocker therapy in patients hospitalized for acute decompensated heart failure. The CIBIS-II, MERIT-HF, and COPERNICUS trials' limited enrollment to patients who were judged to be stable and euvolemic.[1-3] The COPERNICUS trial specifically excluded patients who required intensive care, had marked fluid retention, or were receiving intravenous vasodilators or positive inotropic drugs within 4 days of screening.[3] According to the current practice guidelines for heart failure, patients with current or a recent history of fluid retention should not be prescribed beta-blockers without diuretics because the initiation of beta-blocker therapy can exacerbate fluid retention.[7] The current guidelines also state that it is safe to begin beta-blockers before discharge in patients hospitalized for heart failure if intravenous therapy for heart failure was not required.[7] Therefore, it is understandable that physicians are reluctant to initiate treatment with a beta-blocker during a hospitalization for acute decompensated heart failure.

There is evidence that discontinuation of a beta-blocker when a patient is hospitalized for acute decompensated heart failure may adversely affect outcomes.[8-10] Metra et al[8] reported the outcomes of patients who were hospitalized for decompensated heart failure after enrollment in the Carvedilol or Metoprolol European Trial (COMET). Multivariable analysis showed that a dose reduction or complete withdrawal of beta-blocker therapy was an independent predictor of mortality after discharge (hazard ratio 1.3; 95% CI 1.023–1.656; $P = 0.0318$). Fonarow et al[9] studied the relationship between clinical outcomes and withdrawal or continuation of beta-blocker therapy in patients who were receiving beta-blockers when they were admitted for treatment of acute decompensated heart failure. Withdrawal of beta-blocker therapy was associated with a significantly higher adjusted risk for mortality compared with continuation of beta-blockers (hazard ratio 2.3; 95% CI 1.2–4.6; $P = 0.013$). A small, randomized, controlled, open-label trial compared beta-blockade continuation versus discontinuation during hospitalization for acute decompensated heart failure.[10] After 3 days, dyspnea and well-being were improved in 92.8% of patients who continued beta-blockade compared with 92.3% of patients who stopped beta-blockers. Also, 3 months after discharge, the percentage of patients taking beta-blockers was greater in the continuation group than the discontinuation group (90% vs 76%; $P < 0.05$).

Both metoprolol and carvedilol inhibit the favorable hemodynamic effects of dobutamine in patients with chronic heart failure.[11] After treatment with metoprolol for 9 to 12 months, the decrease in pulmonary capillary wedge during infusion of dobutamine was blunted compared with the baseline response before metoprolol was started. After treatment with carvedilol for 9 to 12 months, the pulmonary capillary wedge pressure, systemic vascular resistance, and pulmonary vascular resistance increased during dobutamine infusion, compared with decreases before carvedilol was begun. Therefore, it is important to understand the impact of beta-blocker therapy on the outcomes of patients who require inotropic therapy during hospitalization for acute decompensated heart failure. Bohm et al[12] attempted to address this question by performing a post hoc analysis of the effects of in-patient beta-blocker therapy on the outcomes of patients who were enrolled in the Survival of Patients with Acute Heart Failure in Need of Intravenous Inotropic Support (SURVIVE) trial. The SURVIVE study was a double-blind, active-controlled, randomized clinical trial that compared levosimendan with dobutamine in hospitalized patients with low-output heart failure who required inotropic therapy.[13] After adjustment for age and comorbidities, there was a signification association between the status of beta-blocker use and survival.[12] All-cause mortality at 31 days and 180 days was lowest among patients who were receiving beta-blockers both at the time of admission and discharge and highest among patients who were taking beta-blockers at the time of admission but not at the time of discharge.[12]

A prospective, randomized trial that enrolled 363 patients who were hospitalized for treatment of decompensated heart failure found that patients who were randomized to initiation of carvedilol before hospital discharge were more likely to be taking carvedilol 60 days later than the patients who were randomized to initiation by the patient's physician after discharge.[14] Among outpatients with chronic heart failure and no contraindications to beta-blockers, the most common reason for the absence of beta-blocker therapy was discontinuation of beta-blocker therapy during a hospitalization.[15] The study by Bohm et al[12] should reassure clinicians that it is safe to maintain beta-blocker therapy in patients who require inotropic therapy for acute decompensated heart failure. Also, maintenance of beta-blocker therapy during hospitalization for acute decompensated heart failure appears to increase the probability that patients with chronic heart failure will experience the proven long-term benefits of beta-blocker therapy.

S. Werns, MD

References

1. The cardiac insufficiency bisoprolol study II (CIBIS-II): a randomised trial. *Lancet.* 1999;353:9-13.

2. Effect of metoprolol CR/XL in chronic heart failure: Metoprolol CR/XL Randomised Intervention Trial in Congestive Heart Failure (MERIT-HF). *Lancet.* 1999; 353:2001-2007.
3. Packer M, Coats AJ, Fowler MB, et al. Effect of carvedilol on survival in severe chronic heart failure. *N Engl J Med.* 2001;344:1651-1658.
4. Hjalmarson A, Goldstein S, Fagerberg B, et al. Effects of controlled-release metoprolol on total mortality, hospitalizations, and well-being in patients with heart failure: the Metoprolol CR/XL Randomized Intervention Trial in congestive heart failure (MERIT-HF). MERIT-HF Study Group. *JAMA.* 2000;283:1295-1302.
5. Packer M, Fowler MB, Roecker EB, et al. Effect of carvedilol on the morbidity of patients with severe chronic heart failure: results of the carvedilol prospective randomized cumulative survival (COPERNICUS) study. *Circulation.* 2002;106: 2194-2199.
6. Brophy JM, Joseph L, Rouleau JL. Beta-blockers in congestive heart failure. A Bayesian meta-analysis. *Ann Intern Med.* 2001;124:550-560.
7. Hunt SA, Abraham WT, Chin MH, et al. 2009 focused update incorporated into the ACC/AHA 2005 guidelines for the diagnosis and management of heart failure in adults: a report of the American College of Cardiology Foundation/American Heart Association Task Force on Practice Guidelines Developed in Collaboration With the International Society for Heart and Lung Transplantation. *J Am Coll Cardiol.* 2009;53:e1-e90.
8. Metra M, Torp-Pedersen C, Cleland JGF, et al. Should beta-blocker therapy be reduced or withdrawn after an episode of decompensated heart failure? Results from COMET. *Eur J Heart Fail.* 2007;9:901-909.
9. Fonarow GC, Abraham WT, Albert NM, et al. Influence of beta-blocker continuation or withdrawal on outcomes in patients hospitalized with heart failure: findings from the OPTIMIZE-HF program. *J Am Coll Cardiol.* 2008;52:190-199.
10. Jondeau G, Neuder Y, Eicher JC, et al. B-CONVINCED: Beta-blocker CONtinuation Vs. INterruption in patients with Congestive heart failure hospitalizED for a decompensation episode. *Eur Heart J.* 2009;30:2186-2192.
11. Metra M, Nodari S, D'Aloia A, et al. Beta-blocker therapy influences the hemodynamic response to inotropic agents in patients with heart failure: a randomized comparison of dobutamine and enoximone before and after chronic treatment with metoprolol or carvedilol. *J Am Coll Cardiol.* 2002;40:1248-1258.
12. Bohm M, Link A, Cai D, et al. Beneficial association of β-blocker therapy on recovery from severe acute heart failure treatment: data from the Survival of Patients With Acute Heart Failure in Need of Intravenous Inotropic Support trial. *Crit Care Med.* 2011;39:940-944.
13. Mebazaa A, Nieminen MS, Packer M, et al. Levosimendan vs dobutamine for patients with acute decompensated heart failure: the SURVIVE Randomized Trial. *JAMA.* 2007;297:1883-1891.
14. Gattis WA, O'Connor CM, Gallup DS, et al. Predischarge initiation of carvedilol in patients hospitalized for decompensated heart failure: results of the Initiation Management Predischarge: Process for Assessment of Carvedilol Therapy in Heart Failure (IMPACT-HF) Trial. *J Am Coll Cardiol.* 2004;43:1534-1541.
15. Parameswaran AC, Tang WH, Francis GS, Gupta R, Young JB. Why do patients fail to receive beta-blockers for chronic heart failure over time? A "real world" single-center, 2-year follow-up experience of beta-blocker therapy in patients with chronic heart failure. *Am Heart J.* 2005;149:921-926.

Diuretic Strategies in Patients with Acute Decompensated Heart Failure

Felker GM, for the NHLBI Heart Failure Clinical Research Network (Duke Univ School of Medicine and Duke Heart Ctr, Durham, NC; et al)

N Engl J Med 364:797-805, 2011

Background.—Loop diuretics are an essential component of therapy for patients with acute decompensated heart failure, but there are few prospective data to guide their use.

Methods.—In a prospective, double-blind, randomized trial, we assigned 308 patients with acute decompensated heart failure to receive furosemide administered intravenously by means of either a bolus every 12 hours or continuous infusion and at either a low dose (equivalent to the patient's previous oral dose) or a high dose (2.5 times the previous oral dose). The protocol allowed specified dose adjustments after 48 hours. The coprimary end points were patients' global assessment of symptoms, quantified as the area under the curve (AUC) of the score on a visual-analogue scale over the course of 72 hours, and the change in the serum creatinine level from baseline to 72 hours.

Results.—In the comparison of bolus with continuous infusion, there was no significant difference in patients' global assessment of symptoms (mean AUC, 4236 ± 1440 and 4373 ± 1404, respectively; $P = 0.47$) or in the mean change in the creatinine level (0.05 ± 0.3 mg per deciliter [4.4 ± 26.5 μmol per liter] and 0.07 ± 0.3 mg per deciliter [6.2 ± 26.5 μmol per liter], respectively; $P = 0.45$). In the comparison of the high-dose strategy with the low-dose strategy, there was a nonsignificant trend toward greater improvement in patients' global assessment of symptoms in the high-dose group (mean AUC, 4430 ± 1401 vs. 4171 ± 1436; $P = 0.06$). There was no significant difference between these groups in the mean change in the creatinine level (0.08 ± 0.3 mg per deciliter [7.1 ± 26.5 μmol per liter] with the high-dose strategy and 0.04 ± 0.3 mg per deciliter [3.5 ± 26.5 μmol per liter] with the low-dose strategy, $P = 0.21$). The high-dose strategy was associated with greater diuresis and more favorable outcomes in some secondary measures but also with transient worsening of renal function.

Conclusions.—Among patients with acute decompensated heart failure, there were no significant differences in patients' global assessment of symptoms or in the change in renal function when diuretic therapy was administered by bolus as compared with continuous infusion or at a high dose as compared with a low dose. (Funded by the National Heart, Lung, and Blood Institute; ClinicalTrials.gov number, NCT00577135.)

► Analysis of a national registry of patients hospitalized with acute decompensated heart failure from 2001 to 2005 found that 88% of the patients were treated with intravenous loop diuretics.[1] Hospitalization for heart failure with evidence of fluid overload is a class I indication for intravenous loop diuretics, according to the American College of Cardiology/American Heart Association Guidelines for the Management of Heart Failure in Adults.[2] Additional class I recommendations include higher doses of loop diuretics or continuous infusion of a loop diuretic when diuresis is inadequate to relieve congestion.[2] Both recommendations, however, are based on expert consensus and are categorized as level of evidence class C because there is a paucity of clinical trial data to support the guidelines, and the results of some observational studies have caused experts to question the efficacy and safety of loop diuretics in the treatment of acute decompensated heart failure.[3]

A randomized trial was performed to compare low-dose intravenous furosemide (average dose 56 mg) plus high-dose intravenous isosorbide dinitrate with high-dose furosemide (average dose 200 mg) plus low-dose intravenous isosorbide dinitrate for the treatment of severe pulmonary edema.[4] The need for mechanical ventilation and the frequency of acute myocardial infarction were both more frequent among the patients who were randomly assigned to the high-dose furosemide/low-dose nitrate group. A case-control study found that higher doses of loop diuretics were an independent predictor of deteriorating renal function.[5] Another observational study reported that the dose of loop diuretics during hospitalization for decompensated heart failure was a multivariate predictor of increased mortality at 6 months.[6] Of course, it is possible that higher doses of diuretics are simply an indicator of greater disease severity, and multivariable adjustment for known predictors of adverse outcomes may not eliminate confounding. A recent study that used propensity-matched analysis found no relationship between the dose of diuretic and short-term mortality among patients who were hospitalized for acute decompensated heart failure.[7] Thus, it remains uncertain whether there is a causal relationship between the dose of diuretics and outcomes.

The theoretical advantages of continuous infusion of loop diuretics include more gradual changes in intravascular volume, less vasoconstriction, and lower peak drug concentrations with less toxicity. A small randomized study in 20 patients suggested that continuous infusion of diuretics compared with intermittent boluses is associated with greater diuresis and less ototoxicity.[8] Another small randomized study compared bolus and continuous infusion of furosemide in 41 patients hospitalized for heart failure.[9] There was no difference in the primary outcome measure, the change in serum creatinine from admission to hospital day 3, or hospital discharge. Also, there was no significant difference in urine output.

The National Heart, Lung, and Blood Institute Heart Failure Clinical Research Network conducted the Diuretic Optimization Strategies Evaluation trial (DOSE) to address 2 issues, diuretic dose, that is, low dose compared with high dose, and the mode of administration, that is, intravenous bolus compared with continuous intravenous infusion.[10] There was no difference in patients' global assessment of symptoms or the mean change in serum creatinine between the group that received boluses every 12 hours and the group that received continuous infusions of diuretic. Compared with the low-dose strategy, the high-dose strategy was associated with greater net fluid loss and relief of dyspnea, but transient increases in serum creatinine more than 0.3 mg/dL were more common. Based on the results of the DOSE trial, there does not appear to be adequate justification for administering furosemide or other loop diruetics via a continuous infusion. The results of the DOSE study provide weak support for a strategy of high-dose loop diuretics in patients with decompensated heart failure. Alternative strategies to relieve fluid overload include the combination of a loop diuretic with a second diuretic such as metolazone or spironolactone,[11] the administration of inotropic agents such as dopamine,[12] and the institution of venovenous ultrafiltration.[13]

S. W. Werns, MD

References

1. Peacock WF, Costanzo MR, De Marco T, et al. Impact of intravenous loop diuretics on outcomes of patients hospitalized with acute decompensated heart failure: insights from the ADHERE registry. *Cardiology.* 2009;113:12-19.
2. Hunt SA, Abraham WT, Chin MH, et al. 2009 Focused update incorporated into the ACC/AHA 2005 guidelines for the Diagnosis and Management of Heart Failure in Adults. A Report of the American College of Cardiology Foundation/American Heart Association Task Force on Practice Guidelines Developed in Collaboration With the International Society for Heart and Lung Transplantation. *J Am Coll Cardiol.* 2009;53:e1-e90.
3. Felker GM, O'Connor CM, Braunwald E. Loop diuretics in acute decompensated heart failure: necessary? Evil? A necessary evil? *Circ Heart Fail.* 2009;2:56-62.
4. Cotter G, Metzkor E, Kaluski E, et al. Randomised trial of high-dose isosorbide dinitrate plus low-dose furosemide versus high-dose furosemide plus low-dose isosorbide dinitrate in severe pulmonary oedema. *Lancet.* 1998;351:389-393.
5. Butler J, Forman DE, Abraham WT, et al. Relationship between heart failure treatment and development of worsening renal function among hospitalized patients. *Am Heart J.* 2004;147:331-338.
6. Hasselblad V, Stough WG, Shah MR, et al. Relation between dose of loop diuretics and outcomes in a heart failure population: results of the ESCAPE trial. *Eur J Heart Fail.* 2007;9:1064-1069.
7. Yilmaz MB, Gayat E, Salem R, et al. Impact of diuretic dosing on mortality in acute heart failure using a propensity-matched analysis. *Eur J Heart Fail.* 2011; 13:1244-1252.
8. Dormans TP, van Meyel JJ, Gerlag PG, et al. Diuretic efficacy of high dose furosemide in severe heart failure: bolus injection versus continuous infusion. *J Am Coll Cardiol.* 1996;28:376-382.
9. Allen LA, Turer AT, DeWald T, et al. Continuous versus bolus dosing of furosemide for patients hospitalized for heart failure. *Am J Cardiol.* 2010;105: 1794-1797.
10. Felker GM, Lee KL, Bull DA, et al. Diuretic strategies in patients with acute decompensated heart failure. *N Engl J Med.* 2011;364:797-805.
11. Channer KS, McLean KA, Lawson-Matthew P, Richardson M. Combination diuretic treatment in severe heart failure: a randomised controlled trial. *Br Heart J.* 1994;71:146-150.
12. Giamouzis G, Butler J, Starling RC, et al. Impact of dopamine infusion on renal function in hospitalized heart failure patients: results of the Dopamine in Acute Decompensated Heart Failure (DAD-HF) Trial. *J Card Fail.* 2010;16:922-930.
13. Costanzo MR, Guglin ME, Saltzberg MT, et al. Ultrafiltration versus intravenous diuretics for patients hospitalized for acute decompensated heart failure. *J Am Coll Cardiol.* 2007;49:675-683.

Standard- vs High-Dose Clopidogrel Based on Platelet Function Testing After Percutaneous Coronary Intervention: The GRAVITAS Randomized Trial

Price MJ, for the GRAVITAS Investigators (Scripps Translational Science Inst, La Jolla, CA; et al)

JAMA 305:1097-1105, 2011

Context.—High platelet reactivity while receiving clopidogrel has been linked to cardiovascular events after percutaneous coronary intervention (PCI), but a treatment strategy for this issue is not well defined.

Objective.—To evaluate the effect of high-dose compared with standard-dose clopidogrel in patients with high on-treatment platelet reactivity after PCI.

Design, Setting, and Patients.—Randomized, double-blind, active-control trial (Gauging Responsiveness with A Verify Now assay—Impact on Thrombosis And Safety [GRAVITAS]) of 2214 patients with high on-treatment reactivity 12 to 24 hours after PCI with drug-eluting stents at 83 centers in North America between July 2008 and April 2010.

Interventions.—High-dose clopidogrel (600-mg initial dose, 150 mg daily thereafter) or standard-dose clopidogrel (no additional loading dose, 75 mg daily) for 6 months.

Main Outcome Measures.—The primary end point was the 6-month incidence of death from cardiovascular causes, nonfatal myocardial infarction, or stent thrombosis. The key safety end point was severe or moderate bleeding according to the Global Utilization of Streptokinase and t-PA for Occluded Coronary Arteries (GUSTO) definition. A key pharmacodynamic end point was the rate of persistently high on-treatment reactivity at 30 days.

Results.—At 6 months, the primary end point had occurred in 25 of 1109 patients (2.3%) receiving high-dose clopidogrel compared with 25 of 1105 patients (2.3%) receiving standard-dose clopidogrel (hazard ratio [HR], 1.01; 95% confidence interval [CI], 0.58-1.76; P=.97). Severe or moderate bleeding was not increased with the high-dose regimen (15 [1.4%] vs 25 [2.3%], HR, 0.59; 95% CI, 0.31-1.11; P=.10). Compared with standard-dose clopidogrel, high-dose clopidogrel provided a 22% (95% CI, 18%-26%) absolute reduction in the rate of high on-treatment reactivity at 30 days (62%; 95% CI, 59%-65% vs 40%; 95% CI, 37%-43%; P<.001).

Conclusions.—Among patients with high on-treatment reactivity after PCI with drug-eluting stents, the use of high-dose clopidogrel compared with standard-dose clopidogrel did not reduce the incidence of death from cardiovascular causes, nonfatal myocardial infarction, or stent thrombosis.

Trial Registration.—clinicaltrials.gov Identifier: NCT00645918.

► It is well established that, compared with aspirin alone, the combination of aspirin and clopidogrel, a thienopyridine antagonist of the P2Y12 receptor, reduces the risk of ischemic events and stent thrombosis in acute coronary syndrome (ACS) patients, with or without ST-segment elevation, whether they are treated medically or with percutaneous coronary intervention (PCI).[1-4]

Therefore, dual antiplatelet therapy with aspirin and an antagonist of the platelet P2Y12 receptor has become the standard of care for patients with ACS with or without ST-segment elevation[5,6] and for patients who undergo PCI.[7]

Unfortunately, there is abundant evidence that common genetic variants are associated with blunting of the platelet inhibitory effect of clopidogrel.[8-10] The enzymatic activities that convert clopidogrel from an inactive pro-drug to an active metabolite are reduced in patients with loss-of-function cytochrome P450 alleles, resulting in increased risk of cardiovascular events, including stent thrombosis and death.[8-10] On March 12, 2010, the US Food and Drug Administration approved a revised label for clopidogrel that included a boxed warning about the decreased effectiveness of clopidogrel in patients with reduced ability to form the active metabolite of clopidogrel.[11] An extensive Clinical Expert Consensus document that was published a few months later included a thorough review of alternative dosing regimens of clopidogrel that have been tested to overcome the decreased efficacy of clopidogrel in patients who are hyporesponders.[12]

Numerous studies have found that a 600-mg loading dose of clopidogrel, compared with a 300-mg loading dose, reduces the risk of major adverse cardiovascular events after PCI without increasing the risk of major bleeding.[13] An increased maintenance dose of clopidogrel also has been investigated. The Clopidogrel and Aspirin Optimal Dose Usage to Reduce Recurrent Events-Seventh Organization to Assess Strategies in Ischemic Syndromes (CURRENT-OASIS 7) Trial was a double-blind, randomized trial that compared 2 regimens of clopidogrel in patients with ACS.[14-16] The double-dose patients received a clopidogrel loading dose of 600 mg and a daily maintenance dose of 150 mg on days 2 through 7, then 75 mg daily. The standard-dose group received a loading dose of 300 mg followed by a daily maintenance dose of 75 mg. The primary results have been published in 2 complementary papers in the September 2, 2010, issue of the *New England Journal of Medicine* (NEJM) and the October 9, 2010, issue of *Lancet*.[15,16] An analysis of the entire enrollment of 25 086 patients, including patients who did not undergo PCI, was described in the NEJM paper, whereas the *Lancet* paper featured a prespecified analysis of the 17 263 patients who underwent PCI. The frequency of major bleeding was greater among the patients who were randomized to the higher dose of clopidogrel.[16] Although the double-dose regimen was associated with a reduction in cardiovascular events and stent thrombosis in ACS patients who underwent PCI, it is uncertain whether the higher maintenance dose that was administered for only 6 days provided any additional benefit beyond the documented benefit of the 600-mg loading dose.

That question may have been answered by the results of the Gauging Responsiveness with A VerifyNow assay-Impact on Thrombosis And Safety (GRAVITAS) trial.[17] High residual platelet reactivity during treatment with clopidogrel is associated with an increased risk of both short- and long-term ischemic events after PCI.[18] The GRAVITAS trial demonstrated that, compared with the standard clopidogrel maintenance dose of 75 mg daily, a clopidogrel maintenance dose of 150 mg daily did not reduce the incidence of cardiovascular death, nonfatal myocardial infarction, or stent thrombosis among patients with high on-treatment platelet reactivity after PCI with drug-eluting stents.[17]

The current ACS and PCI guidelines recommend a clopidogrel maintenance dose of 75 mg daily.[5-7]

Cytochrome P450 genetic polymorphisms do not affect drug metabolite concentrations, inhibition of platelet aggregation, or clinical event rates in patients treated with prasugrel, another thienopyridine,[19,20] or ticagrelor.[21] Also, compared with the combination of aspirin and clopidogrel, the combination of aspirin and ticagrelor reduced the risk of death in patients with ACS.[22] Thus, the Class I recommendations of the most recent updates of the practice guidelines for PCI include both prasugrel and ticagrelor as alternatives to clopidogrel to inhibit the platelet P2Y12 receptor.[7]

S. W. Werns, MD

References

1. Yusuf S, Zhao F, Mehta SR, Chrolavicius S, Tognoni G, Fox KK, The Clopidogrel in Unstable Angina to Prevent Recurrent Events Trial Investigators. Effects of clopidogrel in addition to aspirin in patients with acute coronary syndromes without ST-segment elevation. *N Engl J Med.* 2001;345:494-502.
2. Mehta SR, Yusuf S, Peters RJ, et al. Effects of pretreatment with clopidogrel and aspirin followed by long-term therapy in patients undergoing percutaneous coronary intervention: the PCI-CURE study. *Lancet.* 2001;358:527-533.
3. Sabatine MS, Cannon CP, Gibson CM, et al. Addition of clopidogrel to aspirin and fibrinolytic therapy for myocardial infarction with ST-segment elevation. *N Engl J Med.* 2005;352:1179-1189.
4. Desai NR, Bhatt DL. The state of the periprocedural antiplatelet therapy after recent trials. *JACC Cardiovasc Interv.* 2010;3:571-583.
5. Kushner FG, Hand M, Smith SC Jr, et al. 2009 focused updates: ACC/AHA guidelines for the management of patients with ST-elevation myocardial infarction (updating the 2004 guideline and 2007 focused update) and ACC/AHA/SCAI guidelines on percutaneous coronary intervention (updating the 2005 guideline and 2007 focused update): a report of the American College of Cardiology Foundation/American Heart Association Task Force on Practice Guidelines. *Circulation.* 2009;120:2271-2306.
6. Wright RS, Anderson JL, Adams CD, et al. 2011 ACCF/AHA focused update of the Guidelines for the Management of Patients with Unstable Angina/Non-ST-Elevation Myocardial Infarction (updating the 2007 guideline): a report of the American College of Cardiology Foundation/American Heart Association Task Force on Practice Guidelines developed in collaboration with the American College of Emergency Physicians, Society for Cardiovascular Angiography and Interventions, and Society of Thoracic Surgeons. *J Am Coll Cardiol.* 2011;57:1920-1959.
7. Levine GN, Bates ER, Blankenship JC, et al. 2011 ACCF/AHA/SCAI guideline for percutaneous coronary intervention A report of the American College of Cardiology Foundation/American Heart Association Task Force on Practice Guidelines and the Society for Cardiovascular Angiography and Interventions. *J Am Coll Cardiol.* 2011;58:e44-122.
8. Shuldiner AR, O'Connell JR, Bliden KP, et al. Association of cytochrome P450 2C19 genotype with the antiplatelet effect and clinical efficacy of clopidogrel therapy. *JAMA.* 2009;302:849-857.
9. Mega JL, Close SL, Wiviott SD, et al. Genetic variants in ABCB1 and CYP2C19 and cardiovascular outcomes after treatment with clopidogrel and prasugrel in the TRITON-TIMI 38 trial: a pharmacogenetic analysis. *Lancet.* 2010;376:1312-1319.
10. Mega JL, Simon T, Colleg J-P, et al. Reduced-function CYP2C19 genotype and risk of adverse clinical outcomes among patients treated with clopidogrel predominantly for PCI: a meta-analysis. *JAMA.* 2010;304:1821-1830.

11. FDA Drug Safety Communication: reduced effectiveness of Plavix (clopidogrel) in patients who are poor metabolizers of the drug. http://www.fda.gov/Drugs/DrugSafety/PostmarketDrugSafetyInformationforPatientsandProviders/ucm203888.htm.
12. Holmes DR Jr, Dehmer GJ, Kaul S, et al. ACCF/AHA clopidogrel clinical alert: approaches to the FDA "boxed warning": a report of the American College of Cardiology Foundation Task Force on Clinical Expert Consensus Documents and the American Heart Association endorsed by the Society for Cardiovascular Angiography and Interventions and the Society of Thoracic Surgeons. *J Am Coll Cardiol.* 2010;56:321-341.
13. Siller-Matula JM, Huber K, Christ G, et al. Impact of clopidogrel loading dose on clinical outcome in patients undergoing percutaneous coronary intervention: a systematic review and meta-analysis. *Heart.* 2011;97:98-105.
14. Mehta SR, Bassand JP, Chrolavicius S, et al. Design and rationale of CURRENT-OASIS 7: a randomized, 2 × 2 factorial trial evaluating optimal dosing strategies for clopidogrel and aspirin in patients with ST and non-ST-elevation acute coronary syndromes managed with an early invasive strategy. *Am Heart J.* 2008;156: 1080-1088.
15. The CURRENT-OASIS 7 Investigators, Mehta SR, Bassand JP, Chrolavicius S, et al. Dose comparisons of clopidogrel and aspirin in acute coronary syndromes. *N Engl J Med.* 2010;363:930-942.
16. Mehta SR, Tanguay J-F, Eikelboom JW, et al. Double-dose versus standard-dose clopidogrel and high-dose versus low-dose aspirin in individuals undergoing percutaneous coronary intervention for acute coronary syndromes (CURRENT-OASIS 7): a randomised factorial trial. *Lancet.* 2010;376:1233-1243.
17. Price MJ, Berger PB, Teirstein PS, et al. Standard- vs high-dose clopidogrel based on platelet function testing after percutaneous coronary intervention: the GRAVITAS randomized trial. *JAMA.* 2011;305:1097-1105.
18. Parodi G, Marcucci R, Valenti R, et al. High residual platelet reactivity after clopidogrel loading and long-term cardiovascular events among patients with acute coronary syndromes undergoing PCI. *JAMA.* 2011;306:1215-1223.
19. Varenhorst C, James S, Erlinge D, et al. Genetic variation of CYP2C19 affects both pharmacokinetic and pharmacodynamic responses to clopidogrel but not prasugrel in aspirin-treated patients with coronary artery disease. *Eur Heart J.* 2009;30:1744-1752.
20. Mega JL, Close SL, Wiviott SD, et al. Cytochrome P450 genetic polymorphisms and the response to prasugrel. *Circulation.* 2009;119:2553-2556.
21. Wallentin L, James S, Storey RF, et al. Effect of CYP2C19 and ABCB1 single nucleotide polymorphisms on outcomes of treatment with ticagrelor versus clopidogrel for acute coronary syndromes: a genetic substudy of the PLATO trial. *Lancet.* 2010;376:1320-1328.
22. Wallentin L, Becker RC, Budaz A, et al. Ticagrelor versus clopidogrel in patients with acute coronary syndromes. *N Engl J Med.* 2009;361:1045-1057.

Cardiogenic shock in the setting of severe aortic stenosis: role of intra-aortic balloon pump support

Aksoy O, Yousefzai R, Singh D, et al (Cleveland Clinic, OH)
Heart 97:838-843, 2011

Objective.—To investigate the haemodynamic effects of intra-aortic balloon pump (IABP) support in patients with severe aortic stenosis (AS) presenting in cardiogenic shock (CS).

Design.—Observational cohort study.

Setting.—Tertiary academic centre coronary intensive care unit (CICU).

Patients.—Patients presenting to the CICU in CS with an established diagnosis of AS (n=25 with mean age (±SD) of 73.5±9.5 years). The peak and mean Doppler AV gradients were 67±26.8 mm Hg and 39.8±16.8 mm Hg, respectively, with a mean baseline cardiac index of 1.77±0.38 l/min/m^2).

Interventions.—Utilisation of IABP.

Main Outcome Measures.—Haemodynamic impact of IABP over time.

Results.—With the insertion of an IABP, patients' cardiac index improved from 1.77 l/min/m^2 to 2.18 and 2.36 l/min/m^2 at 6 and 24 h, respectively (p<0.001 for both times points). Systemic vascular resistance was reduced from 1331 dyn/s/cm^5 to 1265 and 1051 dyn/s/cm^5 at 6 and 24 h, respectively (p=0.66 and p=0.005, respectively). The central venous pressure was reduced from 14.8 mm Hg to 13.2 and 10.9 mm Hg at 6 and 24 h, respectively (p=0.12 and p=0.03, respectively). IABP insertion was associated with a complication in 3 of the 25 cases, including a deep vein thrombosis, thrombocytopenia, limb ischaemia, and technical malfunctioning of the device.

Conclusions.—IABP support improves the haemodynamic profile in patients with severe AS who present in CS. IABP utilisation in this critically ill population should be strongly considered as patients are being evaluated for candidacy for advanced interventions.

▶ Symptomatic, severe aortic stenosis (AS) is a Class I indication for aortic valve replacement.[1] Inspection of the surgical literature, however, reveals that aortic valve replacement is not commonly performed in patients with AS and cardiogenic shock. Among 409 904 valve procedures that were performed between 1994 and 2003 and enrolled in the Society of Thoracic Surgeons database, only 3% of patients had cardiogenic shock at the time of surgery.[2] A recent series of 2256 patients who underwent first-time, isolated aortic valve replacement included only 12 patients with cardiogenic shock.[3] Balloon aortic valvuloplasty[4] and transcatheter aortic replacement (TAVR)[5,6] are alternative options for high-risk patients with AS who are not candidates for surgical aortic valve replacement, and recent studies have investigated vasodilator therapy[7] and the intra-aortic balloon pump (IABP)[8] to treat hemodynamic instability in patients with severe AS.

There is a theoretical basis for attempting to reduce afterload in patients with severe AS and decompensated heart failure or cardiogenic shock. It is well documented that patients with severe AS and normal epicardial coronary arteries may have angina pectoris and myocardial ischemia.[9-13] The proposed mechanisms include decreased coronary reserve due to abnormal coronary microcirculatory function, an imbalance between coronary perfusion and left ventricular afterload, and increased wall stress due to inadequate left ventricular hypertrophy.[9-13] Afterload reduction with nitroprusside improved cardiac function in patients with severe AS and severe left ventricular systolic dysfunction.[7] Among a cohort of 25 patients, the cardiac index increased from 1.6 L per minute per square meter (L/min/m^2), to 2.22 L/min/m^2 after 6 hours of nitroprusside infusion ($P < .001$) and 2.52 L/min/m^2 after 24 hours of nitroprusside

($P < .001$; mean dose 128 ± 96 mcg/min). The improvement in cardiac index during nitroprusside contradicts the notion that afterload reduction is contraindicated in patients with severe AS.

Nitroprusside is contraindicated in patients with aortic stenosis and hypotension. Therefore, afterload reduction with an IABP might be an alternative means of improving cardiac function without causing hypotension in patients with AS complicated by cardiogenic shock. Folland et al[14] published a report of 2 patients with severe AS who improved clinically during treatment with an IABP. Simultaneous measurement of aortic and left ventricular pressures before and during treatment with an IABP demonstrated that left ventricular systolic pressure did not decrease, but there was a 32% increase in the diastolic coronary gradient. The authors concluded that the benefit of the IABP was due to relief of myocardial ischemia secondary to the increased diastolic coronary gradient.

Aksoy et al[8] described the outcomes of 25 patients with severe AS (mean aortic valve area 0.64 cm^2) and cardiogenic shock (mean cardiac index 1.77 L/min/m^2 and mean pulmonary capillary wedge pressure 24.6 mm Hg) who were treated with an IABP at the Cleveland Clinic. The mean cardiac index rose to 2.18 and 2.36 L/min/m^2 at 6 and 24 hours, respectively, after insertion of the IABP ($P < .001$). Also, there was a significant decrease in the mean serum concentration of lactic acid after insertion of the IABP. Fifteen patients survived to hospital discharge, 11 after surgical aortic valve replacement, 3 after balloon aortic valvuloplasty, and 1 after medical therapy alone. The results of the study provide convincing evidence that insertion of an IABP may provide sufficient hemodynamic stability to allow patients with severe AS complicated by cardiogenic shock or decompensated heart failure to undergo surgical or percutaneous aortic valve replacement.

S. W. Werns, MD

References

1. Bonow RO, Carabello BA, Chatterjee K, et al. 2008 focused update incorporated into the ACC/AHA 2006 guidelines for the management of patients with valvular heart disease: a report of the American College of Cardiology/American Heart Association Task Force on Practice Guidelines (Writing Committee to revise the 1998 guidelines for the management of patients with valvular heart disease). Endorsed by the Society of Cardiovascular Anesthesiologists, Society for Cardiovascular Angiography and Interventions, and Society of Thoracic Surgeons. *J Am Coll Cardiol.* 2008;52:e1-142.
2. Rankin JS, Hammill BG, Ferguson TB Jr, et al. Determinants of operative mortality in valvular heart surgery. *J Thorac Cardiovasc Surg.* 2006;131:547-557.
3. Di Eusanio M, Fortuna D, De Palma R, et al. Aortic valve replacement: results and predictors of mortality from a contemporary series of 2256 patients. *J Thorac Cardiovasc Surg.* 2011;141:940-947.
4. Moreno PR, Jang IK, Newell JB, Block PC, Palacios IF. The role of percutaneous aortic balloon valvuloplasaty in patients with cardiogenic shock and critical aortic stenosis. *J Am Coll Cardiol.* 1994;23:1071-1075.
5. Leon MB, Smith CR, Mack M, et al. Transcatheter aortic-valve implantation for aortic stenosis in patients who cannot undergo surgery. *N Engl J Med.* 2010;363:1597-1607.

6. Smith CR, Leon MB, Mack MJ, et al. Transcatheter versus surgical aortic-valve replacement in high-risk patients. *N Engl J Med.* 2011;364:2187-2198.
7. Khot UN, Novaro GM, Popović ZB, et al. Nitroprusside in critically ill patients with left ventricular dysfunction and aortic stenosis. *N Engl J Med.* 2003;348: 1756-1763.
8. Aksoy O, Yousefzai R, Singh D, et al. Cardiogenic shock in the setting of severe aortic stenosis: role of intra-aortic balloon pump support. *Heart.* 2011;97: 838-843.
9. Marcus ML, Doty DB, Hiratzka LF, et al. Decreased coronary reserve: a mechanism for angina pectoris in patients with aortic stenosis and normal coronary arteries. *N Engl J Med.* 1982;307:1362-1366.
10. Smucker ML, Tedesco CL, Manning SB, Owen RM, Feldman MD. Demonstration of an imbalance between coronary perfusion and excessive load as a mechanism of ischemia during stress in patients with aortic stenosis. *Circulation.* 1988; 78:573-582.
11. Julius BK, Spillmann M, Vassalli G, et al. Angina pectoris in patients with aortic stenosis and normal coronary arteries. Mechanisms and pathophysiological concepts. *Circulation.* 1997;95:892-898.
12. Rajappan K, Rimoldi OE, Camici PG, et al. Functional changes in coronary microcirculation after valve replacement in patients with aortic stenosis. *Circulation.* 2003;107:3170-3175.
13. Gould KL, Carabello BA. Why angina in aortic stenosis with normal coronary arteriograms? *Circulatioin.* 2003;107:3121-3123.
14. Folland ED, Kempber AJ, Khuri SF, Josa M, Parisi AF. Intraaortic balloon counterpulsation as a temporary support measure in decompensated critical aortic stenosis. *J Am Coll Cardiol.* 1985;5:711-716.

Pulmonary Embolism/Pulmonary Artery

Incidence of Pulmonary Embolus in Combat Casualties With Extremity Amputations and Fractures

Gillern SM, Sheppard FR, Evans KN, et al (Naval Med Res Ctr, Silver Spring, MD; et al)
J Trauma 71:607-613, 2011

Background.—The objective of this retrospective study was to determine the incidence of pulmonary embolism (PE) in casualties of wartime extremity wounds and specifically in casualties with a trauma-associated amputation.

Methods.—Records of all combat-wounded evacuated and admitted between March 1, 2003, and December 31, 2007, were retrospectively reviewed. Continuous and categorical variables were studied with the Student's *t* test, Fisher's exact test or χ^2 test; multivariate analysis was performed using a stepwise regression logistic model.

Results.—A total of 1,213 records were reviewed; 263 casualties met the inclusion criteria. One hundred three (41.5%) had amputations and 145 (58.5%) had long-bone fractures not requiring amputation. The observed rate of PE in these 263 casualties was 5.7%. More casualties with amputations, 10 (3.7%), developed PE than those with long-bone fractures in the absence of amputation, 5 (1.9%) ($p = 0.045$). Casualties with bilateral lower extremity trauma-associated amputations had a significantly higher incidence of PE compared with those sustaining a single amputation

($p = 0.023$), and the presence of bilateral lower extremity amputations was an independent risk factor for development of a PE ($p = 0.007$, odds ratio 5.9) (univariate and multivariate analysis, respectively).

Conclusion.—The cumulative incidence of PE was 5.7%. The incidence of PE is significantly higher with trauma-associated amputation than with extremity long-bone fracture without amputation. Bilateral amputations, multiple long-bone fractures, and pelvic fractures are independent risk factors for the development of PE. The use of aggressive prophylaxis, deep venous thrombosis screening with ultrasound, and use of prophylactic inferior vena cava filters should be considered in this patient population.

▶ This is excellent retrospective data from the trauma registry from contemporary conflicts in the Middle East. The authors effectively indicate the high-risk patient groups for pulmonary emboli. Unfortunately, the quality of prophylaxis is inconsistent, and no routine screening mechanism is described.[1,2]

It is clear that these patients have the classic triad of Virchow. First, there are extended periods of immobility with transportation between various levels of care and the immobility proportional to the severity of fractures sustained. Second, many of these patients receive massive transfusion or other products designed to enhance clotting. Thus, there is a hypocoagulable state. Finally, one can infer that vascular injury has occurred, noting the high Injury Severity Score sustained by these soldiers.

It is imperative that aggressive prophylaxis be implemented.[3-5] This work is now underway. We also need better surveillance. I was surprised to note that only 20% of injured troops had pulmonary embolism and deep vein thrombosis documented together. Whether this reflects surveillance or poorly understood pathophysiology remains unclear.

D. J. Dries, MSE, MD

References

1. Geerts WH, Code KI, Jay RM, Chen E, Szalai JP. A prospective study of venous thromboembolism after major trauma. *N Engl J Med.* 1994;331:1601-1606.
2. Knudson MM, Ikossi DG, Khaw L, Morabito D, Speetzen LS. Thromboembolism after trauma: an analysis of 1602 episodes from the American College of Surgeons National Trauma Data Bank. *Ann Surg.* 2004;240:490-498.
3. Rogers FB, Cipolle MD, Velmahos G, Rozycki G, Luchette FA. Practice management guidelines for the prevention of venous thromboembolism in trauma patients: the EAST practice management guidelines work group. *J Trauma.* 2002;53:142-164.
4. Tapson VF. Acute pulmonary embolism. *N Engl J Med.* 2008;358:1037-1052.
5. Johnson ON 3rd, Gillespie DL, Aidinian G, White PW, Adams E, Fox CJ. The use of retrievable inferior vena cava filters in severely injured military trauma patients. *J Vasc Surg.* 2009;49:410-416.

Three Thousand Seven Hundred Thirty-Eight Posttraumatic Pulmonary Emboli: A New Look At an Old Disease

Knudson MM, Gomez D, Haas B, et al (Univ of California, San Francisco; Univ of Toronto, Ontario, Canada)

Ann Surg 254:625-632, 2011

Objective.—This study was undertaken to determine the current incidence of pulmonary embolism (PE) and its attributable mortality after injury.

Background.—Despite compliance with prophylactic measures, PE remains a threat to postinjury recovery. We hypothesized that the liberal use of chest computed tomography after injury has resulted in an increased rate of detection of PE but that the mortality attributable to PE has decreased over the past decade. We also postulated that the risk factors for posttraumatic PE might be different from those for deep venous thrombosis (DVT).

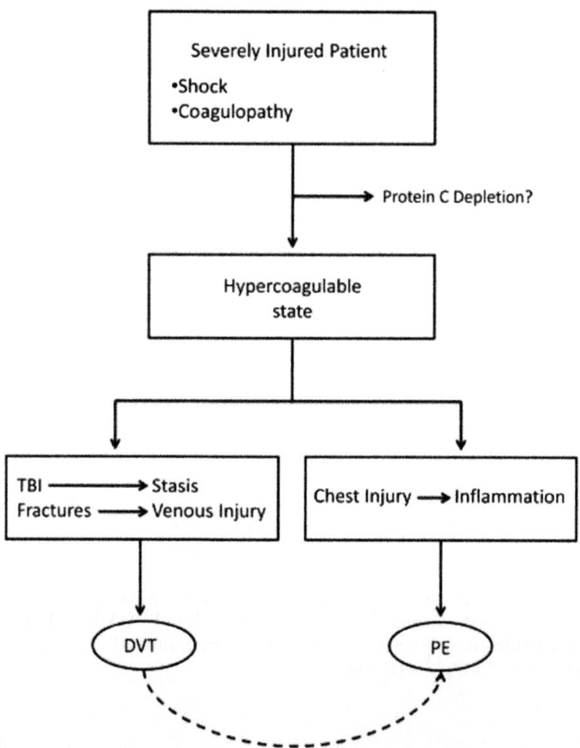

FIGURE 1.—Schematic diagram of factors contributing to the formation of DVT versus PE after trauma, incorporating the 3 arms of Virchow's original triad: stasis; endothelial injury; and hypercoagulability, and adding a fourth: inflammation. (Reprinted from Knudson MM, Gomez D, Haas B, et al. Three thousand seven hundred thirty-eight posttraumatic pulmonary emboli: a new look at an old disease. *Ann Surg*. 2011;254:625-632, with permission from Lippincott Williams & Wilkins.)

Methods.—We examined demographics, injury data, risk factors, and outcomes from patients with DVT and PE compiled in the recent years (2007–2009) in the National Trauma Data Bank (NTDB). For comparison, we used patient data entered into NTDB from 1994 to 2001. Statistical models were created to examine the predictors of DVT and PE and PE-related mortality.

Results.—Among 888,652 patients in the current NTDB cohort, there were 9398 episodes of DVT (1.06%) and 3738 of PE (0.42%). Although many risk factors overlapped, a severe chest injury (Abbreviated Injury Score ≥ 3) conferred a much higher risk of PE than DVT. When comparing results from centers that had contributed to both data sets, there was a more than 2-fold increase in PE occurrence in the current cohort (0.49% vs 0.21%, $P < 0.01$) but with a significant reduction in PE-adjusted mortality (odds ratio, 4.08 vs 2.42).

Conclusions.—The reported incidence of PE after trauma has more than doubled in recent years, while the PE-associated mortality has significantly decreased, suggesting that we are identifying a different disease entity or stage. Chest injuries convey a substantial risk for PE, a risk not likely to be diminished by leg compression devices or vena cava filters (Figs 1-3).

▶ This important study examines the massive National Trauma Data Bank comparing a contemporary cohort (2007 to 2009) to a massive historical cohort from 1994 to 2001.[1] My immediate observation is that practice has changed dramatically during the decades encompassed by this study.

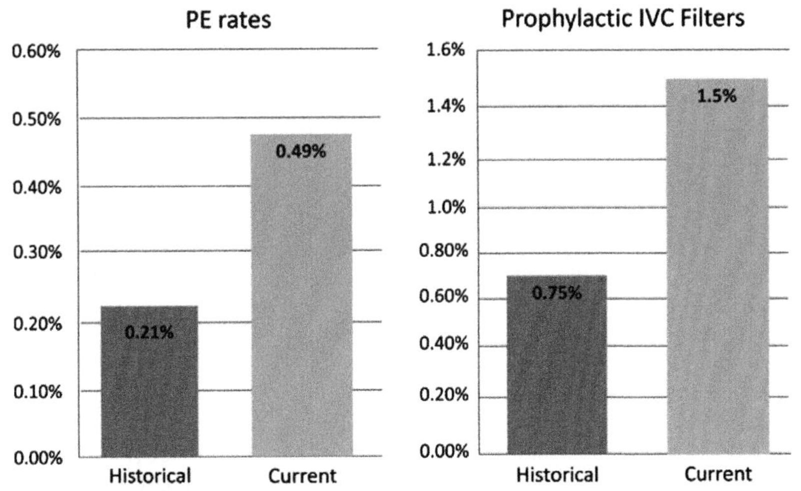

FIGURE 2.—Graphic comparison of PE rates and prophylactic IVC filter insertion rates from our prior study (historic) versus this current study. (Reprinted from Knudson MM, Gomez D, Haas B, et al. Three thousand seven hundred thirty-eight posttraumatic pulmonary emboli: a new look at an old disease. *Ann Surg*. 2011;254:625-632, with permission from Lippincott Williams & Wilkins.)

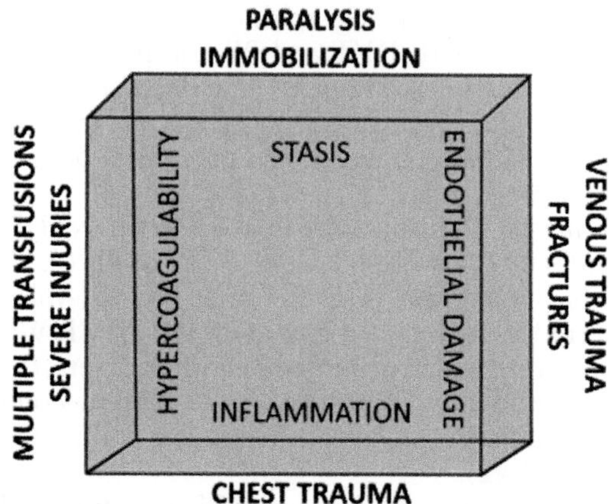

FIGURE 3.—The "Trauma Square" depicting the risk factors for hypercoagulability, as originally described by Virchow, and adding inflammation within the square. The injury patterns outside of the square now include chest trauma (a modification of our previously published trauma triad).[34] *Editor's Note*: Please refer to original journal article for full references. (Reprinted from Knudson MM, Gomez D, Haas B, et al. Three thousand seven hundred thirty-eight posttraumatic pulmonary emboli: a new look at an old disease. *Ann Surg*. 2011;254:625-632, with permission from Lippincott Williams & Wilkins.)

Nonetheless, these results have important implications and obvious limitations. The authors appropriately implicate inflammation, because we now recognize the coincidence of inflammation and hypercoagulable states in the setting of injury (Fig 1). The authors provide attractive diagrams indicating the relationship of the inflammatory component with the classic pieces of Virchow's triad. They also point out the strong correlation between chest injury and pulmonary emboli. A significant number of patients with pulmonary emboli did not have coincident lower extremity clots identified.[2] Although some of this may reflect screening, the authors raise the real possibility that other sources of thoracic clot may be a factor.

A secondary goal is evaluation of vena cava filter use (Fig 2). There is no consistent use of vena cava filters. This dataset does not demonstrate a prophylactic role for vena cava filter implementation. Although more filters are being used, we need additional data to demonstrate their efficacy.[3]

We have become more effective in supporting survival of injured patients, as these data reflect. Our screening technologies also have become much more effective. Therefore, although this paper is presented as benchmark data, until we have consistent screening, these numbers may grossly underestimate the incidence of posttraumatic pulmonary emboli.[4] In addition, resuscitation and other trauma care practices have changed dramatically. We now aggressively use blood component therapy in severely injured patients. This may be an important contributor to reduced overall blood product use and decreased mortality. Massive transfusion may also increase the risk of clot (Fig 3).

D. J. Dries, MSE, MD

References

1. Knudson MM, Ikossi DG, Khaw L, Morabito D, Speetzen LS. Thromboembolism after trauma: an analysis of 1602 episodes from the American College of Surgeons National Trauma Data Bank. *Ann Surg.* 2004;240:490-498.
2. Kucher N. Clinical practice. Deep-vein thrombosis of the upper extremities. *N Engl J Med.* 2011;364:861-869.
3. Velmahos GC, Kern J, Chan LS, Oder D, Murray JA, Shekelle P. Prevention of venous thromboembolism after injury: an evidence-based report—part II: analysis of risk factors and evaluation of the role of vena caval filters. *J Trauma.* 2000;49: 140-144.
4. Pierce CA, Haut ER, Kardooni S, et al. Surveillance bias and deep vein thrombosis in the National Trauma Data Bank: the more we look, the more we find. *J Trauma.* 2008;64:932-937.

3 Hemodynamics and Monitoring

Transthoracic Focused Rapid Echocardiographic Examination: Real-Time Evaluation of Fluid Status in Critically Ill Trauma Patients

Ferrada P, Murthi S, Anand RJ, et al (Virginia Commonwealth Univ, Richmond; Shock Trauma, Baltimore, MD)

J Trauma 70:56-64, 2011

Background.—A transthoracic focused rapid echocardiographic evaluation (FREE) was developed to answer specific questions about treatment direction regarding the use of fluid versus ionotropes in trauma patients. Our objective was to evaluate the clinical utility of the information obtained by this diagnostic test.

Methods.—The FREE was performed by an ultrasonographer or an intensivist and interpreted by a surgical intensivist using a full service portable echo machine (Vivid i; GE Healthcare). The clinical team ordering the examination was surveyed before and after the test was performed.

Results.—During a 9-month study period, the FREE was performed in 53 patients admitted to our trauma critical care units. In 80% of patients, an estimated ejection fraction was obtained. Moderate and severe left ventricular dysfunction was diagnosed in 56% of patients, and right heart dysfunction was found in 25% of the patients. Inferior vena cava (IVC) diameter and IVC respiratory variation was visualized in 80% of patients. In 87% (46 of 53), the FREE was able to answer the clinical question asked by the primary team. Strikingly, in 54% of patients, the plan of care was modified as a result of the FREE examination.

Conclusions.—IVC diameter and IVC respiratory variation was able to be obtained in the majority of cases, giving an estimate of fluid status. Estimation of ejection fraction was useful in guiding the treatment plan regarding the requirement of fluid boluses versus ionotropic support. We conclude that the FREE can provide meaningful data in difficult to image critically ill trauma patients (Fig 3).

▶ The authors demonstrate that a focused echocardiographic examination can provide valuable insight into global ventricular function, sometimes provide an ejection fraction result, and evaluate the vena cava as a surrogate for resuscitation status. The authors suggest that care of patients in a trauma intensive care unit was changed on numerous occasions based on results of the bedside

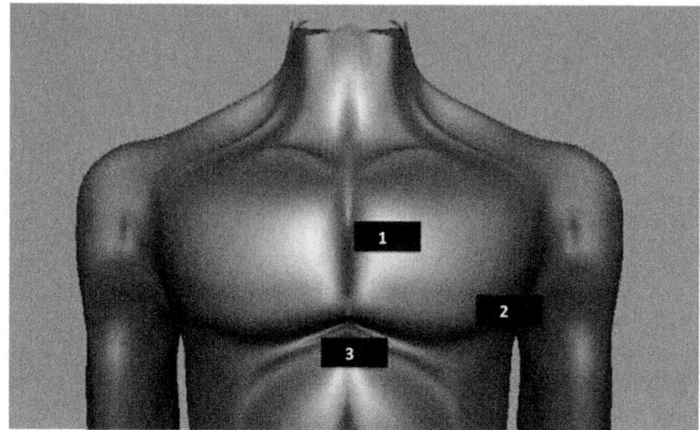

FIGURE 3.—Probe position to obtain the three of the views of the FREE. (1) Parasternal long view and parasternal short. (2) Apical four-chamber view. (3) SX view. (Reprinted from Ferrada P, Murthi S, Anand RJ, et al. Transthoracic focused rapid echocardiographic examination: Real-time evaluation of fluid status in critically ill trauma patients. *J Trauma.* 2011;70:56-64, with permission from Lippincott Williams & Wilkins.)

echocardiogram, which could be performed by trauma or cardiology staff. As a completely noninvasive technique, this approach can be recommended over placement of the pulmonary artery catheter.[1,2]

Parasternal, apical, and subxiphoid views were obtained. Patients studied were older than 60 years, and the majority were male. Mechanism of injury included falls, motor vehicle crashes, and gunshot wounds. Over 70% of patients studied, however, sustained blunt trauma. The authors were able to study patients on mechanical ventilation but note that technically difficult studies were more likely.

I was surprised to see that the average weight of these patients was 78 kg. Obesity may increase the number of suboptimal examinations. Many patients in my hospital weigh far more than this. Surgical clinicians were readily able to adapt this technique and felt that even gross estimation of cardiac function was beneficial.

We need more data to appreciate the full value of focused echocardiography in the hands of surgical intensivists.

D. J. Dries, MSE, MD

References

1. National Heart, Lung, and Blood Institute Acute Respiratory Distress Syndrome (ARDS) Clinical Trials Network, Wheeler AP, Bernard GR, Thompson BT, et al. Pulmonary-artery versus central venous catheter to guide treatment of acute lung injury. *N Engl J Med.* 2006;354:2213-2224.
2. Grissom CK, Morris AH, Lanken PN, et al. Association of physical examination with pulmonary artery catheter parameters in acute lung injury. *Crit Care Med.* 2009;37:2720-2726.

Determination of cardiovascular parameters in burn patients using arterial waveform analysis: A review

Lavrentieva A, Palmieri T (Papanikolaou General Hosp, Thessaloniki, Greece; UC Davis Med Ctr, Sacramento, CA)

Burns 37:196-202, 2011

Optimizing cardiovascular function to ensure adequate tissue oxygen delivery is a key objective in the care of critically ill burn patients. In recent years several less invasive hemodynamic monitoring techniques (arterial waveform analysis techniques) have become available in clinical practice. These alternative techniques provide beat-to-beat cardiac output measurement and permit preload assessment using volumetric parameters. The aim of this article is to review the currently available data regarding to use of less invasive hemodynamic monitoring methods using the pulse wave analysis in burn unit setting.

▶ Lavrentieva's interest and expertise in monitoring burn patients during the sepsis and burns is well known. This is a nice overview of arterial waveform analysis and how it can be evaluated in monitoring critically ill/resuscitating burn patients. The fact remains that current resuscitation strategy endpoints based on urine output with some influence from heart rate/blood pressure data are woefully inadequate. The most invasive monitoring tools are time consuming, expensive, carry risk to the patient, and have not been shown to improve patient outcomes. Using intrathoracic blood volume as an endpoint provides the patient with significantly more fluid than a urine output—based resuscitation without any improved outcomes. Less invasive or noninvasive monitoring tools have the potential to optimize patient outcome while optimizing patient safety during the resuscitation period.

I disagree with Lavrentieva's assertion that using a femoral or brachial artery catheter to monitor the patient is considered less invasive. The location of either catheter is not optimal, and with the upper extremity being the most commonly burned location, placing a catheter here in an end artery is suboptimal.

Studies involving resuscitation and mortality as endpoints should be considered passé, as current mortality rates are so low that thousands of patients would have to be involved in a prospective, randomized, controlled study to show improved outcomes. The development of complications that can be related to resuscitation/monitoring tools would be a better focus for study. We still do not have the answers to resuscitation endpoints, as recent articles regarding fluid creep, opioid creep, and newly discussed ventilator creep aptly demonstrate. Totally noninvasive monitoring techniques requiring only a radial artery catheter may provide the next generation of monitoring tools that provide a leap ahead in understanding burn resuscitation.

B. A. Latenser, MD, FACS

A New Method for Estimation of Involved BSAs for Obese and Normal-Weight Patients With Burn Injury

Neaman KC, Andres LA, McClure AM, et al (Grand Rapids Med Education and Res Ctr/Michigan State Univ Plastic Surgery Residency; Grand Rapids Med Education and Res Ctr/Michigan State Univ General Surgery Residency)
J Burn Care Res 32:421-428, 2011

An accurate measurement of BSA involved in patients injured by burns is critical in determining initial fluid requirements, nutritional needs, and criteria for tertiary center admissions. The rule of nines and the Lund-Browder chart are commonly used to calculate the BSA involved. However, their accuracy in all patient populations, namely obese patients, remains to be proven. Detailed BSA measurements were obtained from 163 adult patients according to linear formulas defined previously for individual body segments. Patients were then grouped based on body mass index (BMI). The contribution of individual body segments to the TBSA was determined based on BMI, and the validity of existing measurement tools was examined. Significant errors were found when comparing all groups with the rule of nines, which overestimated the contribution of the head and arms to the TBSA while underestimating the trunk and legs for all BMI groups. A new rule is proposed to minimize error, assigning 5% of the TBSA to the head and 15% of the TBSA to the arms across all BMI groups, while alternating the contribution of the trunk/legs as follows: normal-weight 35/45%, obese 40/40%, and morbidly obese 45/35%. Current modalities used to determine BSA burned are subject to significant errors, which are magnified as BMI increases. This new method provides increased accuracy in estimating the BSA involved in patients with burn injury regardless of BMI.

▶ In contemporary America, two-thirds of adults are overweight and one-third of adults are obese, and many aspects of how we approach certain aspects of health care need to be reevaluated in light of this fact. Included in this reevaluation is how we calculate the relative weight of each body part as a component of the whole. The Lund-Browder chart continues to be a basis of how a burn size is calculated in most burn centers and is the required form for the National Burn Repository of the American Burn Association. When it was first published in 1944, it was based on patients with a generally normal body mass index (BMI). Sadly, that situation does not exist in the United States today. Because the body surface area (BSA) burned is a key component in calculating fluid resuscitation, a formula in which the trunk and legs are given greater weight in an obese patient would be more accurate.

This is not the first article on burn-size estimation encouraging us to revise the Lund-Browder chart. The current BMI of the average adult American has forced us to revise the Lund-Browder in favor of a more accurate burn diagram. We should do this without delay to improve the accuracy of our burn resuscitations.

B. A. Latenser, MD, FACS

Computerized decision support system improves fluid resuscitation following severe burns: An original study

Salinas J, Chung KK, Mann EA, et al (U.S. Army Inst of Surgical Res, Fort Sam Houston, TX; et al)

Crit Care Med 39:2031-2038, 2011

Objective.—Several formulas have been developed to guide resuscitation in severely burned patients during the initial 48 hrs after injury. These approaches require manual titration of fluid that may result in human error during this process and lead to suboptimal outcomes. The goal of this study was to analyze the efficacy of a computerized open-loop decision support system for burn resuscitation compared to historical controls.

Design.—Fluid infusion rates and urinary output from 39 severely burned patients with >20% total body surface area burns were recorded upon admission (Model group). A fluid-response model based on these data was developed and incorporated into a computerized open-loop algorithm and computer decision support system. The computer decision support system was used to resuscitate 32 subsequent patients with severe burns (computer decision support system group) and compared with the Model group.

Setting.—Burn intensive care unit of a metropolitan Level 1 Trauma center.

Patients.—Acute burn patients with >20% total body surface area requiring active fluid resuscitation during the initial 24 to 48 hours after burn.

Measurements and Main Results.—We found no significant difference between the Model and computer decision support system groups in age, total body surface area, or injury mechanism. Total crystalloid volume during the first 48 hrs post burn, total crystalloid intensive care unit volume, and initial 24-hr crystalloid intensive care unit volume were all lower in the computer decision support system group. Infused volume per kilogram body weight (mL/kg) and per percentage burn (mL/kg/total body surface area) were also lower for the computer decision support system group. The number of patients who met hourly urinary output goals was higher in the computer decision support system group.

Conclusions.—Implementation of a computer decision support system for burn resuscitation in the intensive care unit resulted in improved fluid management of severely burned patients. All measures of crystalloid fluid volume were reduced while patients were maintained within urinary output targets a higher percentage of the time. The addition of computer decision support system technology improved patient care.

▶ Publication of the Parkland Formula for burn resuscitation in 1968 was followed by others with different ideas of what fluids should be used. However, none of the formulas challenged the initial premise of Charlie Baxter and G. Tom Shires's work—namely, how the calculated fluid needs should be divided within that time frame. The schedule of administering half the calculated fluid in the first 8 hours and the other half in the subsequent 16 hours postburn has remained unchallenged until now. The computerized decision support system (CDSS) in this study represents such an improvement over resuscitation formulas and protocols that have historically had problems. The finding that fluid needs crescendo up to hour 13 and then should be gently decreased in a fairly linear manner is exciting, and, I confess, mirrors my bias. We finally have some data with which we can reexamine the 8- and 16-hour divisions that we teach in advanced trauma life support and every other prehospital emergency management course around the world. The authors also address the issue of the current trend in sometimes-severe overresuscitation in burn patients.

The findings in this study may not seem profound, but the implications certainly are. In a mass casualty situation in which experienced burn care providers are not immediately available, a computerized decision tree for burn patients who cannot be treated in burn centers until several days postburn could translate into increased survival for burn victims.

Although it is clear that the practitioners in this study did not always choose to follow the CDSS recommendations, I hope that the authors will make their patented program available to anyone caring for burn patients so that we can improve outcomes.

B. A. Latenser, MD, FACS

The year in burns 2010

Wolf SE, Sterling JP, Hunt JL, et al (Univ of Texas – Southwestern Med Ctr, Dallas)

Burns 37:1275-1287, 2011

For 2010, roughly 1446 original burn research articles were published in scientific journals using the English language. This article reviews those with the most impact on burn treatment according to the Editor of one of the major journals (*Burns*) and his colleagues. As in previous reviews, articles were divided into the following topic areas: epidemiology, demographics of injury, wound characterisation and treatment, critical care, inhalation injury, infection, metabolism and nutrition, psychological considerations, pain and itching management, rehabilitation and long-term outcomes, and burn reconstruction. Each paper is considered very briefly, and the reader is referred to full manuscripts for details.

▶ The authors have once again reviewed all the burn literature published in English-language journals in 2010, and they have chosen those articles that they feel have provided the greatest impact on burn care. Interestingly, burn publications have been increasing at the rate of approximately 75 articles annually since 2003. This review article reveals that epidemiological studies from low-income countries show that scald burns predominate and that women and children are the usual victims. Additionally, burns are a disease of the poor in low-, middle-, and high-income countries. The articles relating to critical care show how it has become an integral part of burn care in high-income countries. The negative impact of hypothermia on outcomes in critically burned patients is discussed. The variability among resuscitation practices throughout the United States was again revealed, with no clear favorites in patient outcomes. Fluid creep and opioid creep, 2 concepts that have garnered some attention, were reviewed. My favorite cited article is the one demonstrating that scalp donor sites do not develop hypertrophic scarring. Nonburn surgeons rarely use the scalp as a donor site, but the color match for any area that requires grafting above the clavicles is perfect when the donor site comes from the face. Although the reviewers do not mention the discomfort from donor sites on the torso or thighs, the scalp donor site seems to be relatively painless. Early excision and grafting was again reviewed and the effect found to be efficacious on cytokine production and insulin resistance. All in all, if the reader is unable to spend the time delving into burn literature, this review article of the year's prior articles is a wonderful global review.

B. A. Latenser, MD, FACS

Another important factor affecting fluid requirement after severe burn: A retrospective study of 166 burn patients in Shanghai

Zhengli C, Kejian Y (Shanghai Jiao Tong Univ School of Medcine, China; the Second Military Med Univ, China)

Burns 37:1145-1149, 2011

Background.—The modified Evans formula is the most often used schema for calculating intravenous resuscitation fluid requirement in burn patients in China, including two parameters: body weight and burnt body surface area (BBS). The aim of this retrospective study was to analyse depth of wound influencing intravenous fluid replacement in addition to these two factors.

Methods.—We reviewed the records of 166 patients admitted in Shanghai Ruijin Hospital during 2000–2008 whose BBS was larger than 25% total body surface area (TBSA). The modified Evans formula was used in all patients. The volume of fluid therapy was determined by urinary output.

Result.—In the first and second 24 h the volume of intravenous fluid resuscitation per bodyweight per BBS (VIWB) showed a significant positive correlation to full-thickness burn size ratio (FBSR: full thickness BBS/total BBS) ($R^2 = 0.138$, $P < 0.001$; $R^2 = 0.108$, $P < 0.001$). The volume of fluid resuscitation was not different than the modified Evans formula in superficial burn only patients. Each 20% increase in full-thickness burn size ratio increased 0.1 in volume infused per bodyweight per BBS in the first 24 h afterburn and 0.06 in the second 24 h.

Conclusion.—Full-thickness burn wounds received more volume of intravenous fluid than superficial burn wounds, especially in the second 24 h afterburn. The formula meets the fluid predictions of different depth of wound by using the modified fluid coefficients.

▶ I find it quite satisfying that this Chinese study revisits the Evans formula, which was first studied and published regarding Chinese patients in the

1960s. Since that time, modifications to the Evans formula make sense, because it is common knowledge that a full-thickness burn sucks up more fluid than a partial-thickness burn. This leads to some insight about the physiology of burn shock. One might presume that a large surface area burn will lead to enhanced fluid loss into dressings, bed linens, and the atmosphere. But the increased fluid requirements of a full-thickness burn, which is dry, desiccated, and leathery, tells us that the fluid losses are intravascular to extravascular, resulting in a need for increased fluid resuscitation. The debate about colloid versus crystalloid in burn resuscitation has not been answered with this study. However, it is nice to know that both the modified Parkland formula, used by more than 90% of US burn centers, and the Evans colloid-based formulas can be successfully modified to meet the requirements of patients with deep full-thickness burns. The question of overresuscitation in recent years is also beyond the scope of this article and better left for a different discussion.

B. A. Latenser, MD, FACS

Comparison of Serial Qualitative and Quantitative Assessments of Caval Index and Left Ventricular Systolic Function During Early Fluid Resuscitation of Hypotensive Emergency Department Patients

Weekes AJ, Tassone HM, Babcock A, et al (Carolinas Med Ctr, Charlotte, NC; et al)

Acad Emerg Med 18:912-921, 2011

Objectives.—The objective was to determine whether serial bedside visual estimates of left ventricular systolic function (LVF) and respiratory variation of the inferior vena cava (IVC) diameter would agree with quantitative measurements of LVF and caval index in hypotensive emergency department (ED) patients during fluid challenges. The authors hypothesized that there would be moderate inter-rater agreement on the visual estimates.

Methods.—This prospective observational study was performed at an urban, regional ED. Patients were eligible for enrollment if they were hypotensive in the ED as defined by a systolic blood pressure (sBP) of <100 mm Hg or mean arterial pressure of ≤65 mm Hg, exhibited signs or symptoms of shock, and the treating physician intended to administer intravenous (IV) fluid boluses for resuscitation. Sonologists performed a sequence of echocardiographic assessments at the beginning, during, and toward the end of fluid challenge. Both caval index and LVF were determined by the sonologist in qualitative then quantitative manners. Deidentified digital video clips of two-dimensional IVC and LVF assessments were later presented, in random order, to an ultrasound (US) fellowship–trained emergency physician using a standardized rating system for review. Statistical analysis included both descriptive statistics and correlation analysis.

Results.—Twenty-four patients were enrolled and yielded 72 caval index and LVF videos that were scored at the bedside prior to any measurements and then reviewed later. Visual estimates of caval index compared to measured caval index yielded a correlation of 0.81 ($p < 0.0001$). Visual estimates of LVF compared to fractional shortening yielded a correlation of 0.84 ($p < 0.0001$). Inter-rater agreement of respiratory variation of IVC diameter and LVF scores had simple kappa values of 0.70 (95% confidence interval [CI] = 0.56 to 0.85) and 0.46 (95% CI = 0.29 to 0.63), respectively. Significant differences in mean values between time 0 and time 2 were found for caval index measurements, the visual scores of IVC diameter variation, and both maximum and minimum IVC diameters.

Conclusions.—This study showed that serial visual estimations of the respiratory variation of IVC diameter and LVF agreed with bedside measurements of caval index and LVF during early fluid challenges to symptomatic hypotensive ED patients. There was moderate inter-rater agreement in both visual estimates. In addition, acute volume loading was associated with detectable acute changes in IVC measurements.

▶ Among the many uses of bedside ultrasound, evaluating an acutely ill patient with hypotension is one of the most valuable. Two critical pieces of this assessment are evaluating left ventricle (LV) function and inferior vena cava (IVC) respiratory variability. This article addressed whether the "eyeball estimate" by clinicians correlated with more formal measurements. The estimate of LV function included categorizing into "severely depressed," "moderately depressed," "normal," or "increased." The categories for IVC respiratory variability (caval index) were "decreased," "normal," and "increased." The encouraging results showed that there was great correlation between estimates and actual measurements (correlation coefficients 0.81 and 0.84). There was also significant change in the IVC measurements and estimations as a patient received fluid boluses. The disconcerting piece of the study showed poor to moderate interobserver agreement and this among quite experienced ultrasonographers. The results generally support the conclusion that clinicians can use a visual estimate when assessing LV function and IVC respiratory variability. It isn't necessary to make detailed measurements. As with all ultrasound, experience counts, and the main limitation of this study is that it included only experienced ultrasonographers.

M. D. Zwank, MD

4 Burns

Burn resuscitation: The results of the ISBI/ABA survey

Greenhalgh DG (Shriners Hosps for Children Northern California, Sacramento, CA)

Burns 36:176-182, 2010

Introduction.—There are valid concerns that burn shock resuscitation is inadequate; a tendency to over-resuscitate the patient seems to exist which may increase complications such as compartment syndrome. The purpose of this study was to survey members of the ISBI and ABA to determine current practices of burn resuscitation.

Methods.—A survey asking for practices of burn shock resuscitation was provided to all participants of a recent ABA meeting. Around the same time, the survey was sent to all members of the ISBI through the internet. The results of the 101 respondents (ABA–59, ISBI–42, approximately a 15% response rate) are described.

Results.—Surveys were returned from all the continents except Africa. Respondents included directors (48%), staff physicians (19%), nurses (23%) and others. Most programs admitted adults (87%) and children (75%) with a mean of 289 admissions per year. The cut off to initiate resuscitation was 15% TBSA and most preferred peripheral IVs (70%) and central lines (47.5%). The Parkland formula was preferred (69.3%) while others were used: Brooke–6.9%, Galveston–8.9%, Warden–5.9%, and colloid 11.9%. Lactated Ringer's (LR) was the preferred solution (91.9%), followed by normal saline–5%, hypertonic saline–4%, albumin–20.8%. FFP–13.9%, and LR/$NaHCO_3$–12.9%. Approximately half (49.5%) added colloid before 24 h. Urine output is the major indicator of success (94.9%) while 22.7% use other monitors. Most (88.8%) feel their protocols work well while 69.8% feel that it provides the right amount of fluid (24%–too much, 7%–too little). Despite this feeling, they still feel that they give more fluid than the formula in 55.1%, less than formula in 12.4% and the right amount in 32.6%. Approximately 1/3 use an oral resuscitation formula and 81.8% feel that an oral formula works for burns < 15% TBSA.

Conclusion.—Large variations exist in resuscitation protocols but the Parkland formula using LR is still the dominant method. Most feel that their resuscitation protocol works well.

▶ Greenhalgh has managed to capture the essential quandary associated with burn resuscitation: What is the best way to accomplish the task? This survey represents the attitudes and practices of burn care professionals from 11 countries on 5 continents. Based on their results, we discover that most of these centers resuscitate patients with a >10% to 20% total body surface area burn using primarily lactated Ringer's and urine output as the main resuscitation guide. And there the similarities end. Some resuscitate only larger burns, some use laboratory values such as lactate or hematocrit, and some use noninvasive monitoring tools such as the LiDCO.

There is agreement that fluid creep is a problem, contributing to the unnecessary development of compartment syndromes, and pulmonary complications and probably worsening the burn depth. The increasing use of opioids is most certainly a contributing factor[1] as is the old adage that more is better when it comes to urine output. The next key piece in the resuscitation puzzle is to determine the impact of these resuscitation issues on outcomes. Once we can answer some of those questions, we can make some statements about best practices related to resuscitation practices. Until then, each burn care practitioner will continue to follow his/her own path.

B. A. Latenser, MD, FACS

Reference

1. Wibbenmeyer LA, Sevier A, Liao J, et al. The impact of opioid administration on resuscitation volumes in thermally injured patients. *J Burn Care Res.* 2010;31: 48-56.

Perioperative use of cuffed endotracheal tubes is advantageous in young pediatric burn patients

Dorsey DP, Bowman SM, Klein MB, et al (Univ of Washington, Seattle; Univ of Arkansas for Med Sciences, Little Rock; et al)

Burns 36:856-860, 2010

Uncuffed endotracheal tubes traditionally have been preferred over cuffed endotracheal tubes in young pediatric patients. However, recent evidence in elective pediatric surgical populations suggests otherwise. Because young pediatric burn patients can pose unique airway and ventilation challenges, we reviewed adverse events associated with the perioperative use of cuffed and uncuffed endotracheal tubes. We retrospectively reviewed 327 cases of operating room endotracheal intubation for general anesthesia in burned children 0–10 years of age over a 10-year period. Clinical airway outcomes were compared using multivariable logistic regression, controlling for relevant patient and injury characteristics. Compared to those receiving cuffed tubes, children receiving uncuffed tubes were significantly more likely to demonstrate clinically significant loss of tidal volume (odds ratio 10.62, 95% confidence interval 2.2–50.5) and require immediate reintubation to change tube size/type (odds ratio 5.54, 95% confidence interval 2.1–13.6). No significant differences were noted for rates of post-extubation stridor. Our data suggest that operating room use of uncuffed endotracheal tubes in such patients is associated with increased rates of tidal volume loss

and reintubation. Due to the frequent challenge of airway management in this population, strategies should emphasize cuffed endotracheal tube use that is associated with lower rates of airway manipulation.

▶ I appreciate this study, as the authors have taken on one of the sacred cows in pediatric burn care, namely, cuffed endotracheal tubes in young patients with pediatric burn. Acute airway management in the severely burned patient may represent one of the most significant challenges in burn care. During preoxygenation, a good seal between the face and the mask may be hampered by a facial burn oozing serum and slimy with the topical antimicrobial in place, not to mention the discomfort of having a mask pressed against a burn. Once the patient is ready for intubation, a posterior neck burn may compromise full neck extension to place the airway in optimal position for instrumentation. Facial and lip edema may hamper the view of the airway by inhibiting full mouth opening. Edema due to inhalation injury and resuscitation may alter the airway anatomy, hindering tube placement and optimal inner-diameter endotracheal tube size. Once the tube is in place, securing the endotracheal tube to the burned face is difficult for the reasons mentioned above, putting the child at risk for tube malposition and either right mainstem intubation or inadvertent extubation. Securing the endotracheal tube to the teeth of the maxilla, while time-consuming, represents a safe and secure airway in this high-risk patient population. Anything that can be done to provide a safer airway for these patients should be actively pursued. The high-volume low-pressure tubes now available represent new technology that should be embraced.

B. A. Latenser, MD, FACS

5 Infectious Disease

Nosocomial/Ventilator-Acquired Pneumonia

Pancreatic Stone Protein: A Marker of Organ Failure and Outcome in Ventilator-Associated Pneumonia

Boeck L, Graf R, Eggimann P, et al (Univ Hosp Basel, Switzerland; Univ Hosp Zürich, Switzerland; et al)

Chest 140:925-932, 2011

Background.—Ventilator-associated pneumonia (VAP) is the most common hospital-acquired, life-threatening infection. Poor outcome and health-care costs of nosocomial pneumonia remain a global burden. Currently, physicians rely on their experience to discriminate patients with good and poor outcome. However, standardized prognostic measures might guide medical decisions in the future. Pancreatic stone protein (PSP)/regenerating protein (reg) is associated with inflammation, infection, and other disease-related stimuli. The prognostic value of PSP/reg among critically ill patients is unknown. The aim of this pilot study was to evaluate PSP/reg in VAP.

Methods.—One hundred one patients with clinically diagnosed VAP were assessed. PSP/reg was retrospectively analyzed using deep-frozen serum samples from VAP onset up to day 7. The main end point was death within 28 days after VAP onset.

Results.—Serum PSP/reg was associated with the sequential organ failure assessment score from VAP onset (Spearman rank correlation coefficient 0.49 $P < .001$) up to day 7. PSP/reg levels at VAP onset were elevated in nonsurvivors (n = 20) as compared with survivors (117.0 ng/mL [36.1-295.3] vs 36.3 ng/mL [21.0-124.0] $P = .011$). The areas under the receiver operating characteristic curves of PSP/reg to predict mortality/survival were 0.69 at VAP onset and 0.76 at day 7. Two PSP/reg cutoffs potentially allow for identification of individuals with a particularly good and poor outcome. Whereas PSP/reg levels below 24 ng/mL at VAP onset were associated with a good chance of survival, levels above 177 ng/mL at day 7 were present in patients with a very poor outcome.

Conclusions.—Serum PSP/reg is a biomarker related to organ failure and outcome in patients with VAP.

Trial Registry.—ISRCTN.org; No.: ISRCTN61015974; URL: www.isrctn.org.

► There has been a virtual explosion in the number of potential biomarkers that may provide important diagnostic, therapeutic, monitoring, or prognostic information for a variety of critically ill patients.[1] The ability of these biomarkers to influence care has so far been rather limited. There have been some interesting and exciting reports detailing procalcitonin in the diagnosis of community-acquired pneumonia, the duration of antibiotic therapy, and in the prognosis of sepsis.[2-4] This report details a preliminary observation on the use of pancreatic stone protein (PSP)/regenerating protein (reg), a 16-kDa polypeptide in the lectin binding protein family, in predicting survival and organ dysfunction in patients with ventilator-associated pneumonia. To the authors' credit, they used a reasonably good definition of ventilator-associated pneumonia (VAP) and found higher mortality in those patients who had higher PSP/reg levels (Fig 2 in the original article). They also noted that the severity and amount of organ failure as measured by sequential organ failure assessment scores was increased in those with higher PSP/reg levels, and when subjects were grouped according to tertiles of PSP/reg level, there was worse survival in those subjects in the highest group (Fig 3 in the original article).

The value and prognostic ability of PSP/reg in patients with sepsis as well as VAP will need to be assessed in a prospective fashion. What will be of most importance will be our ability to alter management and produce improved outcomes by using this biomarker. Only time and future studies will tell us if this is a biomarker worth following.

R. A. Balk, MD

References

1. Marshall JC, Reinhart K. Biomarkers of sepsis. *Crit Care Med.* 2009;37:2290-2298.
2. Schuetz P, Christ-Crain M, Thomann R, et al. Effect of procalcitonin-based guidelines vs standard guidelines on antibiotic use in lower respiratory tract infections: the ProHOSP randomized controlled trial. *JAMA.* 2009;302:1059-1066.
3. Schuetz P, Chiappa V, Briel M, Greenwald JL. Procalcitonin algorithms for antibiotic therapy decisions: a systematic review of randomized controlled trials and recommendations for clinical algorithms. *Arch Intern Med.* 2011;171:1322-1331.
4. Bouadma L, Luyt CE, Tubach F, et al. Use of procalcitonin to reduce patient's exposure to antibiotics in intensive care units (PRORATA trial): a multicentre randomised controlled trial. *Lancet.* 2010;375:463-474.

Intermittent Subglottic Secretion Drainage and Ventilator-associated Pneumonia: A Multicenter Trial

Lacherade J-C, De Jonghe B, Guezennec P, et al (Poissy Saint-Germain Hosp, France; André Mignot Hosp, Le Chesnay, France; et al)

Am J Respir Crit Care Med 182:910-917, 2010

Rationale.—Ventilator-associated pneumonia (VAP) causes substantial morbidity and mortality. The influence of subglottic secretion drainage (SSD) in preventing VAP remains controversial.

Objectives.—To determine whether SSD reduces the overall incidence of microbiologically confirmed VAP.

Methods.—Randomized controlled clinical trial conducted at four French centers. A total of 333 adult patients intubated with a tracheal tube allowing drainage of subglottic secretions and expected to require mechanical ventilation for ≥48 hours was included. Patients were randomly assigned to undergo intermittent SSD (n = 169) or not (n = 164).

Measurements and Main Results.—Primary outcome was the overall incidence of VAP based on quantitative culture of distal pulmonary samplings performed after each clinical suspicion. Other outcomes included incidence of early- and late-onset VAP, duration of mechanical ventilation, and hospital mortality. Microbiologically confirmed VAP occurred in 67 patients, 25 of 169 (14.8%) in the SSD group and 42 of 164 (25.6%) in the control group ($P = 0.02$), yielding a relative risk reduction of 42.2% (95% confidential interval, 10.4–63.1%). Using the Day 5 threshold, the beneficial effect of SSD in reducing VAP was observed in both early-onset VAP (2 of 169 [1.2%] patients undergoing SSD vs. 10 of 164 [6.1%] control patients; $P = 0.02$) and late-onset VAP (23 of 126 [18.6%] patients undergoing SSD vs. 32 of 97 [33.0%] control patients; $P = 0.01$). VAP was clinically suspected at least once in 51 of 169 (30.2%) patients undergoing SSD and 60 of 164 (36.6%) control patients ($P = 0.25$). No significant between group differences were observed in duration of mechanical ventilation and hospital mortality.

Conclusions.—Subglottic secretion drainage during mechanical ventilation results in a significant reduction in VAP, including late-onset VAP.

Clinical trial registered with www.clinicaltrials.gov (NCT00219661).

▶ Ventilator-associated pneumonia (VAP) is a major complication in intensive care unit (ICU) patients requiring mechanical ventilation, with significant associated morbidity, mortality, and cost. It is believed that leakage of oropharyngeal fluids past the endotracheal tube (ETT) cuff and into the lower airways is the major source of bacterial infection. A number of measures are used in an attempt to reduce risk, including semirecumbent body position and optimized ETT cuff designs, materials, and pressures. Aspiration of accumulated subglottic secretions, above the ETT cuff, has long been proposed as another method of reducing the risk of VAP.[1] However, prior trials have been small and conflicting.

The authors performed a multicenter, unblended, randomized, controlled trial looking for benefit from intermittent subglottic secretion drainage. The study has many strengths. The subject group included a mix of patients in a general ICU expected to be intubated for more than 48 hours. A common commercially available ETT tube was used, the Mallinckrodt Hi-Lo Evac ETT, that incorporates a drain above the ETT cuff. The primary outcome showed a significant reduction in microbiologically confirmed VAP, with a number needed to treat of approximately 10. Subgroup analysis supported a significant reduction in both early- and late-onset VAP. The lack of reduction in antibiotic use is notable. While mortality was not reduced, the study was vastly underpowered to detect a potential reduction, which may be on the order of 1%.

Overall, this study supports the use of intermittent subglottic secretion drainage using a specific ETT, with the proviso that mortality, cost, and antibiotic-reduction benefits remain unclear. The choice of intermittent versus continuous drainage remains a question, with continuous drainage proposed to cause more tracheal trauma.

Finally, it must be noted that while this study looked at a single ETT model, newer ETT designs incorporating subglottic drainage, but also featuring thinner, tapered cuffs, which supposedly form a better seal with the tracheal wall, are now being marketed and are beginning to have similar evidence supporting their use.[2] Randomized comparisons of different cuff designs have not yet been done.

U. M. Unligil, MD, PhD
A. Kumar, MD

References

1. Mahul P, Auboyer C, Jospe R, et al. Prevention of nosocomial pneumonia in intubated patients: respective role of mechanical subglottic secretions drainage and stress ulcer prophylaxis. *Intensive Care Med.* 1992;18:20-25.
2. Lorente L, Lecuona M, Jiménez A, Mora ML, Sierra A. Influence of an endotracheal tube with polyurethane cuff and subglottic secretion drainage on pneumonia. *Am J Respir Crit Care Med.* 2007;176:1079-1083.

Use of a Simple Criteria Set for Guiding Echocardiography in Nosocomial ***Staphylococcus aureus*** Bacteremia

Kaasch AJ, Fowler VG Jr, Rieg S, et al (Univ of Cologne, Germany; Duke Univ Durham, NC; Univ Hosp of Freiburg, Germany)
Clin Infect Dis 53:1-9, 2011

Background.—Infective endocarditis (IE) is a severe complication in patients with nosocomial *Staphylococcus aureus* bacteremia (SAB). We sought to develop and validate criteria to identify patients at low risk for the development of IE in whom transesophageal echocardiography (TEE) might be dispensable.

Methods.—Consecutive patients with nosocomial SAB from independent cohorts in Europe (Invasive S. aureus Infection Cohort [INSTINCT]) and North America (*S. aureus* Bacteremia Group [SABG]) were evaluated for the presence of clinical criteria predicting an increased risk for the development of IE (ie, prolonged bacteremia of >4 days' duration, presence of a permanent intracardiac device, hemodialysis dependency, spinal infection, and nonvertebral osteomyelitis). Patients were observed closely for clinical signs and symptoms of IE during hospitalization and a 3-month follow-up period.

Results.—IE was present in 13 (4.3%) of 304 patients in the INSTINCT cohort and in 40 (9.3%) of 432 patients in the SABG cohort. Within 14 days after the first positive blood culture result, echocardiography was performed in 39.8% and 57.4% of patients in the INSTINCT and SABG cohorts, respectively. In patients with IE, the most common clinical prediction criteria present were prolonged bacteremia (69.2% vs 90% for INSTINCT vs SABG, respectively) and presence of a permanent intracardiac device (53.8% vs 32.5%). In total, 13 of 13 patients in the INSTINCT cohort and 39 of 40 patients in the SABG cohort with documented IE fulfilled at least 1 criterion (sensitivity, 100% vs. 97.5%; negative predictive value, 100% vs 99.2%).

Conclusions.—A simple criteria set for patients with nosocomial SAB can identify patients at low risk of IE. Patients who meet these criteria may not routinely require TEE.

▶ *Staphylococcus aureus* bacteremia remains a serious problem and is the second leading cause of bacteremia worldwide.[1] Identifying the focus of *S. aureus* bacteremia (SAB) is a challenge for clinicians. Because a clear focus of infection is only found in 60% to 80% of cases,[2] with infectious endocarditis (IE) occurring in about 17%, it has been suggested that all patients with SAB undergo transesophageal echocardiography (TEE). TEE is superior to transthoracic echocardiography (TTE) for detection of vegetations on heart valves. TEE is more invasive, and complications such as airway compromise and esophageal perforation have been reported.[3] Ideally, only patients at high risk for endocarditis should be screened with TEE. The purpose of the study by Kaasch et al was to develop simple criteria to guide the decision to perform a TEE in patients with SAB.

The authors utilized data from 2 preexisting published cohorts comprising a total of 738 SAB patients to develop criteria for predicting increased risk of IE. Infectious endocarditis was present in approximately 5% to 10% of cohorts.

Clinical criteria that suggested the presence of IE were prolonged bacteremia (defined as a subsequent positive blood culture between days 1 and 4 after the initial positive blood culture) and the presence of a permanent intracardiac device (such as a pacemaker, implanted cardioverter/defibrillator, or prosthetic heart valve).

The sensitivity of the clinical criteria approximated 100% in the combined cohort; specificity, however, was low (approximately 30%). The negative predictive value of these criteria was, therefore, high, approaching 100%.

Limitations to this study include the retrospective nature of how the criteria were defined. Also, there were low rates of TTE and TEE in both groups, which may have led to fewer cases of IE being diagnosed. This study will need to be completed in a prospective fashion to ensure the clinical criteria from the derivation cohort are applicable in real-world situations. However, based on this study, patients who do not have prolonged bacteremia and who do not have a permanent intracardiac device can probably forgo TEE to rule out endocarditis.

D. Funk, MD
A. Kumar, MD

References

1. Wisplinghoff H, Bischoff T, Tallent SM, Seifert H, Wenzel RP, Edmond MB. Nosocomial bloodstream infections in US hospitals: analysis of 24,179 cases from a prospective nationwide surveillance study. *Clin Infect Dis.* 2004;39:309-317.

2. Hill PC, Birch M, Chambers S, et al. Prospective study of 424 cases of *Staphylococcus aureus* bacteraemia: determination of factors affecting incidence and mortality. *Intern Med J*. 2001;31:97-103.
3. Côté G, Denault A. Transesophageal echocardiography-related complications. *Can J Anaesth*. 2008;55:622-647.

Linezolid vs Glycopeptide Antibiotics for the Treatment of Suspected Methicillin-Resistant *Staphylococcus aureus* Nosocomial Pneumonia: A Meta-analysis of Randomized Controlled Trials

Walkey AJ, O'Donnell MR, Wiener RS (Boston Univ School of Medicine, MA; Albert Einstein College of Medicine, Bronx, NY; Edith Nourse Rogers Memorial VA Hosp, Bedford, MA)

Chest 139:1148-1155, 2011

Background.—Methicillin-resistant *Staphylococcus aureus* (MRSA) is an important cause of nosocomial pneumonia. Societal guidelines suggest linezolid may be the preferred treatment of MRSA nosocomial pneumonia. We investigated the efficacy of linezolid compared with glycopeptide antibiotics (vancomycin or teicoplanin) for nosocomial pneumonia.

Methods.—This was a systematic review and meta-analysis of English language, randomized, controlled trials comparing linezolid to glycopeptide antibiotics for suspected MRSA pneumonia in subjects > 12 years of age. A highly sensitive search of PubMed MEDLINE and Cochrane Central Register of Controlled Trials databases identified relevant studies.

Results.—Eight trials encompassing 1,641 subjects met entry criteria. Linezolid was not superior to glycopeptide antibiotics for end points of clinical success (relative risk [RR] linezolid vs glycopeptide, 1.04; 95% CI, 0.97-1.11; *P* =.28), microbiologic success (RR, 1.13; 95% CI, 0.97-1.31; *P* =.12), or mortality (RR, 0.91; 95% CI, 0.69-1.18; *P* =.47). In addition, clinical success in the subgroup of subjects with MRSA-positive respiratory tract culture (RR, 1.23; 95% CI, 0.97-1.57; *P* =.09) was not significantly different from those without MRSA (RR, 0.95; 95% CI, 0.83-1.09; *P* =.48), P for interaction, 0.07. The risk for adverse events was not different between the two antibiotic classes (RR, 0.96; 95% CI, 0.86-1.07; *P* =.48).

Conclusion.—Randomized controlled trials do not support superiority of linezolid over glycopeptide antibiotics for the treatment of nosocomial pneumonia. We recommend that decisions between linezolid or glycopeptide antibiotics for empirical or MRSA-directed therapy of nosocomial pneumonia depend on local availability, antibiotic resistance patterns, preferred routes of delivery, and cost, rather than presumed differences in efficacy.

► Methicillin-resistant *Staphylococcal aureus* (MRSA) is the most common cause of nosocomial pneumonia,[1] which is associated with longer hospital stays, increased costs, and increased morbidity. Current Infectious Disease

Society of America (IDSA) guidelines suggest the superiority of oxazolidinone antibiotics (linezolid) compared with glycopeptides (vancomycin and teicoplanin) for treatment of MRSA pneumonia.[2] This recommendation was based on a post hoc analysis of 1 trial that found a survival advantage of linezolid over glycopeptides in patients with documented MRSA pneumonia.[3] However, there is an approximately 10-fold increase in cost with the use of linezolid versus glycopeptides along with a higher incidence of thrombocytopenia. This meta-analysis was performed to determine the efficacy and adverse effect profile of linezolid versus glycopeptides in the treatment of MRSA pneumonia.

All trials in patients over the age of 12 with MRSA pneumonia were included. In total, 8 trials encompassing 1641 patients met the entry criteria. Linezolid was not found to be superior to glycopeptide antibiotics for endpoints of clinical or microbiological success. The risk of adverse events was similar in both groups. All trials were of relatively small size. Because of the increased cost of linezolid, and the lack of improved clinical efficacy, one can question whether linezolid should be recommended in place of glycopeptides for MRSA pneumonia.

Ongoing larger randomized clinical trials will hopefully shed further light on the clinical difference (if any) between these 2 antibiotics. For now, the clinician treating patients with nosocomial MRSA pneumonia should choose antibiotics based on local resistance patterns, route of delivery, and cost, rather than purported efficacy differences, as this study demonstrated clinical equivalence of the 2 drugs based on the meta-analysis of current randomized, controlled trials.

D. Funk, MD
A. Kumar, MD

References

1. Kollef MH, Shorr A, Tabak YP, Gupta V, Liu LZ, Johannes RS. Epidemiology and outcomes of health-care-associated pneumonia: results from a large US database of culture-positive pneumonia. *Chest.* 2005;128:3854-3862.
2. American Thoracic Society; Infectious Diseases Society of America. Guidelines for the management of adults with hospital-acquired, ventilator-associated, and healthcare-associated pneumonia. *Am J Respir Crit Care Med.* 2005;171:388-416.
3. Wunderink RG, Rello J, Cammarata SK, Croos-Dabrera RV, Kollef MH. Linezolid vs vancomycin: analysis of two double-blind studies of patients with methicillin-resistant *Staphylococcus aureus* nosocomial pneumonia. *Chest.* 2003;124:1789-1797.

Incidence of and Risk Factors for Colistin-Associated Nephrotoxicity in a Large Academic Health System

Pogue JM, Lee J, Marchaim D, et al (Detroit Med Ctr, MI; Wayne State Univ School of Medicine, Detroit, MI; et al)
Clin Infect Dis 53:879-884, 2011

Background.—Colistin, originally abandoned due to high rates of nephrotoxicity, has been recently reintroduced due to activity against carbapenem-resistant Gram-negative organisms. Recent literature, largely obtained from outside the United States, suggests a lower rate of nephrotoxicity than historically reported.

Methods.—A retrospective cohort of all patients who received colistin for ≥48 hours at the Detroit Medical Center over a 5-year period was performed to determine the rate of colistin-associated nephrotoxicity as defined by the RIFLE criteria.

Results.—Fifty-four (43%) patients in the cohort developed nephrotoxicity. Patients who experienced nephrotoxicity after colistin administration were in the Risk (13%), Injury (17%), or Failure (13%) categories per RIFLE criteria. Patients who developed nephrotoxicity received significantly higher mean doses than those who did not (5.48 mg/kg per day vs 3.95 mg/kg per day; $P < .001$), and the toxicity occurred in a dose-dependent fashion. Independent predictors for nephrotoxicity were a colistin dose of ≥5.0 mg/kg per day of ideal body weight (odds ratio [OR], 23.41; 95% confidence interval [CI], 5.3–103.55), receipt of concomitant rifampin (OR, 3.81; 95% CI, 1.42–10.2), and coadministration of ≥3 concomitant nephrotoxins (OR, 6.80; 95% CI, 1.42–32.49).

Conclusions.—In this retrospective cohort, nephrotoxicity (as defined by RIFLE criteria) occurred among 43% of treated patients in a dose-dependent manner. Higher colistin doses, similar to those commonly used in the United States, led to a relatively high rate of nephrotoxicity. These data raise important questions regarding the safe use of colistin in the treatment of multidrug-resistant pathogens.

▶ As the incidence of infections (primarily nosocomial) with highly resistant Gram-negative pathogens increases, the use of antimicrobials with previously limited utility has soared. Colistin (polymyxin E), a polymyxin antibiotic composed of a mix of the cyclic polypeptides A and B, is a case in point. This antibiotic, discovered more than 50 years ago, saw relatively little use during that period owing to its significant, recognized nephrotoxic potential and the development of more effective, less toxic alternatives such as advanced β-lactams. Nonetheless, in the current environment in which multiresistant Gram-negative pathogens (*Pseudomonas aeruginosa, Acinetobacter baumanni, Klebsiella pneumoniae*, etc) are increasingly frequent and the development of new antibiotics has rapidly slowed, colistin has been pressed into common service as the only active available antimicrobial, often in salvage situations in the intensive care unit (ICU).

Unfortunately, because colistin was approved before the current highly controlled regulatory conditions, relatively few data on its pharmacologic/pharmacodynamic effects, particularly in the ICU population, are available. This retrospective study assessed the incidence and risk factors for nephrotoxicity in a cohort of patients receiving colistin for serious, resistant Gram-negative infections. This issue is particularly important because it is well-recognized that the occurrence of nephrotoxicity and renal failure in the ICU is associated with a marked increase in mortality risk.[1] The incidence of development of nephrotoxicity was startlingly high at 43%, although the baseline risk of nephrotoxicity in this group is unclear. Risk was dose-dependent and independently associated with the administration of other nephrotoxic agents.

These data only begin to address the need to develop an improved understanding of the role and risks associated with colistin use in seriously ill patients. The next step would be to determine the incremental risk of colistin in seriously ill patients. However, until better options are developed, other choices may be limited.

A. Kumar, MD

Reference

1. Brivet FG, Kleinknecht DJ, Loirat P, Landais PJ. Acute renal failure in intensive care units—causes, outcome, and prognostic factors of hospital mortality; a prospective, multicenter study. French Study Group on Acute Renal Failure. *Crit Care Med.* 1996;24:192-198.

Other

Use of a Simple Criteria Set for Guiding Echocardiography in Nosocomial *Staphylococcus aureus* Bacteremia

Kaasch AJ, Fowler VG Jr, Rieg S, et al (Univ of Cologne, Germany; Duke Univ Durham, NC; Univ Hosp of Freiburg, Germany)

Clin Infect Dis 53:1-9, 2011

Background.—Infective endocarditis (IE) is a severe complication in patients with nosocomial *Staphylococcus aureus* bacteremia (SAB). We sought to develop and validate criteria to identify patients at low risk for the development of IE in whom transesophageal echocardiography (TEE) might be dispensable.

Methods.—Consecutive patients with nosocomial SAB from independent cohorts in Europe (Invasive *S. aureus* Infection Cohort [INSTINCT]) and North America (*S. aureus* Bacteremia Group [SABG]) were evaluated for the presence of clinical criteria predicting an increased risk for the development of IE (ie, prolonged bacteremia of >4 days' duration, presence of a permanent intracardiac device, hemodialysis dependency, spinal infection, and nonvertebral osteomyelitis). Patients were observed closely for clinical signs and symptoms of IE during hospitalization and a 3-month follow-up period.

Results.—IE was present in 13 (4.3%) of 304 patients in the INSTINCT cohort and in 40 (9.3%) of 432 patients in the SABG cohort. Within 14 days after the first positive blood culture result, echocardiography was performed in 39.8% and 57.4% of patients in the INSTINCT and SABG cohorts, respectively. In patients with IE, the most common clinical prediction criteria present were prolonged bacteremia (69.2% vs 90% for INSTINCT vs SABG, respectively) and presence of a permanent intracardiac device (53.8% vs 32.5%). In total, 13 of 13 patients in the INSTINCT cohort and 39 of 40 patients in the SABG cohort with documented IE fulfilled at least 1 criterion (sensitivity, 100% vs. 97.5%; negative predictive value, 100% vs 99.2%).

Conclusions.—A simple criteria set for patients with nosocomial SAB can identify patients at low risk of IE. Patients who meet these criteria may not routinely require TEE.

▶ *Staphylococcus aureus* bacteremia (SAB) is the second most common nosocomial bloodstream infection and is associated with a 30-day case fatality rate of approximately 20% to 30%. Because of the frequency of SAB infections and the potential for endocarditis, transesophageal echocardiograms (TEEs) have been recommended to guide therapy in all patients with catheter-elated SAB. However, a paucity of data exists about the need for invasive testing criteria for SAB. The authors analyzed 2 independent prospective trials in an attempt to address this gap in the medical literature.

The 2 trials were the European, Invasive Staphylococcus Aureus Infection Cohort trial (INSTINCT) and the American, *Staphyloccocus Aureus* Bacteremia Group (SABG). A nosocomial SAB infection was defined as an infection with clinical symptoms that developed more than 48 hours after hospital admission. Both populations were similar except that the SABG group was both more ethnically diverse and had a higher rate of methicillin-resistant *S aureus* (65.7% vs 15.5%). The authors applied a clinical prediction criteria with 5 variables, 6 to 8 days after SAB was noted, to these 2 trials. The variables were prolonged bacteremia (which meant greater than 4 days elapsed prior to a negative blood culture for SAB), the presence of an intracardiac device, hemodialysis dependence, spinal infection, and nonvertebral osteomyelitis. Infective endocarditis was found in 13 of 309 patients (4.3%) of INSTINCT and 40 of 459 patients (9.3%) of SABG. In patients positive for 1 clinical criterion the sensitivity was 100% in INSTINCT and 97.5% in SABG. The negative predictive value of both trials was 99.5% with only 1 patient with infective endocarditis being missed using this criteria. Yet, more than 50% of patients in both trials fulfilled 1 clinical criteria, and the majority of patients in both trials did not have TEEs. The authors tried to compensate for this defect by following patients for 3 months after their initial diagnosis of SAB. This study is important, because, if followed, it would lead to a significant reductions in the use of TEEs for SAB. The advantages of decreasing the use of TEEs are its limited availability dependent on practice location, the expense of the procedure, and the associated risks of any invasive procedure. Because of the retrospective nature of the study, it is hypothesis-generating, and prospective studies are needed to confirm these results.

N. Puri, MD
S. L. Zanotti-Cavazzoni, MD

Prediction of Serious Infection During Prehospital Emergency Care

Suffoletto B, Frisch A, Prabhu A, et al (Univ of Pittsburgh, PA)

Prehosp Emerg Care 15:325-330, 2011

Background.—Regionalization of emergency care for patients with serious infections has the potential to improve outcomes, but is not feasible without accurate identification of patients in the prehospital environment.

Objective.—To determine the incremental predictive value of provider judgment in addition to prehospital physiologic variables for identifying patients who have serious infections.

Methods.—We conducted a prospective study at a single teaching tertiary-care emergency department (ED) where a convenience sample of emergency medical services (EMS) providers and ED clinicians completed a questionnaire about the same patients. Prehospital providers provided limited demographics and work history about themselves. They also reported the presence of abnormal prehospital physiology for each patient (heart rate >90 beats/min, systolic blood pressure <100 mmHg, respiratory rate >20 breaths/min, pulse oximetry <95%, history of fever, altered mental status) and their judgment about whether the patient had an infection. At the end of formal evaluation in the ED, the physician was asked to complete a survey describing the same patient factors in addition to patient disposition. The primary outcome of serious infection was defined as the presence of both 1) ED report of acute infection and 2) patient admission. We included prehospital factors associated with serious infection in the prediction models. Operating characteristics for various cutoffs and the area under the curve (AUC) were calculated and reported with 95% confidence intervals (95% CIs).

Results.—Serious infection occurred in 32 (16%) of 199 patients transported by EMS, 50% of whom were septic, and 16% of whom were admitted to the intensive care unit. Prehospital systolic blood pressure <100 mmHg, EMS-elicited history or suspicion of fever, and prehospital judgment of infection were associated with primary outcome. Presence of any one of these resulted in a sensitivity of 0.59 (95% CI 0.40–0.76) and a specificity of 0.81 (95% CI 0.74–0.86). The AUC for the model was 0.71.

Conclusions.—Including prehospital provider impression to objective physiologic factors identified three more patients with infection at the cost of overtriaging five. Future research should determine the effect of training or diagnostic aids for improving the sensitivity of prehospital identification of patients with serious infection.

▶ Accurate prehospital identification of serious infection could expedite the delivery of early resuscitation. Furthermore, it would be an important step to facilitate regionalization of sepsis care, similar to the management of major trauma, ST elevation myocardial infarction, and stroke. Regionalizing treatment for sepsis is contingent on accurate recognition of serious infection by emergency medical service (EMS) providers in the prehospital setting.

In this prospective, observational study, the authors sought to identify subjective and objective predictors to aid EMS detection of patients with serious infection. Serious infections were defined as the presence of both emergency department assessment of acute infection and subsequent hospital admission. Both prehospital providers and emergency medicine physicians blinded to prehospital assessment completed a questionnaire eliciting the presence of abnormal objective physiologic parameters (heart rate > 80 beats/min, systolic blood pressure < 100 mg Hg, respiratory rate > 20 breaths/min, pulse oximetry < 95%, altered mental status, suspicion of fever) and subjective suspicion of new infection. Objective predictors, specifically systolic blood pressure < 100 and history of fever, in addition to subjective prehospital provider suspicion for infection, were associated with the primary outcome of serious infection. The presence of each factor was assigned 1 point and scored from 0 to 3 points. The authors identified that a threshold score of 1 predicted the presence of serious infection with a sensitivity of 0.59 and specificity of 0.81.

The algorithm used in the current study would miss nearly 40% of patients with serious infection, presenting a substantial obstacle to initiating prehospital resuscitation and regionalizing treatment for patients with serious infection. Based on these data and prior studies, regionalization of sepsis care has yet to be substantiated. Currently, no outcome improvement has been shown by diverting patients with sepsis to regional centers with a threshold volume of experience. Before pursuing regionalized sepsis management, an algorithm must be developed to enhance the accuracy of prehospital identification of serious infection in the field by EMS providers. In addition, there must be stronger evidence that patient outcome benefit exceeds the detriment of prolonging EMS transport times and delaying initiation of resuscitation.

E. Damuth, MD
S. L. Zanotti-Cavazzoni, MD

Procalcitonin Algorithms for Antibiotic Therapy Decisions: A Systematic Review of Randomized Controlled Trials and Recommendations for Clinical Algorithms

Schuetz P, Chiappa V, Briel M, et al (Harvard School of Public Health, Boston, MA; Massachusetts General Hosp, Boston; McMaster Univ, Hamilton, Ontario, Canada)

Arch Intern Med 171:1322-1331, 2011

Previous randomized controlled trials suggest that using clinical algorithms based on procalcitonin levels, a marker of bacterial infections, results in reduced antibiotic use without a deleterious effect on clinical outcomes. However, algorithms differed among trials and were embedded primarily within the European health care setting. Herein, we summarize the design, efficacy, and safety of previous randomized controlled trials and propose adapted algorithms for US settings. We performed a systematic search and included all 14 randomized controlled trials (N=4467 patients) that investigated procalcitonin algorithms for antibiotic treatment decisions in adult patients with respiratory tract infections and sepsis from primary care, emergency department (ED), and intensive care unit settings. We found no significant difference in mortality between procalcitonin-treated and control patients overall (odds ratio, 0.91; 95% confidence interval, 0.73-1.14) or in primary care (0.13; 0-6.64), ED (0.95; 0.67-1.36), and intensive care unit (0.89; 0.66-1.20) settings individually. A consistent reduction was observed in antibiotic prescription and/or duration of therapy, mainly owing to lower prescribing rates in low-acuity primary care and ED patients, and shorter duration of therapy in moderate- and high-acuity ED and intensive care unit patients. Measurement of procalcitonin levels for antibiotic decisions in patients with respiratory tract infections and sepsis appears to reduce antibiotic exposure without worsening the mortality rate. We propose specific procalcitonin algorithms for low-, moderate-, and high-acuity patients as a basis for future trials aiming at reducing antibiotic overconsumption.

▶ The overuse of antibiotics, which is well documented, leads to antimicrobial resistance, increasing hospital stays by anywhere between 6 and 12 days. Potentially, the right biomarker could help guide antimicrobial therapy. A growing body of literature shows that procalcitonin (PCT) maybe elevated in bacterial infections but not in nonbacterial infection. The authors performed a systemic review to summarize the randomized controlled trial evidence for the use of PCT in respiratory tract infections and sepsis in guiding antibiotic therapy. They used the results of their review to develop an algorithm for use in clinical practice in the United States because most of the studies have been done in Europe.

Fourteen studies met the authors' eligibility criteria for the systemic review. The studies came from disparate clinical locations ranging from primary care to emergency departments to intensive care units. In total, only 3 of the studies were considered low risk for bias. No significant difference in mortality was observed in the PCT- versus the non-PCT-guided therapy groups. There were 6 trials in the critically ill, with 3 trials focused on postoperative patients, 1 trial focused on ventilator-associated pneumonia patients, and 2 trials focused on septic patients. In the critically ill, PCT was used mostly to de-escalate antibiotic therapy, which was different from in the primary care and emergency department setting, where it was also used to determine the need for antibiotics. Procalcitonin was measured twice, and if it reduced significantly, antibiotics were discontinued. If PCT was used to guide antibiotic therapy in the critically ill, there was no statistical difference in mortality, and in 5 out of 6 trials, antibiotic exposure was reduced.

The authors use their systemic review of PCT to develop an algorithm for future randomized clinical trials in the United States. Their study is subject to the same limitations as all meta-analysis. The inherent flaws in the individual trials are not ameliorated by combing them together but may compound erroneous analysis. Caution needs to be exercised in the clinical use of PCT in the United States because of the lack of adequate literature. There are also potential problems with the proposed algorithm. The high level of bias in their selected studies and the combining of 3 clinically different populations may cause the wrong variables to be studied in future randomized controlled trials. More studies are needed to further our knowledge of the potential role of PCT in guiding antibiotic therapy in the critically ill.

N. Puri, MD
S. L. Zanotti-Cavazzoni, MD

Procalcitonin-guided interventions against infections to increase early appropriate antibiotics and improve survival in the intensive care unit: A randomized trial

Jensen JU, for The Procalcitonin And Survival Study (PASS) Group (Univ of Copenhagen, Denmark; et al)

Crit Care Med 39:2048-2058, 2011

Objective.—For patients in intensive care units, sepsis is a common and potentially deadly complication and prompt initiation of appropriate antimicrobial therapy improves prognosis. The objective of this trial was to determine whether a strategy of antimicrobial spectrum escalation, guided by daily measurements of the biomarker procalcitonin, could reduce the time to appropriate therapy, thus improving survival.

Design.—Randomized controlled open-label trial.

Setting.—Nine multidisciplinary intensive care units across Denmark.

Patients.—A total of 1,200 critically ill patients were included after meeting the following eligibility requirements: expected intensive care unit stay of ≥24 hrs, nonpregnant, judged to not be harmed by blood sampling, bilirubin <40 mg/dL, and triglycerides <1000 mg/dL (not suspensive).

Interventions.—Patients were randomized either to the "standard-of-care-only arm," receiving treatment according to the current international guidelines and blinded to procalcitonin levels, or to the "procalcitonin arm," in which current guidelines were supplemented with a drug-escalation algorithm and intensified diagnostics based on daily procalcitonin measurements.

Measurements and Main Results.—The primary end point was death from any cause at day 28; this occurred for 31.5% (190 of 604) patients in the procalcitonin arm and for 32.0% (191 of 596) patients in the standard-of-care-only arm (absolute risk reduction, 0.6%; 95% confidence interval [CI] −4.7% to 5.9%). Length of stay in the intensive care unit was increased by one day ($p = .004$) in the procalcitonin arm, the rate of mechanical ventilation per day in the intensive care unit increased 4.9% (95% CI, 3.0–6.7%), and the relative risk of days with estimated glomerular filtration rate <60 mL/min/1.73 m was 1.21 (95% CI, 1.15–1.27).

Conclusions.—Procalcitonin-guided antimicrobial escalation in the intensive care unit did not improve survival and did lead to organ-related harm and prolonged admission to the intensive care unit. The procalcitonin strategy like the one used in this trial cannot be recommended.

▶ The treatment of severe infections and sepsis in the modern era has been greatly enhanced by the knowledge that prompt initiation of appropriate antimicrobials improves patient mortality.[1] Procalcitonin has emerged in recent years as a possible biologic marker for severe sepsis. Its use is supported mostly in the context of lower respiratory tract infection,[2] although its application to early sepsis due to a variety of infections is under investigation. This large study shows that daily measurement of procalcitonin levels for purposes of guiding escalations of antimicrobial therapy prolonged intensive care unit length of stay, increased ventilator days, and increased use of broad-spectrum antimicrobials. The lack of a survival benefit with the potential for harm is concerning and should lead intensivists to reconsider how they use this costly assay.

A recent study suggests that overly aggressive antimicrobial use in patients with lower severity of illness is harmful,[3] a potential reason for the lack of survival benefit seen in the current study. While the use of procalcitonin as a marker of bacterial infection has shown promise in certain clinical settings,[4] this important trial should encourage intensivists using this test as a guide for empiric escalation of antimicrobial therapy, as opposed to de-escalation, to reevaluate how best to use this test. Current biomarker studies are looking at the potential for guided de-escalation in antimicrobial therapy and perhaps will be a more clinically relevant tool for the practicing intensivist.

M. Blouw, MD
S. Kethireddy, MD
A. Kumar, MD

References

1. Kumar A, Roberts D, Wood KE, et al. Duration of hypotension before initiation of effective antimicrobial therapy is the critical determinant of survival in human septic shock. *Crit Care Med.* 2006;34:1589-1596.
2. Schuetz P, Christ-Crain M, Thomann R, et al. Effect of procalcitonin-based guidelines vs standard guidelines on antibiotic use in lower respiratory tract infections: the ProHOSP randomized controlled trial. *JAMA.* 2009;302:1059-1066.
3. Kumar A, Safdar N, Kethireddy S, Chateau D. A survival benefit of combination antibiotic therapy for serious infections associated with sepsis and septic shock is contingent on the risk of death: a meta-analytic/meta-regression study. *Crit Care Med.* 2010;38:1651-1664.
4. Heyland DK, Johnson AP, Reynolds SC, Muscedere J. Procalcitonin for reduced antibiotic exposure in the critical care setting: a systematic review and an economic evaluation. *Crit Care Med.* 2011;39:1792-1799.

Fidaxomicin versus Vancomycin for *Clostridium difficile* Infection

Louie TJ, for the OPT-80-003 Clinical Study Group (Univ of Calgary, Alberta, Canada; et al)
N Engl J Med 364:422-431, 2011

Background.—Clostridium difficile infection is a serious diarrheal illness associated with substantial morbidity and mortality. Patients generally have a response to oral vancomycin or metronidazole; however, the rate of recurrence is high. This phase 3 clinical trial compared the efficacy and safety of fidaxomicin with those of vancomycin in treating *C. difficile* infection.

Methods.—Adults with acute symptoms of *C. difficile* infection and a positive result on a stool toxin test were eligible for study entry. We randomly assigned patients to receive fidaxomicin (200 mg twice daily) or vancomycin (125 mg four times daily) orally for 10 days. The primary end point was clinical cure (resolution of symptoms and no need for further therapy for C. *difficile* infection as of the second day after the end of the course of therapy). The secondary end points were recurrence of C. *difficile* infection (diarrhea and a positive result on a stool toxin test within 4 weeks after treatment) and global cure (i.e., cure with no recurrence).

Results.—A total of 629 patients were enrolled, of whom 548 (87.1%) could be evaluated for the per-protocol analysis. The rates of clinical cure with fidaxomicin were noninferior to those with vancomycin in both the modified intention-to-treat analysis (88.2% with fidaxomicin and 85.8% with vancomycin) and the per-protocol analysis (92.1% and 89.8%, respectively). Significantly fewer patients in the fidaxomicin group than in the vancomycin group had a recurrence of the infection, in both the modified intention-to-treat analysis (15.4% vs. 25.3%, P = 0.005) and the per-protocol analysis (13.3% vs. 24.0%, P = 0.004). The lower rate of recurrence was seen in patients with non–North American Pulsed Field type 1 strains. The adverse-event profile was similar for the two therapies.

Conclusions.—The rates of clinical cure after treatment with fidaxomicin were noninferior to those after treatment with vancomycin. Fidaxomicin was associated with a significantly lower rate of recurrence of C. *difficile* infection associated with non–North American Pulsed Field type 1 strains. (Funded by Optimer Pharmaceuticals; ClinicalTrials.gov number, NCT00314951.)

▶ Until recently, metronidazole and vancomycin have been the main antimicrobial agents used in the treatment of *Clostridium difficile*–associated diarrhea (CDAD). The changing epidemiology, high disease recurrence rates (20%–80%), and the tremendous health care costs attributed to CDAD require continued research into newer therapies that could decrease the overall impact of this disease among hospitalized patients.[1] The Food and Drug Administration's approval of fidaxomicin (OPT-80, Dificid) was based on the results of 2 double-blind randomized controlled noninferiority trials (including this study) comparing fidaxomicin 200 mg twice a day for 10 days to vancomycin 125 mg 4 times a day.[2] Although the clinical cure rates were similar between both groups, the current published study found a significant 10% relative reduction in relapse rates among patients in the fidaxomicin arm.

Fidaxomicin is a narrow-spectrum, bactericidal, macrocyclic antibiotic that acts by inhibiting bacterial RNA polymerase. It may offer advantages over established treatment options because of its demonstrated activity against hypervirulent *C difficile*, limited impact on normal intestinal flora, and high retention in the gut. Although encouraging, the data from the published studies to date mostly reflect an advantage over vancomycin in reducing relapse rates among non–North American Pulse Field type 1 strains and among patients receiving concomitant antibiotics. Intensivists should recognize that patients with life-threatening infections and toxic megacolon were excluded from the studies. In this study by Louie et al, the authors mention that subgroup analysis did not identify any difference in clinical cure between either drug according to baseline severity of illness. At this time, vancomycin should still be considered first-line antibiotic therapy for severe life-threatening CDAD infections in the intensive care unit (ICU) until further studies can examine this issue. It remains unclear what role fidaxomicin will have in the treatment paradigm among ICU patients. A direct cost-benefit analysis has not been conducted and, given the substantial projected cost of fidaxomicin (nearly $3000) for a 10-day course, further studies will be needed to identify how this drug should be used in critically ill patients.[3]

A. Kumar, MD

References

1. Venugopal AA, Johnson S. Fidaxomicin: a novel macrocyclic antibiotic approved for treatment of clostridium difficile infection. *Clin Infect Dis.* 2011 Dec 7 [Epub ahead of print].
2. Crook D, Weiss K, Cornerly OA, et al. Randomized clinical trial (RCT) in *Clostridium difficile* infection (CDI) confirms equivalent cure rate and lower recurrence rate of fidaxomicin (FDX) versus vanomycin. European Congress of Clinical Microbiology and Infectious Diseases (ECCMID). 2010:10-13.
3. Ghaffarian S, Fox E. *New Drug Bulletin.* Fidaxomicin University of Utah Hospitals and Clinics New Drug Bulletin. 2011:1-2.

Dexamethasone and length of hospital stay in patients with community-acquired pneumonia: a randomised, double-blind, placebo-controlled trial

Meijvis SCA, Hardeman H, Remmelts HHF, et al (St Antonius Hosp, Nieuwegein, Netherlands; et al)

Lancet 377:2023-2030, 2011

Background.—Whether addition of corticosteroids to antibiotic treatment benefits patients with community-acquired pneumonia who are not in intensive care units is unclear. We aimed to assess effect of addition of dexamethasone on length of stay in this group, which might result in earlier resolution of pneumonia through dampening of systemic inflammation.

Methods.—In our double-blind, placebo-controlled trial, we randomly assigned adults aged 18 years or older with confirmed community-acquired pneumonia who presented to emergency departments of two teaching hospitals in the Netherlands to receive intravenous dexamethasone (5 mg once a day) or placebo for 4 days from admission. Patients were ineligible if they were immunocompromised, needed immediate transfer to an intensive-care unit, or were already receiving corticosteroids or immunosuppressive drugs. We randomly allocated patients on a one-to-one basis to treatment groups with a computerised randomisation allocation sequence in blocks of 20. The primary outcome was length of hospital stay in all enrolled patients. This study is registered with ClinicalTrials.gov, number NCT00471640.

Findings.—Between November, 2007, and September, 2010, we enrolled 304 patients and randomly allocated 153 to the placebo group and 151 to the dexamethasone group. 143 (47%) of 304 enrolled patients had pneumonia of pneumonia severity index class 4–5 (79 [52%] patients in the dexamethasone group and 64 [42%] controls). Median length of stay was 6·5 days (IQR 5·0–9·0) in the dexamethasone group compared with 7·5 days (5·3–11·5) in the placebo group (95% CI of difference in medians 0–2 days; p=0·0480). In-hospital mortality and severe adverse events were infrequent and rates did not differ between groups, although 67 (44%) of 151 patients in the dexamethasone group had hyperglycaemia compared with 35 (23%) of 153 controls (p<0·0001).

Interpretation.—Dexamethasone can reduce length of hospital stay when added to antibiotic treatment in nonimmunocompromised patients with community-acquired pneumonia.

▶ Community-acquired pneumonia results in approximately 1 million hospitalizations in the United States at a cost of nearly $9 billion dollars annually, costs mostly related to the length of hospitalization.[1] Early antimicrobial therapy and scoring systems to reliably predict those in need of hospitalization are invaluable management aspects both to improve mortality and to limit costs due to community-acquired pneumonia. The use of steroids as adjunctive therapy to further reduce length of stay and improve survival has been controversial.

The current trial from the Netherlands randomized 300 patients to receive either placebo or low-dose dexamethasone (5 mg/day) for 3 days. The authors conclude that patients receiving low-dose steroids at the time of admission had shorter lengths of stay. The conclusions of this trial have several limitations that intensivists should recognize before considering adopting this into practice. First, and perhaps the most concerning, is that patients subsequently requiring intensive care unit (ICU) care were omitted from the primary outcome analysis. The study points out nonstatistically significant trends toward shorter time to death, delay in ICU admission, and longer ICU length of stay among patients in the dexamethasone arm. Furthermore, the authors acknowledge that 11 patients violated protocol and were given steroids by the attending physician, 7 for what appeared to be chronic obstructive pulmonary disorder (COPD) exacerbations. It is unclear from this study how many patients not admitted to the ICU simply had COPD exacerbations or viral pneumonias thought to be bacterial in origin. The higher rate of empyemas in the steroid arm is concerning given that a recent study suggests that the incidence pneumococcal empyema has nearly doubled following the introduction of widespread vaccination.[2] Two recent clinical trials examining adjunctive steroid use in both community-acquired pneumonia and severe H1N1 pneumonia found the intervention to be of no benefit and potentially harmful.[3,4] Using steroids in community-acquired pneumonia, based on the current best literature, is not a practice that can be recommended for universal adoption.

M. Blouw, MD
S. Kethireddy, MD
A. Kumar, MD

References

1. Halm EA, Teirstein AS. Management of community-acquired pneumonia. *N Engl J Med*. 2002;347:2039-2045.

2. Burgos J, Lujan M, Falcó V, et al. The spectrum of pneumococcal empyema in adults in the early 21st century. *Clin Infect Dis.* 2011;53:254-261.
3. Snijders D, Daniels JM, de Graaff CS, van der Werf TS, Boersma WG. Efficacy of corticosteroids in community-acquired pneumonia: a randomized double-blinded clinical trial. *Am J Respir Crit Care Med.* 2010;81:975-982.
4. Brun-Buisson C, Richard JC, Mercat A, Thiébaut ACM, Brochard L. Early corticosteroids in severe influenza A/H1N1 pneumonia and acute respiratory distress syndrome. *Am J Respir Crit Care Med.* 2011;183:1200-1206.

Procalcitonin and C-Reactive Protein in Hospitalized Adult Patients With Community-Acquired Pneumonia or Exacerbation of Asthma or COPD

Bafadhel M, Clark TW, Reid C, et al (Univ of Leicester, England; et al)
Chest 139:1410-1418, 2011

Background.—Antibiotic overuse in respiratory illness is common and is associated with drug resistance and hospital-acquired infection. Biomarkers that can identify bacterial infections may reduce antibiotic prescription. We aimed to compare the usefulness of the biomarkers procalcitonin and C-reactive protein (CRP) in patients with pneumonia or exacerbations of asthma or COPD.

Methods.—Patients with a diagnosis of community-acquired pneumonia or exacerbation of asthma or COPD were recruited during the winter months of 2006 to 2008. Demographics, clinical data, and blood samples were collected. Procalcitonin and CRP concentrations were measured from available sera.

Results.—Sixty-two patients with pneumonia, 96 with asthma, and 161 with COPD were studied. Serum procalcitonin and CRP concentrations were strongly correlated (Spearman rank correlation coefficient [*rs*] = 0.56, $P < .001$). Patients with pneumonia had increased procalcitonin and CRP levels (median [interquartile range] 1.27 ng/mL [2.36], 191 mg/L [159]) compared with those with asthma (0.03 ng/mL [0.04], 9 mg/L [21]) and COPD (0.05 ng/mL [0.06], 16 mg/L [34]). The area under the receiver operating characteristic curve (95% CI) for distinguishing between patients with pneumonia (antibiotics required) and exacerbations of asthma (antibiotics not required), for procalcitonin and CRP was 0.93 (0.88-0.98) and 0.96 (0.93-1.00). A CRP value >48 mg/L had a sensitivity of 91% (95% CI, 80%-97%) and specificity of 93% (95% CI, 86%-98%) for identifying patients with pneumonia.

Conclusions.—Procalcitonin and CRP levels can both independently distinguish pneumonia from exacerbations of asthma. CRP levels could be used to guide antibiotic therapy and reduce antibiotic overuse in hospitalized patients with acute respiratory illness.

▶ In recent years, there has been a surge of interest in the use of biological markers to detect bacterial infection and guide subsequent prescription of antimicrobials in intensive care units. With globally increasing rates of antibiotic resistance, it is becoming ever more important to limit the unnecessary prescription of antimicrobials.

This study adds to a growing body of literature examining the relative efficacy of C-reactive protein (CRP) and procalcitonin (PCT) levels to predict which patients are more likely to benefit from de-escalation of antimicrobial therapy. This study demonstrates that in a population of patients with mild to moderate lower respiratory tract infection (LRTI) symptoms, these biomarkers can effectively identify those patients who do not require antimicrobial therapy. Other studies have shown that inappropriate use of broad-spectrum antimicrobials in patients with mild illness can be harmful[1] and that withdrawal of antibiotics from cases of bacterial LRTI associated with low levels of biomarkers is not detrimental to patient outcomes.[2] It is important for intensivists to note that the use of PCT in the early identification of sepsis and for determining when to escalate antimicrobial therapy has been shown to result in overuse of antimicrobial agents as well as a substantial increase in mortality.[3] The results of the current trial suggest that the use of the costly PCT assay is comparable to the less expensive CRP test as a guide to antimicrobial de-escalation or discontinuation in cases of mild to moderate LRTI.

M. Blouw, MD
S. Kethireddy, MD
A. Kumar, MD

References

1. Kumar A, Safdar N, Kethireddy S, Chateau D. A survival benefit of combination antibiotic therapy for serious infections associated with sepsis and septic shock is contingent on the risk of death: a meta-analytic/meta-regression study. *Crit Care Med.* 2010;38:1651-1664.
2. Christ-Crain M, Stolz D, Bingisser R, et al. Procalcitonin guidance of antibiotic therapy in community-acquired pneumonia: a randomized trial. *Am J Respir Crit Care Med.* 2006;174:84-93.
3. Jensen JU, Hein L, Lundgren B, et al. Procalcitonin-guided interventions against infections to increase early appropriate antibiotics and improve survival in the intensive care unit: a randomized trial. *Crit Care Med.* 2011;39:2048-2058.

Community-Acquired Respiratory Coinfection in Critically Ill Patients With Pandemic 2009 Influenza A(H1N1) Virus

Martín-Loeches I, H1N1 SEMICYUC Working Group (Univ Rovira i Virgili, Tarragona, Spain; et al)
Chest 139:555-562, 2011

Background.—Little is known about the impact of community-acquired respiratory coinfection in patients with pandemic 2009 influenza A(H1N1) virus infection.

Methods.—This was a prospective, observational, multicenter study conducted in 148 Spanish ICUs.

Results.—Severe respiratory syndrome was present in 645 ICU patients. Coinfection occurred in 113 (17.5%) of patients. *Streptococcus pneumoniae* (in 62 patients [54.8%]) was identified as the most prevalent bacteria. Patients with coinfection at ICU admission were older (47.5 ± 15.7 vs 43.8 ± 14.2 years, $P < .05$) and presented a higher APACHE (Acute Physiology and Chronic Health Evaluation) II score (16.1 ± 7.3 vs 13.3 ± 7.1, $P < .05$) and Sequential Organ Failure Assessment (SOFA) score (7.0 ± 3.8 vs 5.2 ± 3.5, $P < .05$). No differences in comorbidities were observed. Patients who had coinfection required vasopressors (63.7% vs 39.3%, $P < .05$) and invasive mechanical ventilation (69% vs 58.5%, $P < .05$) more frequently. ICU length of stay was 3 days longer in patients who had coinfection than in patients who did not (11 [interquartile range, 5-23] vs 8 [interquartile range 4-17], $P = .01$). Coinfection was associated with increased ICU mortality (26.2% vs 15.5%; OR, 1.94; 95% CI, 1.21-3.09), but Cox regression analysis adjusted by potential confounders did not confirm a significant association between coinfection and ICU mortality.

Conclusions.—During the 2009 pandemics, the role played by bacterial coinfection in bringing patients to the ICU was not clear, *S pneumoniae* being the most common pathogen. This work provides clear evidence that bacterial coinfection is a contributor to increased consumption of health resources by critical patients infected with the virus and is the virus that causes critical illness in the vast majority of cases.

▶ The World Health Organization reported that the 2009 Influenza A (H1N1) viral pandemic resulted in at least 17 000 deaths worldwide by March 2010.[1] Secondary bacterial pneumonia reportedly occurred in 25% to 38% of fatal cases.[1] Kash and colleagues[2] postulated that the lethal synergism between pneumococcus and pandemic influenza may be related to the loss or impairment of lung repair processes. Autopsy studies have also reported that a substantial number of influenza-related deaths were associated with the pathologic findings of secondary bacterial infection.[3] This study is different from prior epidemiologic studies in that the authors sought to identify the direct clinical impact that community-acquired bacterial coinfection had on influenza-related mortality.

In this observational study, less than a quarter of patients identified presented with bacterial coinfection, much less than in other series.[4] Though coinfected patients had higher mean APACHE II scores and more often required hemodynamic support and mechanical ventilation (nearly 30% more often relative to patients with isolated influenza infection), the authors were unable to identify a risk-adjusted mortality difference between groups. Perhaps the inability to identify a particular mortality difference reflects the fact that all patients potentially received empiric antimicrobial therapy early enough so as to provide a survival advantage. Typical community-acquired pathogens like *Streptococcus pneumoniae* (54.8%) and methicillin-susceptible *Staphylococcus aureus* (8%) comprised a large number of the identified organisms, organisms that would be covered by a wide variety of empiric antimicrobial regimens.

The occurrence of invasive pulmonary aspergillosis in nearly 8% of patients is unusual and may not be generalizable to other populations. The findings of this single study should be interpreted in context with a larger body of evidence suggesting an important role in secondary bacterial infection in poor outcomes in influenza-infected patients. Early aggressive antimicrobial therapy in addition to antiviral therapy may be the most effective way to minimize the risk of death after severe influenza infection.

M. Blouw, MD
S. Kethireddy, MD
A. Kumar, MD

References

1. Writing Committee of the WHO Consultation on Clinical Aspects of Pandemic (H1N1) 2009 Influenza, Bautista E, Chotpitayasunondh T, Gao Z, et al. Clinical aspects of pandemic 2009 influenza A (H1N1) virus infection. *N Engl J Med.* 2010;362:1708-1719.
2. Kash JC, Walters KA, Davis SA, et al. Lethal synergism of 2009 pandemic H1N1 influenza virus and streptococcus pneumoniae coinfection is associated with loss of murine lung repair responses. *MBio.* 2011;2:e00171-e00172.
3. Shieh W, Blau DM, Denison AM, et al. 2009 pandemic influenza A (H1N1): pathology and pathogenesis of 100 fatal cases in the United States. *Am J Pathol.* 2010;177:166-175.
4. Kumar A, Zarychanski R, Pinto R, Cook DJ, et al. Critically ill patients with 2009 influenza A(H1N1) infection in Canada. *JAMA.* 2009;302:1872-1879.

Impact of Vancomycin Exposure on Outcomes in Patients With Methicillin-Resistant *Staphylococcus aureus* Bacteremia: Support for Consensus Guidelines Suggested Targets

Kullar R, Davis SL, Levine DP, et al (Wayne State Univ, Detroit, MI)
Clin Infect Dis 52:975-981, 2011

Background.—High rates of vancomycin failure in methicillin-resistant *Staphylococcus aureus* (MRSA) infections have been increasingly reported over time. The primary objective of our study was to determine the impact of vancomycin exposure and outcomes in patients with MRSA bacteremia initially treated with vancomycin.

Methods.—This was a single-center retrospective analysis of 320 patients with documented MRSA bacteremia initially treated with vancomycin from January 2005 through April 2010. Two methods of susceptibility, Etest and broth microdilution, were performed for all isolates to determine the correlation of susceptibility testing to patient outcomes.

Results.—Among a cohort of 320 patients, more than half (52.5%) experienced vancomycin failure. Independent predictors of vancomycin failure in logistic regression included infective endocarditis (adjusted odds ratio [AOR], 4.55; 95% confidence interval [CI], 2.26–9.15), nosocomial-acquired infection (AOR, 2.19; 95% CI, 1.21–3.97), initial vancomycin trough <15 mg/L (AOR, 2.00; 95% CI, 1.25–3.22), and vancomycin minimum inhibitory concentration (MIC) >1 mg/L by Etest (AOR, 1.52; 95% CI, 1.09–2.49). With use of Classification and Regression Tree (CART) analysis, patients with vancomycin area under the curve at 24 h (AUC_{24h}) to MIC ratios <421 were found to have significantly higher rates of failure, compared with patients with AUC_{24h} to MIC ratios >421 (61.2% vs 48.6%; $P=.038$)

Conclusions.—In light of the high failure rates associated with this antimicrobial, optimizing the pharmacokinetic/pharmacodynamic properties of vancomycin by targeting higher trough values of 15–20 mg/L and AUC_{24h}/MIC ratios ≥400 in selected patients should be considered.

▶ Prior observational studies have described the association between vancomycin minimal inhibitory concentrations (MICs) of 1 to 2 μg/mL and reduced clinical efficacy.[1] Soriano et al brought further attention to the importance of increasing vancomycin MICs through their prospective study of methicillin-resistant *Staphylococcus aureus* (MRSA) bacteremia in which they identified an association between MICs greater than 1 μg/mL and increased mortality.[2]

This single-center retrospective study of MRSA bacteremia isolates further demonstrates that a vancomycin MIC greater than 1 μg/mL in *S aureus* is associated with clinical failure. In addition, the authors identified several other important predictors of vancomycin failure. Optimized vancomycin pharmacokinetic/pharmacodynamic parameters, specifically area under the curve at 24 hours/MIC ratios greater than 400 and vancomycin trough values of 15 to 20 μg/mL, appear to be associated with lower rates of clinical failure. Similar rates of failure were found among patients with MRSA pneumonia with high vancomycin MICs.[3] Of concern in this study, more than half of patients treated with vancomycin experienced clinical failure, with the majority of patients experiencing prolonged bacteremia.

Intensivists should note that although clinical failure was associated with longer hospitalization, achieving optimal vancomycin levels could lead to higher rates of nephrotoxicity. Thus aggressive vancomycin dosing is not a strategy that should be adopted for all MRSA infections. Clinicians should consider the risks and benefits of top-end dosing with respect to the severity of illness, type of infection, and the probability of a clinical isolate exhibiting high MICs. Lubin et al developed a simple scoring system with good negative predictive values to guide intensivists in decision making.[4]

S. Kethireddy, MD
A. Kumar, MD

References

1. Sakoulas G, Moise-Broder PA, Schentag J, Forrest A, Moellering RC Jr, Eliopoulos GM. Relationship of MIC and bactericidal activity to efficacy of vancomycin for treatment of methicillin-resistant *Staphylococcus aureus* bacteremia. *J Clin Microbiol.* 2004;42:2398-2402.
2. Soriano A, Marco F, Martinez JA, et al. Influence of vancomycin minimum inhibitory concentration on the treatment of methicillin-resistant *Staphylococcus aureus* bacteremia. *Clin Infect Dis.* 2008;46:193-200.

3. Choi EY, Huh JW, Lim CM, et al. Relationship between the MIC of vancomycin and clinical outcome in patients with MRSA nosocomial pneumonia. *Intensive Care Med.* 2011;37:639-647.
4. Lubin AS, Snydman DR, Ruthazer R, Bide P, Golan Y. Predicting high vancomycin minimum inhibitory concentration in methicillin-resistant *Staphylococcus aureus* bloodstream infections. *Clin Infect Dis.* 2011;52:997-1002.

Timing of Oseltamivir Administration and Outcomes in Hospitalized Adults With Pandemic 2009 Influenza A(H1N1) Virus Infection

Viasus D, for the Novel Influenza A(H1N1) Study Group of the Spanish Network for Research in Infectious Diseases (REIPI) (Univ of Barcelona, Spain; et al)
Chest 140:1025-1032, 2011

Background.—Data on the clinical effectiveness of oseltamivir in patients with pandemic 2009 influenza A(H1N1) (A[H1N1]) virus infection are scarce. We aimed to determine the effect of timing of oseltamivir administration on outcomes in hospitalized adults with A(H1N1).

Methods.—Observational analysis of a prospective cohort of adults hospitalized with laboratory confirmed A(H1N1) was performed at 13 Spanish hospitals. Time from onset of symptoms to oseltamivir administration was the independent variable. Outcomes were duration of fever, hospital length of stay (LOS), need for mechanical ventilation, and mortality during hospitalization. Multivariate logistic regression was used to describe the association between the independent variable and the outcomes.

Results.—Five hundred thirty-eight hospitalized patients with A(H1N1) were studied. The median time from onset of symptoms to oseltamivir administration was 3 days (interquartile range [IQR], 2-5 days). With regard to outcomes, the median duration of fever was 2 days (IQR, 1-3 days), the median LOS was 5 days (IQR, 3-8 days), 49 patients (9.1%) underwent mechanical ventilation, and 11 patients (2%) died during hospitalization. In univariate analysis, prolonged duration of fever (above the median), prolonged LOS (above the median), need for mechanical ventilation, and mortality all increased with time to oseltamivir administration (χ^2 test for trend $P = .001$, $P \leq .001$, $P = .008$, and $P = .001$, respectively). After adjustment for confounding factors, time from onset of symptoms to oseltamivir administration (+1-day increase) was associated with a prolonged duration of fever (OR, 1.10; 95% CI, 1.02-1.19), prolonged LOS (OR, 1.07; 95% CI, 1.00-1.15), and higher mortality (OR, 1.20; 95% CI, 1.06-1.35).

Conclusions.—Timely oseltamivir administration has a beneficial effect on outcomes in hospitalized adults with A(H1N1), even in those who are admitted beyond 48 h after onset of symptoms.

▶ Despite the large body of epidemiologic data describing the characteristics of pandemic influenza A (H1N1), controversy regarding the utility of early administration of oseltamivir to hospitalized patients has persisted. A previous study by Jain and colleagues observed that early antiviral treatment within 48 hours of symptoms could be beneficial for hospitalized patients.[1] Zarychanski and colleagues have similarly demonstrated that delays in initiation of antiviral therapy relative to symptom onset are associated with greater severity of illness.[2] Nonetheless, as the authors correctly state, randomized control trials and subsequent meta-analyses do not provide clarity regarding the importance of timing of antiviral therapy on survival.

The most striking observation of the current study suggests that delayed antiviral therapy (administered after 24 hours of hospitalization) is associated with a 4-fold increased odds of death (when compared with therapy administered within 24 hours). The results of this study should encourage intensivists to institute early antiviral therapy when there is a high index of suspicion for influenza even if polymerase chain reaction results are not rapidly available, as was the case in 25% of patients in this study.

Certain limitations in this study are noteworthy. Most important, the authors did not clearly stratify patients and outcomes based on conventional severity of illness indices. The results of the multivariate analysis, although impressive, similarly did not adjust for severity of illness. Despite these limitations, the findings of this study are informative. Antiviral therapy has been shown to be safe and reduce influenza-related complications.[3] The benefits observed in this study and supportive analyses from review of the subject should lead clinicians to consider early antiviral therapy when influenza is suspected clinically upon hospitalization, a paradigm similar to early initiation of antimicrobial therapy for community-acquired bacterial pneumonia requiring hospitalization.

S. Kethireddy, MD
A. Kumar, MD

References

1. Jain S, Kamimoto L, Bramley AM, et al. Hospitalized patients with 2009 H1N1 influenza in the United States, April-June 2009. *N Engl J Med*. 2009;361:1935-1944.
2. Zarychanski R, Stuart TL, Kumar A, et al. Correlates of severe disease in patients with 2009 pandemic influenza (H1N1) virus infection. *CMAJ*. 2010;182:257-264.
3. Falagas ME, Koletsi PK, Vouloumanou EK, Rafailidis PI, et al. Effectiveness and safety of neuraminidase inhibitors in reducing influenza complications: a met-analysis of randomized controlled trials. *J Antimicrob Chemother*. 2010; 65:1330-1346.

Early-Onset Pneumonia after Cardiac Arrest: Characteristics, Risk Factors and Influence on Prognosis

Perbet S, Mongardon N, Dumas F, et al (Cochin Hosp, Paris, France; Hôtel-Dieu Hosp, Paris, France; et al)

Am J Respir Crit Care Med 184:1048-1054, 2011

Rationale.—Although frequent, little is known about early-onset pneumonia that occurs in the postresus citation period. Although induced hypothermia is recommended as a method of improving neurological outcome, its influence on the occurrence of early-onset pneumonia is not well defined.

Objectives.—To describe the incidence, risk factors, causative agents, and impact on outcome of early-onset pneumonia occurring within 3 days after out-of-hospital cardiac arrest (OHCA).

Methods.—Retrospective analysis of a large cohort study of all patients successfully resuscitated after OHCA and admitted from July 2002 to March 2008 in two medical intensive care units (ICUs). Patients who presented accidental hypothermia or a known pneumonia before OHCA, or patients who died within the first 24 hours, were excluded.

Measurements and Main Results.—During this 6-year period, 845 patients were admitted after OHCA, and 641 consecutive patients were included. A total of 500 patients (78%) were treated with therapeutic hypothermia. In the first 3 days, 419 (65%) presented early-onset pneumonia. Multivariate analysis disclosed therapeutic hypothermia as the single independent risk factor of early-onset pneumonia (odds ratio, 1.90; 95% confidence interval, 1.28–2.80; $P = 0.001$). Early-onset pneumonia increased length of mechanical ventilation (5.7 ± 5.9 vs. 4.7 ± 6.2 d; $P = 0.001$) and ICU stay (7.9 ± 7.2 versus 6.7 ± 7.6 d; $P = 0.001$), but did not influence incidence of ventilator-associated pneumonia ($P = 0.25$), favorable neurologic outcome ($P = 0.35$), or ICU mortality ($P = 0.26$).

Conclusions.—After OHCA, therapeutic hypothermia is associated with an increased risk of early-onset pneumonia. This complication was associated with prolonged respiratory support and ICU stay, but did not significantly influence ICU mortality.

► One of the risks of therapeutic hypothermia for out-of-hospital cardiac arrests is infection. Hypothermia's impairment of the inflammatory response acts as a double-edged sword: it constitutes part of the mechanism of neuroprotection but also leads to the inhibition of the immune functions required to fight off pathogenic microbes. Indeed, cardiac arrest and resuscitation themselves set the patient up for infection: the loss of airway protection, along with the effects of cardiopulmonary resuscitation, bag-mask ventilation, and intubation, put the patient at particular risk for aspiration of both oropharyngeal and gastric contents. Complicating the situation is the obfuscation of our usual markers of infection, including fever, changes in white blood cell counts, hemodynamics, and inflammatory markers.

Here, the authors follow up on their previous work on the infectious complications of therapeutic hypothermia,[1] this time focusing on early-onset pneumonia. This cohort study shows that 65% of cardiac arrest patients treated with therapeutic hypothermia developed early-onset pneumonia. Their multivariate analysis shows therapeutic hypothermia to be the single significant independent risk factor for the occurrence of pneumonia. Interestingly, although they did identify a significantly increased length of mechanical ventilation and intensive care unit (ICU) stay, they found no influence on neurologic outcome or ICU mortality. Overall, this article provides us with some needed basic data regarding postarrest early-onset pneumonia and its consequences and serves to generate discussion in regard to its diagnosis and treatment.

U. M. Unligil, MD, PhD
A. Kumar, MD

Reference

1. Mongardon N, Perbet S, Lemiale V, et al. Infectious complications in out-of-hospital cardiac arrest patients in the therapeutic hypothermia era. *Crit Care Med.* 2011;39:1359-1364.

Impact of herpes simplex virus detection in respiratory specimens of patients with suspected viral pneumonia

Scheithauer S, Manemann AK, Krüger S, et al (Univ Hosp Aachen, Germany)
Infection 38:401-405, 2010

Background.—Respiratory infection and failure is a commonly encountered problem in intensive care unit (ICU) patients. However, despite the accumulating body of evidence to suggest that herpes simplex virus type 1 (HSV-1) is associated with pneumonia, the exact role played by this virus in this process is still not fully understood. Therefore, to identify patients at risk, we have conducted a case-control study to characterize patients with HSV-1-positive pneumonia.

Patients and Methods.—Between 2007 and 2009, all patients with suspected viral pneumonia were tested for the presence of herpes viruses using a PCR assay approach with respiratory specimens. To identify possible associations, risk factors, and impact of HSV, HSV-1-positive ICU patients ($n = 51$) were compared to age-, gender-, and department and season-matched HSV-negative patients ($n = 52$).

Results.—HSV-positive patients differed significantly from the HSV-negative ones only in terms of time of mechanical ventilation (13 vs. 6 days, respectively; $p = 0.002$). Subgroup analysis in the patients aged >60 years and in those without bacterial detection revealed a similar trend ($p = 0.01$ and $p = 0.004$, respectively). Mortality did not differ between the groups or between the HSV-1-positive patients treated with acyclovir and those who were not. A viral load >10E+05 geq/ml was associated with mechanical ventilation (20/21 vs. 17/29; $p = 0.004$), acute respiratory distress syndrome (ARDS; 19/21 vs. 18/29; $p = 0.005$), sepsis (18/21 vs. 14/29; $p = 0.008$), detection of a bacterial pathogen in the same specimen (10/21 vs. 4/29; $p = 0.01$) and longer ICU stay (25 vs. 30 days; $p = 0.04$).

Conclusion.—Despite several associations with high viral load, the clinical outcome of HSV-1-positive ICU patients did not differ significantly from the clinical outcome of HSV-negative patients. This finding indicates that HSV-1 viral loads in respiratory specimens are a symptom of a clinically poor condition rather than a cause of it. Longitudinal and therapy studies are therefore needed to distinguish between HSV-1 as a causative pathogen and HSV-1 as a bystander of pneumonia/ARDS.

▶ Herpes simplex viral (HSV) infections in the intensive care unit (ICU) can present a dilemma in both immunocompromised and immunocompetent patients. Whether viral loads identified in serum, bronchial,[1] or gastrointestinal fluids of the critically ill patient represent significant infection or whether they represent bystander viral replication with little clinical effect is difficult to assess. If treatment is implemented, then the question of potential viral resistance to acyclovir complicates the situation.

In this article, the authors attempt to shed some light on herpes simplex in patients with suspected viral pneumonia by conducting a case-controlled study on HSV-1—infected ICU patients, matched against HSV-negative patients. Despite looking at 24 different clinical parameters, only duration of mechanical ventilation was found to significantly differ between the 2 groups, with the HSV-1—positive patients having a median of 9 days, and the HSV-1—negative patients having a median of 1 day. Notably, however, mortality did not differ between the groups or among HSV-positive patients based on treatment with acyclovir. The acyclovir results, while intriguing, are of little importance given the baseline differences between the 2 nonrandomized groups of patients. A properly executed randomized trial would be needed to address the issue of utility of acyclovir therapy in this context.

A viral load of 105 geq/mL was used to stratify patients in a subgroup analysis of HSV-positive patients. As expected, increased loads do appear to correlate with worse clinical status (more acute respiratory distress syndrome, sepsis, mechanical ventilation) but cannot suggest causality.

Overall, the results do little to clarify the role of HSV infection in ICU patients, but they do provide a starting point for the design of future randomized, controlled trials.

U. M. Unligil, MD, PhD
A. Kumar, MD

Reference

1. Linssen CFM, Jacobs JA, Stelma FF, et al. Herpes simplex virus load in bronchoalveolar lavage fluid is related to poor outcome in critically ill patients. *Intensive Care Med.* 2008;34:2202-2209.

Use of early corticosteroid therapy on ICU admission in patients affected by severe pandemic (H1N1)v influenza A infection

Martin-Loeches I, The ESICM H1N1 Registry Contributors (Univ Rovira i Virgili, Tarragona, Spain; et al)
Intensive Care Med 37:272-283, 2011

Introduction.—Early use of corticosteroids in patients affected by pandemic (H1N1)v influenza A infection, although relatively common, remains controversial.

Methods.—Prospective, observational, multicenter study from 23 June 2009 through 11 February 2010, reported in the European Society of Intensive Care Medicine (ESICM) H1N1 registry.

Results.—Two hundred twenty patients admitted to an intensive care unit (ICU) with completed outcome data were analyzed. Invasive mechanical ventilation was used in 155 (70.5%). Sixty-seven (30.5%) of the patients died in ICU and 75 (34.1%) whilst in hospital. One hundred twenty-six (57.3%) patients received corticosteroid therapy on admission to ICU. Patients who received corticosteroids were significantly older and were more likely to have coexisting asthma, chronic obstructive pulmonary disease (COPD), and chronic steroid use. These patients receiving corticosteroids had increased likelihood of developing hospital-acquired pneumonia (HAP) [26.2% versus 13.8%, $p < 0.05$; odds ratio (OR) 2.2, confidence interval (CI) 1.1–4.5]. Patients who received corticosteroids had significantly higher ICU mortality than patients who did not (46.0% versus 18.1%, $p < 0.01$; OR 3.8, CI 2.1–7.2). Cox regression analysis adjusted for severity and potential confounding factors identified that early use of corticosteroids was not significantly associated with mortality [hazard ratio (HR) 1.3, 95% CI 0.7–2.4, $p = 0.4$] but was still associated with an increased rate of HAP (OR 2.2, 95% CI 1.0–4.8, $p < 0.05$). When only patients developing acute respiratory distress syndrome (ARDS) were analyzed, similar results were observed.

Conclusions.—Early use of corticosteroids in patients affected by pandemic (H1N1)v influenza A infection did not result in better outcomes and was associated with increased risk of superinfections.

▶ Pandemic 2009 influenza A (H1N1) was associated with disproportionately high hospitalization rates among the young and case fatality rates highest among pregnant women and those older than 50 years, demographics much different than seen with seasonal H1N1 influenza.[1] Epidemiologic data have shown that early antiviral therapy of this infection is associated with less severe illness and improved survival.[2-4] Early steroid therapy, although controversial for presumed viral pneumonias,[5] has also been used for treatment of critically ill patients with severe respiratory failure caused by H1N1. This study, along with data from 2 other contemporary studies,[6,7] strongly dispute this practice.

This study shows that the practice of steroid use for severe pandemic influenza infection among European intensive care units was fairly common. However, adjusted multivariate analysis did not show a mortality benefit. In fact, steroid use was associated with harm; specifically a 2-fold higher odds of developing nosocomial pneumonia. A similar study by Kim and colleagues[6] with slightly higher numbers of patients also found that corticosteroids use resulted in higher mortality and nosocomial pneumonia rates. Both articles included patients who received fairly low doses of corticosteroids and neither found a mortality difference when evaluating patients with acute respiratory distress syndrome (ARDS) who received steroids. Another study by Brun-Buisson and colleagues[7] shows that early use of high-dose steroids (median doses of 270 mg of hydrocortisone per day) for influenza-associated ARDS is associated with a nearly 3-fold increased risk of death. Current best evidence strongly suggests that the use of corticosteroids in this particular setting should be avoided.

S. Kethireddy, MD
A. Kumar, MD

References

1. Writing Committee of the WHO Consultation on Clinical Aspects of Pandemic (H1N1) 2009 Influenza, Bautista E, Chotpitayasunondh T, Gao Z. Clinical aspects of pandemic 2009 influenza A (H1N1) virus infection. *N Engl J Med.* 2010;362: 1708-1719.
2. Jain S, Kamimoto L, Bramley AM, et al. Hospitalized patients with 2009 H1N1 influenza in the United States, April-June 2009. *N Engl J Med.* 2009;361:1935-1944.
3. Zarychanski R, Stuart TL, Kumar A, et al. Correlates of severe disease in patients with 2009 pandemic influenza (H1N1) virus infection. *CMAJ.* 2010;182:257-264.
4. Kumar A. Early versus late oseltamivir treatment in severely ill patients with 2009 pandemic influenza A (H1N1): speed is life. *J Antimicrob Chemother.* 2011;66: 959-963.
5. Cheng VCC, Tang BS, Wu AK, Chu CM, Yuen KY. Medical treatment of viral pneumonia including SARS in immunocompetent adult. *J Infect.* 2004;49:262-273.
6. Kim SH, Hong SB, Yun SC, et al. Corticosteroid treatment in critically ill patients with pandemic influenza A/H1N1 2009 infection: analytic strategy using propensity scores. *Am J Respir Crit Care Med.* 2011;183:1207-1214.
7. Brun-Buisson C, Richard JCM, Mercat A, et al. Early corticosteroids in severe influenza A/H1N1 pneumonia and acute respiratory distress syndrome. *Am J Respir Crit Care Med.* 2011;183:1200-1206.

Epidemiology and Risk Factors for Hospital-Acquired Methicillin-Resistant *Staphylococcus aureus* Among Burn Patients

Kaiser ML, Thompson DJ, Malinoski D, et al (Univ of California, Irvine, Orange)
J Burn Care Res 32:429-434, 2011

Methicillin-resistant *Staphylococcus aureus* (MRSA) is a substantial source of morbidity among burn patients. The objectives of this study were to determine the feasibility and efficacy of surveillance cultures and isolation precautions on limiting the transmission of MRSA among burn patients and to determine risk factors for the development of hospital-acquired MRSA (HA-MRSA). All patients admitted to the burn service from January 2007 to June 2009 were screened by nasal swab culture on admission and weekly thereafter. Other sites were cultured based on clinical suspicion. Patients with MRSA were immediately placed on isolation precautions. Community-acquired MRSA (CA-MRSA) and HA-MRSA were defined as identification of the organism <72 hours from admission (CA-MRSA) or ≥72 hours after admission (HA-MRSA). Charts were retrospectively analyzed to identify risk factors for development of HA. Screening compliance was 100%. Seventy MRSA cases were identified in 752 admissions (9% incidence), including 30 cases of CA-MRSA and 40 cases of HA-MRSA. Over the 30-month study period, HA-MRSA incidence decreased according to a significant linear trend. Independent risk factors for the development of HA-MRSA on multivariate analysis included length of stay >7 days (odds ratio [OR] 12.0, 95% confidence interval [CI] 1.6–91), TBSA affected >10% (OR 6.1, CI 2.6–14.2), age >30 years (OR 4.9, CI 2.0–12.0), and inhalation injury (OR 3.5, CI 1.0–11.7). Surveillance cultures with isolation precautions are practical and effective for preventing HA-MRSA among burn patients. Older patients with prolonged hospital stays, large wounds, and inhalation injury are at greatest risk.

▶ Methicillin-resistant *Staphylococcus aureus* (MRSA) continues to be an important pathogen in hospitalized burn patients. In addition to the septicemia and skin graft loss noted by the authors, bloodstream infections, pneumonias, and even urinary tract infections have been noted in a recent work by Wibbenmeyer et al.[1] The current authors work in an 8-bed burn unit, and the isolation practice in their unit involved instituting contact precautions only after a positive nasal swab for MRSA was obtained. Because colonization with MRSA often precedes invasive infections, it makes sense to prevent the vulnerable burn population from ever acquiring these organisms. In our burn center (16 beds), all patients are placed in contact precautions (gowns and gloves) until the results from the polymerase chain reaction (PCR) for the MRSA nasal swab are available, generally within 4 to 6 hours of admission. Because not all patients who get MRSA infections have positive nares PCR, wounds must also be cultured. Although it might seem to needlessly increase the cost of health care in the burn unit, surveillance cultures done on a routine basis are easy to do and effective in identifying exposure to MRSA during the hospital stay. Because you cannot predict who has community-acquired MRSA, the most cost-effective strategy, in addition to rigorous hand washing, is to place all admitted patients in a burn center in contact precautions until the results of the MRSA nasal swab has returned. Prevention is better than subsequent treatment, with all the possible sequelae that entails.

B. A. Latenser, MD, FACS

Reference

1. Wibbenmeyer L, Williams I, Ward M, et al. Risk factors for acquiring vancomycin-resistant Enterococcus and methicillin-resistant Staphylococcus aureus on a burn surgery step-down unit. *J Burn care Res.* 2010;31:269-279.

Impact of Diabetes on Burn Injury: Preliminary Results From Prospective Study

Schwartz SB, Rothrock M, Barron-Vaya Y, et al (The Joan and Sanford I. Weill Med College of Cornell Univ, NY; et al)
J Burn Care Res 32:435-441, 2011

Reducing diabetes mellitus complications has been a major focus for Healthy People 2010. A prior retrospective cohort of our burn center's admissions revealed worse outcomes among diabetic patients, that is, increased infection rates, grafting and graft complications, and increased length of hospital stay. Therefore, a prospective study has been designed to carefully assess wound repair and recovery of diabetic and nondiabetic burn patients. Our long-term aim is to determine the characteristics of the wound milieu along with global responses to injury that may predict poor outcome among diabetic patients. This is an initial phase of a larger observational study of in-hospital diabetic (types 1 and 2) and nondiabetic patients, prospectively matched for age (18–70 and >70 years) and burn size (<5, 5–15, and 16–25%). Time (days) to complete index wound closure, documented through serial photography, is the main outcome measure. Secondary measures compare delays in presentation, prevalence of infections, graft rates, wound and graft complications, adverse events, and length of hospital stay. Detailed history, physical, and baseline hemoglobin A1C are elicited from all subjects who are assessed daily over the initial 72 hours poststudy entry, then weekly until complete index wound closure, and finally monthly through 3 months. Forty subjects are presented herein, 24 diabetic and 16 nondiabetic patients. Time to index wound closure was significantly prolonged in diabetic patients, despite increased grafting. These findings suggest that excision and grafting in diabetic patients may not alone be sufficient to ensure rapid closure, as graft complications may contribute to protracted closure. Evaluating graft need may be more complex among diabetic patients, suggesting the need for alternative management strategies. The current prospective study confirms our previous retrospective analysis, notably manifested by significant delays in index wound closure. Our efforts continue in identifying the most important predictors of outcome, especially modifiable factors that would create a basis of intervention to improve care.

▶ Schwartz et al have looked at the first small cohort from their prospective study comparing burn wound healing in diabetic and nondiabetic patients. The main outcome was time to complete wound closure, the same endpoint recommended for all wound healing studies. Not surprisingly, burn wounds in diabetic patients took longer to heal. That finding is not new, as diabetic burn patients have previously been shown to experience more burn wound infections as well as nonburn infections, bacteremia, and sepsis.[1] Glycemic control (represented by HbA1C in the longer term and absolute blood glucose measurements in the shorter term) have also been shown to play a role, regardless of whether the patient is diabetic.[2]

One study weakness is that we don't have information regarding blood glucose management strategies in this patient population. Hopefully, the authors will provide more details about it in future, along with more complete data analyses. The unexpected finding in this study is that burn wounds in diabetic patients took longer to heal regardless of whether they were treated to excision and grafting. Unfortunately, there is a great deal about wound management strategies for which we have no information: time to actually decide whether to excise and graft a wound, specific wound management strategies, systemic antibiotic strategies, and, as mentioned before, glycemic control strategies. We also do not know if the diabetic patients had a higher body mass index, another confounder when discussing wound healing. However, the single finding that even grafted wounds fared much worse in the diabetic population must lead us to question our current burn wound management strategies in diabetic patients. With the increased wound infections and length of stay in diabetic burn patients, modifiable patient care factors will certainly play a role in improving outcomes while decreasing patient care costs. Look for the more complete study from this group to help refine some of the answers in this patient population.

B. A. Latenser, MD, FACS

References

1. Memmel H, Kowal-Vern A, Latenser BA. Infections in diabetic burn patients. *Diabetes Care*. 2004;27:229-233.
2. Hemmila MR, Taddonio MA, Arbabi S, Maggio PM, Wahl WL. Intensive insulin therapy is associated with reduced infectious complications in burn patients. *Surgery*. 2008;144:629-637.

Is Prophylactic Acyclovir Treatment Warranted for Prevention of Herpes Simplex Virus Infections in Facial Burns? A Review of the Literature

Haik J, Weissman O, Stavrou D, et al (Tel-Aviv Univ, Tel-Hashomer, Israel)

J Burn Care Res 32:358-362, 2011

Both cosmetic facial resurfacing and facial burns cause an injury to the dermal layer of the skin. This injury renders the patient susceptible to primary herpes simplex virus (HSV) infection or, more commonly, to HSV reactivation. This in turn can lead to bacterial superinfection, possibly resulting in scarring and systemic dissemination in the immunosuppressed burn patient. HSV reactivation rates have been reported to be up to 50% in cosmetic procedures without acyclovir prophylaxis and up to 25% in patients with burn injury. Currently, acyclovir prophylaxis is a common practice in facial resurfacing, but no such recommendations have been issued for patients with burn injury. HSV usually presents in a febrile burn patient between the first and third postburn weeks as a cluster of small, umbilicated vesicles or vesicopustules on an erythematous base found within or around the margins of healing partial-thickness wounds. Diagnosis is confirmed through viral culture from the base of an unroofed vesicle, and treatment is begun with intravenous acyclovir. Antiviral prophylaxis should be strongly considered for HSV infection prevention in patients with major burn injury, particularly with burns involving the face. Acyclovir is the primary drug of choice, and contact precautions should be practiced. High suspicion levels and alertness to this entity can help prompt diagnosis and timely treatment while alleviating late complications.

▶ Herpes simplex infections in burn patients are an unfortunate but common occurrence in patients with burns that are large enough to be a systemic event (eg, ~20% total body surface area burn). Although burn care practitioners are familiar with the event, the existing literature is sparse, with many citations being case reports. This review presents the practical aspects of diagnosing and treating a patient with a herpetic outbreak, usually in the setting of partial-thickness facial burns, 1 to 3 weeks after burn injury. Because the herpetic lesions are symptomatic, they are worth treating. Preventing spread to other patients in the unit must also be a consideration in caring for the patient with active lesions.

The only portion of this article I disagree with is when the authors state that surgical procedures must be delayed until symptoms have resolved or lesions crusted over, a process that can take more than a week. If the patient has a significant full-thickness burn injury and it has not yet been completely excised, it could be potentially dangerous to delay excision. If the patient cannot wait for full-thickness burn wound excision, the surgeons should strongly consider excision and allografting and avoid creating a donor site, which would be the prime target for further herpes simplex virus infections. Missing the diagnosis altogether could prove fatal, so be aware that this is probably a more common occurrence than we think.

B. A. Latenser, MD, FACS

An Open, Parallel, Randomized, Comparative, Multicenter Study to Evaluate the Cost-Effectiveness, Performance, Tolerance, and Safety of a Silver-Containing Soft Silicone Foam Dressing (Intervention) vs Silver Sulfadiazine Cream

Silverstein P, Heimbach D, Meites H, et al (Paul Silverstein Burn Ctr, Oklahoma City, OK; Harborview Med Ctr, Seattle, WA; et al)
J Burn Care Res 32:617-626, 2011

An open, parallel, randomized, comparative, multicenter study was implemented to evaluate the cost-effectiveness, performance, tolerance, and safety of a silver-containing soft silicone foam dressing (Mepilex Ag) vs silver sulfadiazine cream (control) in the treatment of partial-thickness thermal burns. Individuals aged 5 years and older with partial-thickness thermal burns (2.5–20% BSA) were randomized into two groups and treated with the trial products for 21 days or until healed, whichever occurred first. Data were obtained and analyzed on cost (direct and indirect), healing rates, pain, comfort, ease of product use, and adverse events. A total of 101 subjects were recruited. There were no significant differences in burn area profiles within the groups. The cost of dressing-related analgesia was lower in the intervention group ($P = .03$) as was the cost of background analgesia ($P = .07$). The mean total cost of treatment was $309 vs $513 in the control ($P < .001$). The average cost-effectiveness per treatment regime was $381 lower in the intervention product, producing an incremental cost-effectiveness ratio of $1688 in favor of the soft silicone foam dressing. Mean healing rates were 71.7 vs 60.8% at final visit, and the number of dressing changes were 2.2 vs 12.4 in the treatment and control groups, respectively. Subjects reported significantly less pain at application

(P =.02) and during wear (P =.048) of the Mepilex Ag dressing in the acute stages of wound healing. Clinicians reported the intervention dressing was significantly easier to use (P =.03) and flexible (P =.04). Both treatments were well tolerated; however, the total incidence of adverse events was higher in the control group. The silver-containing soft silicone foam dressing was as effective in the treatment of patients as the standard care (silver sulfadiazine). In addition, the group of patients treated with the soft silicone foam dressing demonstrated decreased pain and lower costs associated with treatment.

▶ This study involved 10 US burn centers using standard US Food and Drug Administration criteria for wound evaluation (eg, time to wound closure). The thing that makes this study quite unique is that it was designed by the participating burn surgeons in a way that was clinically meaningful. My participation in the study was predicated on the unbiased nature of the study and the guarantee that we would publish the results, regardless of the outcome. The silicone foam dressing used in the study, Mepilex AG, is just one of many silver-containing products currently on the market. The real costs described in the study are even more significant when you consider that time away from work for the patient or the family, the costs associated with driving to the hospital, parking, and time taken to perform the wound care were not factored into the financial impact of this dressing. If they had been, the dramatically fewer dressing changes required per patient would have made the financial findings even more pronounced. Additionally, the cost of pain is immeasurable. In adults, one can work with the patient to provide intellectual reasoning when one has to perform a painful procedure, but in young children, the pain and subsequent emotional trauma may persist beyond the dressing change. We know that pain and acute stress disorder (ASD) and posttraumatic stress disorder (PTSD) are related; therefore, anything we can do to decrease the pain in the early postburn period will decrease the ASD/PTSD later. Silver sulfadiazine was also related to delayed wound healing in this study, a finding that has been known to burn care practitioners for some time. Early wound closure in burn care is always the goal, as every day that a burn wound stays open is a day toward scarring. Silver-impregnated compounds are clearly the way to go for wound healing. Anything that provides less pain and more rapid healing and is easier for the patient to use gets my vote.

B. A. Latenser, MD, FACS

β-D-Glucan Assay for the Diagnosis of Invasive Fungal Infections: A Meta-analysis

Karageorgopoulos DE, Vouloumanou EK, Ntziora F, et al (Henry Dunant Hosp, Athens, Greece)

Clin Infect Dis 52:750-770, 2011

We aimed to assess the accuracy of measuring serum or plasma (1→3)-β-D-glucan (BDG) for the diagnosis of invasive fungal infections (IFIs) by means of a meta-analysis of relevant studies. We searched in bibliographic databases for relevant cohort or case-control studies. We primarily compared BDG between patients with proven or probable IFIs (excluding *Pneumocystis jiroveci* infections), according to the criteria of the European Organization for Research and Treatment of Cancer/Mycoses Study Group or similar criteria, and patients without IFIs (excluding healthy individuals as controls). A total of 2979 patients (594 with proven or probable IFIs), included in 16 studies, were analyzed. The pooled sensitivity of BDG was 76.8% (95% confidence interval [CI], 67.1%–84.3%), and the specificity was 85.3% (95% CI, 79.6%–89.7%). The area under the summary receiver operating characteristic curve was 0.89. Marked statistical heterogeneity was noted. BDG has good diagnostic accuracy for distinguishing proven or probable IFIs from no IFIs. It can be useful in clinical practice, if implemented in the proper setting and interpreted after consideration of its limitations.

▶ The survival benefit following early, appropriate treatment of candidemia and candida septic shock has been described in several studies.[1] The ongoing challenge for intensivists remains identifying those high-risk patients who would benefit from early or preemptive antifungal therapy. Candida colonization indices, candida scoring systems, and biomarkers have been developed to aid clinicians in identifying these patients without overtreating patients at low risk.[2] Despite the excellent negative predictive value of some of these methods, poor positive predictive values may result in unnecessary treatment. Bioassays identifying the presence of (1→3)-β-D-glucan, a cell wall constituent of many fungi, represents a complementary diagnostic aid to the current predictive systems.

The current meta-analysis, the largest to date, describes the operating characteristics of this serum assay for both proven invasive candidiasis and aspergillosis. Despite the heterogeneity in study methodology and assays used, this study supports using a (1→3)-β-D-glucan bioassay for early detection of invasive fungal infections primarily among high-risk hematologic-oncologic patients. Although potentially applicable to intensive care unit (ICU) patients, the role of this assay remains undefined. The pooled sensitivity of 77% described in this study suggests that a substantial number of patients with significant infections could be missed using this assay alone. However, as Posteraro and colleagues recently reported, a combined approach using both scoring systems and assay levels could prove cost-effective and more accurately identify those at high risk for developing invasive fungal infections in the ICU.[3] If this assay is used, intensivists will need to recognize that it may yield false-positive (specificity of 85%) results during the first 3 days of ICU care or following surgery, as well as from cross-reactivity with hemodialysis membranes, surgical gauze, certain blood products, immunoglobulin therapy, and some antimicrobial agents.[2]

S. Kethireddy, MD
A. Kumar, MD

References

1. Kumar A, Roberts D, Wood KE, et al. Duration of hypotension before initiation of effective antimicrobial therapy is the critical determinant of survival in human septic shock. *Crit Care Med.* 2006;34:1589-1596.
2. Ostrosky-Zeichner L, Kullberg BJ, Bow EJ, et al. Early treatment of candidemia in adults: a review. *Med Mycol.* 2011;49:113-120.
3. Posteraro B, DePascale G, Tumbarello M, et al. Early diagnosis of candidemia in intensive care unit patients with sepsis: a prospective comparison of (1→3)-β-D-glucan assay, candida score, and colonization index. *Crit Care.* 2011;15:R249.

6 Postoperative Management

Cardiovascular Surgery

Impact of pulmonary hypertension on outcomes after aortic valve replacement for aortic valve stenosis

Melby SJ, Moon MR, Lindman BR, et al (Washington Univ School of Medicine, St Louis, MO)

J Thorac Cardiovasc Surg 141:1424-1430, 2011

Objective.—The presence of pulmonary hypertension historically has been considered a significant risk factor affecting early and late outcomes after valve replacement. Given the number of recent advances in the management of pulmonary hypertension after cardiac surgery, a better understanding of its impact on outcomes may assist in the clinical management of these patients. The purpose of this study was to determine whether pulmonary hypertension remains a risk factor in the modern era for adverse outcomes after aortic valve replacement for aortic valve stenosis.

Methods.—From January 1996 to June 2009, a total of 1080 patients underwent aortic valve replacement for primary aortic valve stenosis, of whom 574 (53%) had normal systolic pulmonary artery pressures (sPAP) and 506 (47%) had pulmonary hypertension. Pulmonary hypertension was defined as mild (sPAP 35–44 mm Hg), moderate (45–59 mm Hg), or severe (≥ 60 mm Hg). In the group of patients with pulmonary hypertension, 204 had postoperative echocardiograms.

Results.—Operative mortality was significantly higher in patients with pulmonary hypertension (47/506, 9%, vs 31/574, 5%, $P = .02$). The incidence of postoperative stroke was similar ($P = .14$), but patients with pulmonary hypertension had an increased median hospital length of stay (8 vs 7 days, $P = .001$) and an increased incidence of prolonged ventilation (26% vs 17%, $P < .001$). Preoperative pulmonary hypertension was an independent risk factor for decreased long-term survival (relative risk 1.7, $P = .02$). Those with persistent pulmonary hypertension postoperatively had decreased survival. Five-year survival (Kaplan–Meier) was 78% ± 6% with normal sPAP and 77% ± 7% with mild pulmonary hypertension postoperatively, compared with 64% ± 8% with moderate and 45% ± 12% with severe pulmonary hypertension ($P < .001$).

Conclusions.—In patients undergoing aortic valve replacement, preoperative pulmonary hypertension increased operative mortality and decreased long-term survival. Patients with persistent moderate or severe pulmonary hypertension after aortic valve replacement had decreased long-term survival. These data suggest that pulmonary hypertension had a significant impact on outcomes in patients undergoing aortic valve replacement and should be considered in preoperative risk assessment (Fig 1, Table 2).

▶ Pulmonary hypertension (PH) is a condition regarded as an important risk factor for complications and poor outcomes in the perioperative setting. In a cohort of general surgery patients, PH was found to be associated with an excess mortality risk of 7%.[1] It would seem then that patients with pulmonary hypertension undergoing cardiac surgery would also be at risk for worse outcomes. This may be especially true in patients undergoing surgery for aortic stenosis, because it has been shown that those patients with aortic stenosis (AS) and PH are more likely to also have impaired left ventricular function, mitral regurgitation, and increased left ventricular end-diastolic pressure. Each of these characteristics would presumably increase their risk compared with patients with AS and no PH. Surprisingly, the assessment of the added perioperative risk of PH in patients undergoing aortic valve replacement (AVR) for AS has not been performed before, despite the increasing prevalence of PH in these patients.

In this retrospective observational study in 1080 patients from a single center, the authors delineate this important increased risk. In a multivariable logistic regression, they found that in patients who underwent an AVR with or without

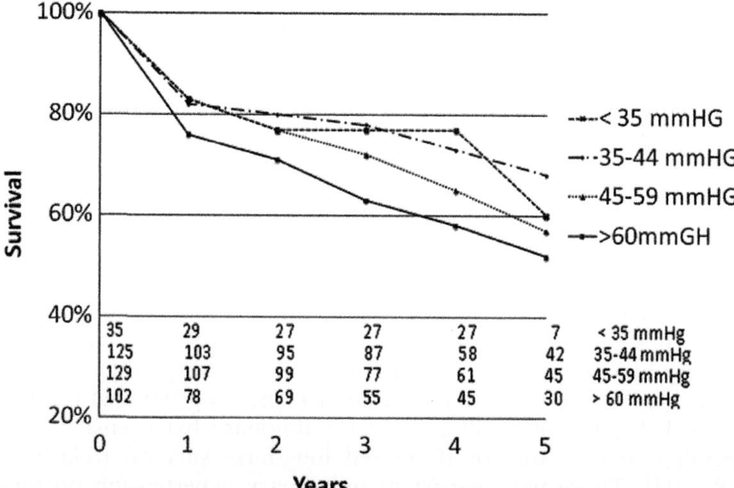

FIGURE 1.—Kaplan–Meier survival curve based on preoperative pulmonary artery pressure. Number at each time point is depicted at the bottom of the graph. (Reprinted from the Journal of Thoracic and Cardiovascular Surgery, Melby SJ, Moon MR, Lindman BR, et al. Impact of pulmonary hypertension on outcomes after aortic valve replacement for aortic valve stenosis. *J Thorac Cardiovasc Surg*. 2011;141:1424-1430. Copyright 2011 with permission from The American Association for Thoracic Surgery.)

TABLE 2.—Multivariate Cox Regression Analysis of Risk Factors for Decreased Survival After AVR for Aortic Stenosis (n = 1080)

Variable	N	RR	95% CI	*P* Value
Pulmonary hypertension	506	1.51	1.160–1.965	.002
Age (y)	1080	1.036	1.020–1.051	<.001
Diabetes	317	1.697	1.120–3.875	<.001
Renal failure	93	2.505	1.613–3.890	<.001
Dialysis	40	2.083	1.308–2.202	.020
NYHA class III or IV	728	1.507	1.101–2.061	.010
LVEF (%)	876	0.991	0.983–1.000	.049
Previous cardiopulmonary bypass	195	1.631	1.210–2.198	.001

Factors found to trend toward significance (gender, age, pulmonary hypertension, isolated aortic valve replacement *[AVR]*, New York Heart Association *[NYHA]* class III or IV, myocardial infarction, stroke, left ventricular ejection fraction *[LVEF]*, systemic hypertension, diabetes, renal failure, dialysis, atrial fibrillation, hypercholesterolemia, chronic obstructive pulmonary disease, previous cardiac surgery requiring cardiopulmonary bypass, body surface area) by univariate testing ($P \leq .10$) were analyzed. Gender, isolated aortic valve replacement, myocardial infarction, stroke, systemic hypertension, atrial fibrillation, hypercholesterolemia, chronic obstructive pulmonary disease, and body surface area were not found to be significant independent predictors for lower survival after aortic valve replacement for aortic stenosis in the mitral valve model. *RR*, Relative risk; *CI*, confidence intervals.

concomitant procedures, the relative risk (RR) of mortality associated with pulmonary hypertension was 1.5 (95% confidence interval 1.160–1.965). Factors included in this adjusted analysis were those that in the univariate analysis had a $P = .1$. These factors were age, gender, isolated AVR, New York Heart Association class III or IV, myocardial infarction, stroke, left ventricular ejection fraction, systemic hypertension, diabetes, renal failure, dialysis, atrial fibrillation, hypercholesterolemia, chronic obstructive pulmonary disease, previous cardiac surgery requiring cardiopulmonary bypass, and body surface area. Those risk factors that remained statistically significant in the multivariate logistic regression and are associated with mortality are shown in Table 2. In this analysis, PH was defined as a systolic pulmonary artery pressure of 35 mm Hg or higher. However, the authors also looked at classes of pulmonary hypertension based on severity: no PH (systemic pulmonary arterial pressure [sPAP] < 35 mmHg), mild PH (sPAP 35–44 mm Hg), moderate PH (sPAP 45–59 mm Hg), and severe PH (sPAP > 60 mm Hg). To further strengthen the association between PH and outcomes, they demonstrated a dose-response curve with the severity of preoperative PH and mortality. They report that the Kaplan-Meier survival analysis of patients with preoperative PH was statistically significantly worse in the more severe PH groups ($P = .020$; Fig 1).

Although this study has important limitations inherent to its retrospective design, it highlights an important risk factor that affects outcomes in patients undergoing aortic valve surgery for aortic stenosis. One important limitation is the potential confounder of having mitral disease. However, they addressed this by performing a subgroup analysis excluding patients with mitral disease. When patients with mitral disease were excluded, the qualitative findings were similar: there was still an increased risk associated with PH, although this increased risk was no longer statistically significant.

Importantly, PH is not included as a risk factor in the Society of Thoracic Surgeons (STS) risk calculator[2] for postoperative complications and mortality, and this may limit our ability to give patients an honest and accurate risk assessment for them to be able to make an informed decision and to discuss their likely postoperative course. For example, using the STS risk calculator, an average male aged 60 years will have an operative mortality risk of 0.6% and 7.9% risk of any postoperative morbidity or mortality for an isolated AVR; his added risk with pulmonary hypertension may be much greater. When determining appropriateness of procedures and informed consent, these factors are extremely important. Adding pulmonary hypertension to the STS risk calculation should be considered.

E. A. Martinez, MD, MHS

References

1. Ramakrishna G, Sprung J, Ravi BS, Chandrasekaran K, McGoon MD. Impact of pulmonary hypertension on the outcomes of noncardiac surgery: predictors of perioperative morbidity and mortality. *J Am Coll Cardiol.* 2005;45:1691-1699.
2. Society of Thoracic Surgeons. Online STS Risk Calculator. http://209.220.160.181/STSWebRiskCalc261/. Accessed December 18, 2011.

Surveillance and epidemiology of surgical site infections after cardiothoracic surgery in The Netherlands, 2002–2007

Manniën J, Wille JC, Kloek JJ, et al (Natl Inst for Public Health and the Environment (RIVM), Bilthoven, The Netherlands; Dutch Inst for Healthcare Improvement (CBO), Utrecht, The Netherlands; Univ of Amsterdam, The Netherlands)

J Thorac Cardiovasc Surg 141:899-904, 2011

Objective.—Surgical site infections after cardiothoracic surgery substantially increase the risk for illness, mortality, and costs. Surveillance of surgical site infections might assist in the prevention of these infections. This study describes the Dutch surveillance methods and results of data collected between 2002 and 2007.

Methods.—Three cardiothoracic procedures were included: coronary artery bypass graft procedures, valve surgery, and a combination of coronary artery bypass graft procedures with concomitant valve surgery. The surgical site infections were divided into sternal and harvest-site infections. Postdischarge surveillance of surgical site infections was mandatory for sternal wounds and elective for harvest-site wounds, with a follow-up period of 42 postoperative days. Multivariate logistic regression was used for risk factor analysis of coronary artery bypass grafts, with adjustment for random variation among hospitals.

Results.—Eight of the 16 Dutch cardiothoracic centers participated and collected data on 4066 procedures and 183 surgical site infections, revealing a surgical site infection rate of 2.4% for sternal wounds and 3.2% for harvest sites. Sixty-one percent of all surgical site infections were recorded after discharge. For sternal surgical site infections after coronary artery bypass graft procedures, the significant risk factors were rethoracotomy, diabetes, preoperative length of stay, and obesity; for harvest-site infections, the most relevant risk factor was a long time on extracorporeal circulation. Adjusted surgical site infection rates regarding coronary artery bypass graft procedures varied between hospitals from 0.0% to 9.7%.

Conclusions.—Large differences were found in surgical site infection rates between Dutch hospitals, which indicate room for improvement. The follow-up of patients after hospital discharge reduces underestimation of surgical site infection rates (Table 4).

▶ Nosocomial infections pose a significant risk to hospitalized patients. In the perioperative setting, surgical site infections (SSIs) are associated with increased morbidity, mortality, and cost. In the setting of postcardiac surgery, the additional costs are estimated at anywhere between \$8000 and \$26 000 and increased length of stay of approximately 20 days.[1] The study by Manniën and colleagues evaluated the epidemiology of SSIs after cardiac surgery in The Netherlands between 2002 and 2007. In their cohort of more than 4000 patients, 183 patients developed an SSI. Of these, 53 were deep sternal infections, 44 were superficial sternal infections, and in the patients with a harvest site, 86 of 2691 developed an SSI. While the standardized criteria that are used by the US Centers for Disease Control and Prevention were applied to define the SSIs, they did not adopt the American National Nosocomial Infections Surveillance (NNIS, now National Healthcare Safety Network) risk index, which includes the American Society of Anesthesiologists physical status classification, wound contamination class, and duration of the operation. Instead, they included more granular data: age, sex, insulin-dependent diabetes, obesity (body mass index ≥ 30), preoperative duration of hospitalization, whether the operation was emergent, use of internal thoracic arteries, use of cardiopulmonary bypass (CPB), time on CPB, lowest body temperature, duration of intensive care unit admission, and rethoracotomy (if not performed because of an infection). These risks were included based on a literature review. Of these, 5 were included in the multilevel (hierarchical) multivariable analysis for isolated coronary artery bypass graft (CABG) procedures (Table 4).

They identified that the number of procedures per hospital varied significantly from 108 to 1146, as did the rates of SSIs: 0.0% to 9.7% for the isolated CABG procedures (the incidence of sternal SSIs ranged from 0.0% to 4.5% and for harvest sites, 0.4% to 6.9%). The authors appropriately acknowledge that the

TABLE 4.—Multilevel Multivariate Risk Factor Analyses for CABG Procedures

Type of SSI	Risk Factor	Odds Ratio	95% CI	*P* Value
Sternal SSIs	Rethoracotomy	5.2	2.5–10.6	.001
	Diabetes	2.5	1.1–5.5	.03
	Preoperative LOS >3 d	2.1	1.1–4.1	.04
	Obesity	2.0	1.0–3.8	.04
Harvest-site SSIs	ECC time >123 min	1.8	0.9–3.7	.08

Based on 2732 procedures for sternal SSIs and 2289 procedures for harvest-site SSIs.

CABG, Coronary artery bypass graft; *SSI*, surgical site infection; *CI*, confidence interval; *LOS*, length of stay; *ECC*, time on extracorporeal circulation (75th percentile = 123 minutes).

surveillance for the harvest sites varied, specifically, that postdischarge surveillance was optional for the harvest site compared with being mandatory for the sternal site. This identifies a very important issue when reporting patient-level outcomes: surveillance bias. Surveillance bias is an extremely important consideration when tracking patient complications, especially when they are publicly reported, as they are in the United States.[2] For example, those sites that have a robust postdischarge surveillance in place will likely identify more SSIs and, therefore, their rates of infection would be higher. Thus, they could be penalized for doing a better job. This is in contrast to those hospitals that do not have a robust postdischarge system; those hospitals would likely not identify all of the attributable SSIs, and therefore would appear to have better outcomes when, in fact, they have worse surveillance capacity. In this study, 61% of all SSIs were identified postdischarge. If we are to have public reporting and pay for performance metrics, it is important to not only robustly define and standardize the numerator and denominator (cases and population at risk); it is also very important to robustly define the surveillance process so we can develop accurate and reliable methods for comparing patient-level outcomes (eg, apples to apples) and inform patient decision making.

E. A. Martinez, MD, MHS

References

1. Graf K, Ott E, Vonberg RP, et al. Surgical site infections—economic consequences for the health care system. *Langenbecks Arch Surg*. 2011;396:453-459.
2. Haut ER, Pronovost PJ. Surveillance bias in outcomes reporting. *JAMA*. 2011; 305:2462-2463.

A Method to Evaluate Cardiac Surgery Mortality: Phase of Care Mortality Analysis

Shannon FL, for the Michigan Society of Thoracic and Cardiovascular Surgeons (William Beaumont Hosp, Royal Oak, MI; et al)
Ann Thorac Surg 93:36-43, 2012

Background.—This is a study of a method of mortality review, adopted by the Michigan Society of Thoracic and Cardiovascular Surgeons, to enhance understanding of mortality and potentially avoidable deaths after cardiac surgery, utilizing a voluntary statewide database.

Methods.—A system to categorize mortality was developed utilizing a phase of care mortality analysis approach as well as providing criteria to classify mortality as potentially "avoidable." For each mortality, the operating surgeon categorized a cardiac surgery mortality trigger into 1 of 5 time frames: preoperative, intraoperative, intensive care unit (ICU), postoperative floor, and discharge.

Results.—A total of 53,674 adult cardiac operations were performed from January 1, 2006 to June 30, 2010 with a crude mortality of 3.5% (1,905 of 53,674). Of the mortalities analyzed, 35% (618 of 1,780) were preoperative, 25% (451 of 1,780) were ICU, 19% (333 of 1,780) were intraoperative, 11% (198 of 1,780) were floor, and 10% (180 of 1,780) were discharge phase. “Avoidable” mortality triggers occurred in 53% (174 of 333) of the intraoperative, 41% (253 of 618) and (184 of 451) of the preoperative and ICU phases, 42% (83 of 198) of the floor, and 19% (35 of 180) of the discharge phase. Overall potentially avoidable mortality was 41% (729 of 1780). Thirty-six percent (644 of 1,780) of the mortalities were coronary artery bypass grafting patients and 29% (188 of 644) of these were in the preoperative phase, with a mean predicted risk of 16%.

Conclusions.—This analysis identifies the recurrence of potentially avoidable mortalities in the 4 hospital phases of care, with the largest absolute number of avoidable mortalities occurring in the preoperative phase. A focus on these phases of care provides significant opportunity for quality improvement initiatives. Utilizing phase of care mortality analysis stimulates surgeons and hospitals to develop and refine mortality reviews and provides a structured statewide platform for discussion, education, quality improvement, and enhanced outcomes (Fig 1).

▶ Beyond reviewing morbidity and mortality cases, learning from these to prevent a subsequent event is the key to improving patient safety. This article by Shannon and colleagues presents a novel approach adopted by the Michigan Society of Thoracic Cardiovascular Surgeons statewide collaborative to review

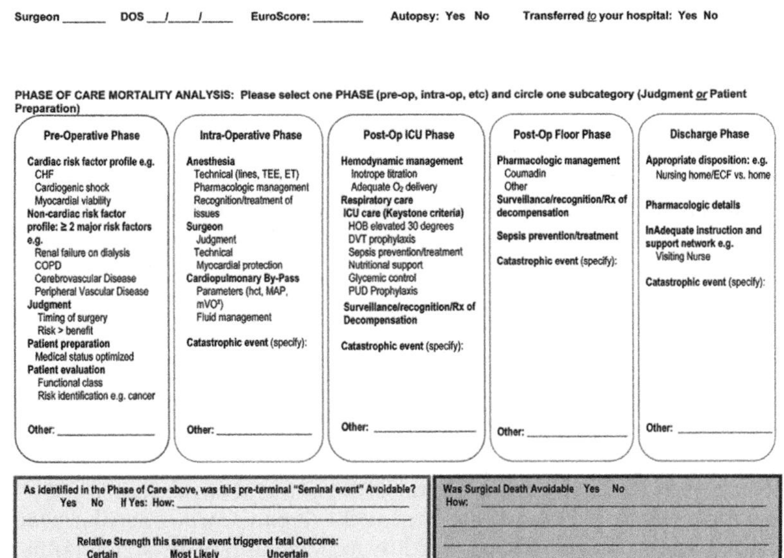

Surgeon ______ **DOS** __/____/____ **EuroScore:** ________ **Autopsy: Yes No** **Transferred *to* your hospital: Yes No**

PHASE OF CARE MORTALITY ANALYSIS: Please select one PHASE (pre-op, intra-op, etc) and circle one subcategory (Judgment *or* Patient Preparation)

Pre-Operative Phase	Intra-Operative Phase	Post-Op ICU Phase	Post-Op Floor Phase	Discharge Phase
Cardiac risk factor profile e.g. CHF Cardiogenic shock Myocardial viability **Non-cardiac risk factor profile: ≥ 2 major risk factors e.g.** Renal failure on dialysis COPD Cerebrovascular Disease Peripheral Vascular Disease **Judgment** Timing of surgery Risk > benefit **Patient preparation** Medical status optimized **Patient evaluation** Functional class Risk identification e.g. cancer **Other:** ________	**Anesthesia** Technical (lines, TEE, ET) Pharmacologic management Recognition/treatment of issues **Surgeon** Judgment Technical Myocardial protection **Cardiopulmonary By-Pass** Parameters (hct, MAP, mVO²) Fluid management **Catastrophic event** (specify): **Other:** ________	**Hemodynamic management** Inotrope titration Adequate O_2 delivery **Respiratory care** **ICU care (Keystone criteria)** HOB elevated 30 degrees DVT prophylaxis Sepsis prevention/treatment Nutritional support Glycemic control PUD Prophylaxis **Surveillance/recognition/Rx of Decompensation** **Catastrophic event** (specify): **Other:** ________	**Pharmacologic management** Coumadin Other **Surveillance/recognition/Rx of decompensation** **Sepsis prevention/treatment** **Catastrophic event** (specify): **Other:** ________	**Appropriate disposition: e.g.** Nursing home/ECF vs. home **Pharmacologic details** **InAdequate instruction and support network e.g.** Visiting Nurse **Catastrophic event** (specify): **Other:** ________

As identified in the Phase of Care above, was this pre-terminal “Seminal event” Avoidable?
Yes No If Yes: How: ________________

Relative Strength this seminal event triggered fatal Outcome:
Certain Most Likely Uncertain

Was Surgical Death Avoidable Yes No
How: ________________

FIGURE 1.—Phase of care mortality analysis form. (CHF = congestive heart failure; COPD = chronic obstructive pulmonary disease; DVT = deep vein thrombosis; ECF = extended care facility; ET = endotracheal; HCT = hematocrit; HOB = head of bed; ICU = intensive care unit; MAP = mean arterial pressure; mVO^2 = myocardial oxygen consumption; PUD = peptic ulcer disease; TEE = transesophageal echocardiography.) (Reprinted from Shannon FL, for the Michigan Society of Thoracic and Cardiovascular Surgeons. A method to evaluate cardiac surgery mortality: phase of care mortality analysis. *Ann Thorac Surg*. 2012;93:36-43, with permission from The Society of Thoracic Surgeons.)

and learn from every patient death. They developed and pilot-tested a mortality assessment tool that was based on the concept that all cardiac surgical deaths are initiated by a seminal event that triggers a cascade of deterioration culminating in death. It was pilot-tested at a single hospital and then rolled out across the state. The roll-out included educational tools for teams to understand the structured review tool and perform the analysis. The tool is called the Phase of Care Mortality Analysis tool (Fig 1) and includes a list of mortality triggers that were developed for each phase of care and represents the most likely seminal event or trigger. These were reviewed locally and, if a case was equivocal, a central team reviewed it. Statewide results were also reviewed annually and frequently became sources for statewide and local quality improvement and education.

Upon review of the statewide database, it was identified that 41% of deaths were potentially avoidable and that these were distributed throughout the perioperative period as described in the abstract. The authors note that while the overall outcomes for cardiac surgery are excellent, there remains significant room for improvement.

While this study has important limitations because of its observational nature, there are some very important lessons. First, it takes time to build trust: prior to sharing data about mortality across the hospitals, there was a period of trust building across the Michigan cardiovascular centers through sharing of other, perhaps less controversial, data and quality improvement programs. Second, implementing a systematic approach to reviewing morbidity and mortality makes the process more objective and, importantly, sets the stage for actionable next steps and shared learning that will improve the care of the patients that undergo cardiac surgery in Michigan.

E. A. Martinez, MD, MHS

Cardiovascular surgery risk prediction from the patient's perspective

Miyata H, for the Japan Cardiovascular Surgery Database (Japan Cardiovascular Surgery Database, Tokyo)

J Thorac Cardiovasc Surg 142:e71-e76, 2011

Objective.—Previous studies have developed cardiovascular surgery outcome prediction models using only patient risk factors, but surgery outcomes from the patient's perspective seem to differ between hospitals. We have developed outcome prediction models that incorporate preoperative patient risks, as well as hospital processes and structure.

Methods.—Data were collected from the Japan Cardiovascular Database for patients scheduled for cardiovascular surgery between January 2005 and December 2007.We analyzed 33,821 procedures in 102 hospitals. Logistic regression was used to generate risk models, which were then validated through split-sample validation.

Results.—Odds ratios, 95% confidence intervals, and *P* values for structures and processes in the mortality prediction model were as follows:

"hospital annual adult cardiac surgery volume (continuous; every 1 procedure increase per year)" (odds ratio, 0.998; confidence interval, 0.997–0.999; $P < .001$); "recommended staffing and equipment" (odds ratio, 0.75; confidence interval, 0.64–0.87; $P < .001$); "daily conferences with cardiologists" (odds ratio, 0.79; confidence interval, 0.60–1.02; $P = .073$); "intensivists involved in postsurgical management" (odds ratio, 0.89; confidence interval, 0.77–1.02; $P = .90$); "public hospitals" (odds ratio, 0.80; confidence interval, 0.70–0.93; $P = .003$); "surgeons lacking miscellaneous duties" (odds ratio, 0.80; confidence interval, 0.70–0.93; $P = .003$); and "surgeons who work no more than 32 hours per week" (odds ratio, 0.55; confidence interval, 0.32–0.95; $P = .032$). The mortality prediction model had a C-index of 0.85 and a Hosmer–Lemeshow P value of .79.

Conclusions.—Our models yielded good discrimination and calibration, so they may prove useful for hospital selection based on individual patient risks and circumstances. Improved surgeon work environments were also shown to be important for both surgeons and patients (Table 2).

▶ Public reporting of outcomes in cardiac surgery is nothing new.[1,2] While the goals of public reporting may be multiple, a primary goal is commonly to

TABLE 2.—Characteristics of Hospital (N = 102)

Hospital Annual Adult Cardiac Surgery Volume, Median (25–75)	115.3 (70.8–168.1) n	%
Public hospital	55	53.9
University hospital	46	45.1
General hospital	91	89.2
Recommended staffing and equipment*	65	63.7
Autologous blood transfusion system	88	86.3
Have an infection control team	90	88.2
Conference with cardiovascular surgeons (every day)	49	48.0
Conference with cardiovascular surgeons (≥1/wk)	99	97.1
Conference with cardiologists (every day)	7	6.9
Conference with cardiologists (≥1/wk)	74	72.5
Conference with nurse (≥1/wk)	47	46.1
Conference with anesthesiologist (≥1/wk)	40	39.2
Intensivists involved in postsurgical management	54	52.9
Have some protocols regarding drug selection	37	36.3
Have some protocols regarding drug dilution method	70	68.6
Have some protocols regarding patients' rehabilitation	49	48.0
Routinely check head and aortic wall CT scan	78	76.5
Preoperative beta-blocker use for CABG surgery (first choice)	5	4.9
Discharge beta-blocker use for CABG surgery (first choice)	12	11.8
Discharge antiplatelet use for CABG surgery (first choice)	92	90.2
Discharge anti-lipid use for CABG surgery (first choice)	15	14.7
ITA use for CABG surgery (first choice)	99	97.1
Off-pump procedure for CABG surgery (first choice)	49	48.0
Surgeons do not have miscellaneous duties	59	57.8
Surgeons do not have >32-h labor	4	3.9

CT, Computed tomography; *ITA*, internal thoracic artery; *CABG*, coronary artery bypass grafting.

*Recommended staffing and equipment were ">4 CV surgeons," ">2 expert CV surgeons," ">4 cardiologists," ">2 anesthesiologists," ">2 clinical engineers," "have an intensive-care unit facility," "have a hemodialysis unit," and ">2 heart-lung machines."

increase the transparency of the quality of programs and to inform patients in their selection of surgeons or hospitals. In this article by Miyata and colleagues, the authors sought to develop a risk prediction model that expands beyond the typical patient-level parameters that go into such risk models. Their goal was to identify hospital-level factors that could be modifiable. They sought to include hospital characteristics that patients might look for in the decision process above just the overall outcomes of a hospital or surgeon. This, in theory, would help patients identify specific characteristics to ask about and potentially guide their selection.

The Japan Adult Cardiovascular Surgery Database (JACVSD) that was used to develop this risk model is very similar to the Society of Thoracic Surgeons (STS) database in the United States. Approximately 50% of the Japanese cardiovascular programs submit data to this national database, and the accuracy of the data is supported by monthly audits at each center comparing the database elements with the clinical charts. Nonpatient-level parameters that they included in the model are staffing and equipment criteria (that they report were recommended by previous research in Japan). These parameters included having more than 4 cardiovascular surgeons, more than 2 expert CV surgeons, more than 4 cardiologists, more than 2 anesthesiologists, more than 2 clinical engineers, an intensive-care unit facility, a hemodialysis unit, and more than 2 heart-lung machines. In addition, they included additional hospital characteristics that are shown Table 2. Using a multivariable logistic regression, they identified that many of these hospital-level characteristics impact outcomes (see abstract results).

However, there are some important methodological concerns with this study. While they report these hospital-level predictors, they do not report how these data were ascertained. It does not appear to this reviewer that these elements are included in the JACVSD. These parameters are not included in the US STS database either. In addition, they refer to the previous research in Japan that supported the inclusion of the specific hospital-level parameters, yet there is no reference to how those were developed or evaluated. Finally, they report using a logistic regression model. In this type of analysis, a hierarchical model may be more appropriate to account for the similarities of patients within a hospital. However, these issues do not discount the potential importance of such hospital-level characteristics and their impact on patient outcomes. Finally, while this is a step in the right direction to further to delineate what factors impact outcomes and how a patient can become a better informed consumer of health care, this study fails to present a usable model for consumers based on their specific risks and those of the hospital in question.

E. A. Martinez, MD, MHS

References

1. Shahian DM, Edwards FH, Jacobs JP, et al. Public reporting of cardiac surgery performance: part 1—history, rationale, consequences. *Ann Thorac Surg.* 2011; 92:S2-S11.
2. Shahian DM. Public reporting of cardiac surgery performance: introduction. *Ann Thorac Surg.* 2011;92:S1.

First-line Therapy with Coagulation Factor Concentrates Combined with Point-of-Care Coagulation Testing Is Associated with Decreased Allogeneic Blood Transfusion in Cardiovascular Surgery: A Retrospective, Single-center Cohort Study

Görlinger K, Dirkmann D, Hanke AA, et al (Universitätsklinikum Essen, Germany; et al)

Anesthesiology 115:1179-1191, 2011

Introduction.—Blood transfusion is associated with increased morbidity and mortality. We developed and implemented an algorithm for coagulation management in cardiovascular surgery based on first-line administration of coagulation factor concentrates combined with point-of-care thromboelastometry/impedance aggregometry.

Methods.—In a retrospective cohort study including 3,865 patients, we analyzed the incidence of intraoperative allogeneic blood transfusions (primary endpoints) before and after algorithm implementation.

Results.—Following algorithm implementation, the incidence of any allogeneic blood transfusion (52.5 *vs.* 42.2%; $P < 0.0001$), packed red blood cells (49.7 *vs.* 40.4%; $P < 0.0001$), and fresh frozen plasma (19.4 *vs.* 1.1%; $P < 0.0001$) decreased, whereas platelet transfusion increased (10.1 *vs.* 13.0%; $P = 0.0041$). Yearly transfusion of packed red blood cells (3,276 *vs.* 2,959 units; $P < 0.0001$) and fresh frozen plasma (1986 *vs.* 102 units; $P < 0.0001$) decreased, as did the median number of packed red blood cells and fresh frozen plasma per patient. The incidence of fibrinogen concentrate (3.73 *vs.* 10.01%; $P < 0.0001$) and prothrombin complex concentrate administration (4.42 *vs.* 8.9%; $P < 0.0001$) increased, as did their amount administered per year (179 *vs.* 702 g; $P = 0.0008$ and 162×10^3 U *vs.* 388×10^3 U; $P = 0.0184$, respectively). Despite a switch from aprotinin to tranexamic acid, an increase in use of dual antiplatelet therapy (2.7 *vs.* 13.7%; $P < 0.0001$), patients' age, proportion of females, emergency cases, and more complex surgery, the incidence of massive transfusion [($\geq$10 units packed red blood cells), (2.5 *vs.* 1.26%; $P = 0.0057$)] and unplanned reexploration (4.19 *vs.* 2.24%; $P = 0.0007$) decreased. Composite thrombotic/thromboembolic events (3.19 *vs.* 1.77%; $P = 0.0115$) decreased, but in-hospital mortality did not change (5.24 *vs.* 5.22%; $P = 0.98$).

Conclusions.—First-line administration of coagulation factor concentrates combined with point-of-care testing was associated with decreased incidence of blood transfusion and thrombotic/thromboembolic events (Table 2).

▶ Görlinger and colleagues present a single-center retrospective cohort study that shows the impact of a coagulation management protocol. The main principles of this protocol were the implementation of a standardized protocol for transfusion and the introduction of point-of-care testing including thromboelastometry with EXTEM®, FIBTEM®, and APTEM® assays, and whole blood impedance aggregometry. The formal protocol is complex, and the specific algorithms for use and

TABLE 2.—Primary and Secondary Binary Endpoints: Transfusion and Outcome

	Before Implementation of Point-of-Care-Supported Coagulation Management (2004)	After Implementation of Point-of-Care-Supported Coagulation Management (2009)	*P* Value	Relative Risk of Cohort 2009 Compared with Cohort 2004
Primary binary endpoints: Incidence of transfusion				
Any allogeneic blood product transfusion (n, %)	902/1,718 (52.5%)	906/2,147 (42.2%)	<0.0001	0.804 (0.752–0.859)
PRBC transfusion (n, %)	854/1,718 (49.7%)	868/2,147 (40.4%)	<0.0001	0.813 (0.758–0.872)
FFP transfusion (n, %)	333/1,718 (19.4%)	24/2,147 (1.1%)	<0.0001	0.058 (0.038–0.087)
Platelet transfusion (n, %)	173/1,718 (10.1%)	280/2,147 (13%)	0.0041	1.295 (1.083–1.548)
Massive transfusion (≥10 units of PRBC) (n, %)	43/1,718 (2.50%)	27/2,147 (1.26%)	0.0057	0.502 (0.312–0.81)
Secondary binary endpoints: Factor concentrates, adverse events, and mortality				
Fibrinogen concentrate administration (n, %)	64/1,718 (3.73%)	215/2,147 (10.01%)	<0.0001	2.688 (2.048–3.528)
PCC administration (n, %)	76/1,718 (4.42%)	191/2,147 (8.9%)	<0.0001	2.011 (1.553–2.603)
AT administration (n, %)	148/1,718 (8.61%)	170/2,147 (7.92%)	0.4689	0.919 (0.744–1.135)
FXIII administration (n, %)	10/1,718 (0.58%)	0/2,147 (0%)	0.0013	0
rFVIIa administration (n, %)	1/1,718 (0.06%)	0/2,147 (0%)	0.9111	0
Reexploration rate (unscheduled within 48 h) (n, %)	72/1,718 (4.19%)	48/2,147 (2.24%)	0.0007	0.533 (0.372–0.764)
Venous thrombosis (n, %)	14/1,441 (0.97%)	9/1,582 (0.57%)	0.2032	0.586 (0.254–1.349)
Pulmonary embolism (n, %)	5/1,441 (0.35%)	1/1,582 (0.57%)	0.08	0.182 (0.021–1.558)
Other arterial embolism (n, %)	3/1,441 (0.35%)	2/1,582 (0.13%)	0.5806	0.607 (0.102–3.629)
Stroke (n, %)	12/1,441 (0.83%)	7/1,582 (0.44%)	0.1751	0.531 (0.21–1.346)
Coronary bypass graft occlusion (n, %)	12/1,441 (0.83%)	9/1,582 (0.57%)	0.3830	0.683 (0.289–1.617)
Composite thrombotic/thromboembolic adverse events (n, %)	46/1,441 (3.19%)	28/1,582 (1.77%)	0.0115	0.554 (0.348–0.882)
Renal replacement therapy (n, %)	122/1,441 (8.47%)	127/1,582 (8.03%)	0.6614	0.948 (0.747–1.203)
In-hospital mortality (n, %)	90/1,718 (5.24%)	112/2,147 (5.22%)	0.9756	0.996 (0.760–1.305)

Data are presented as numbers (%), relative risk (95% CI of relative risk).

AT = antithrombin concentrate; FFP = fresh frozen plasma; FXIII = factor XIII concentrate; PCC = prothrombin complex concentrate; platelet = platelet concentrate; PRBC = packed red blood cells; rFVIIa = recombinant activated factor VII.

interpretation of each point-of-care measure and use of coagulation factors are fully outlined in the article. The authors show that, with the combined implementation of the protocol and thrombelastography, the number of allogeneic blood products transfused was significantly reduced. In accordance with the protocol, the use of fibrinogen concentrate and prothrombin complex concentrate administration was increased. Importantly, with the introduction of these prothrombotic products, there was no change in the incidence of unintended consequences, namely, thrombotic or thromboembolic events. The overall balance of costs, with the reduction of allogeneic products and the increased use of coagulation factor concentrates, was a net reduction of 6.5% (mean cost of $357.79 per patient in the prephase compared with $334.56 per patient in the postphase). This translates into a substantial savings of approximately $300 000 per 1 000 patients. The overall impact of the protocol is shown in Table 2. The overall impact of the protocol could be substantially greater if it incorporated a hemoglobin trigger of 7 g/dL instead of 8–10 g/dL.

This report of the local implementation of a blood conservation protocol is one more in a series of reports showing that the implementation of a protocol or point-of-care testing can impact the costs associated with transfusions and reduce the exposure of patients to the risk of transfusion. What this study does not tell is the incremental impact of the protocol, the specific factor concentrates, or point-of-care testing on the outcomes.

In 2007, the Society of Thoracic Surgeons and the Society of Cardiovascular Anesthesiologists published a guideline for blood transfusion and conservation in cardiac surgery.[1] In 2009, Likosky and colleagues[2] performed a survey to understand current practices among cardiac anesthesiologists and perfusionists. They identified that there was wide variation in clinical transfusion practices and, importantly, that there was little adoption and little change in clinical practices following the publication of the guidelines.[3] This low adoption rate was despite growing evidence that transfusions, especially of packed red blood cells, are associated with increased morbidity and mortality. The study by Likosky and colleagues highlights the importance of understanding the barriers that the front-line providers have to adoption and implementation of evidence-based practices. It would be very enlightening to understand how Görlinger and colleagues successfully implemented their complex protocol.

E. A. Martinez, MD, MHS

References

1. Ferraris VA, Ferraris SP, Saha SP, et al. Perioperative blood transfusion and blood conservation in cardiac surgery: the Society of Thoracic Surgeons and The Society of Cardiovascular Anesthesiologists clinical practice guideline. *Ann Thorac Surg.* 2007;83:S27-S86.
2. Likosky DS, FitzGerald DC, Groom RC, et al. Effect of the perioperative blood transfusion and blood conservation in cardiac surgery clinical practice guidelines of the Society of Thoracic Surgeons and the Society of Cardiovascular Anesthesiologists upon clinical practices. *Anesth Analg.* 2011;111:316-323.

Influence of Low Tidal Volume Ventilation on Time to Extubation in Cardiac Surgical Patients

Sundar S, Novack V, Jervis K, et al (Beth Israel Deaconess Med Ctr, Boston, MA; et al)

Anesthesiology 114:1102-1110, 2011

Background.—Low tidal volumes have been associated with improved outcomes in patients with established acute lung injury. The role of low tidal volume ventilation in patients without lung injury is still unresolved. We hypothesized that such a strategy in patients undergoing elective surgery would reduce ventilator-associated lung injury and that this improvement would lead to a shortened time to extubation.

Methods.—A single-center randomized controlled trial was undertaken in 149 patients undergoing elective cardiac surgery. Ventilation with 6 *versus* 10 ml/kg tidal volume was compared. Ventilator settings were applied immediately after anesthesia induction and continued throughout surgery and the subsequent intensive care unit stay. The primary endpoint of the study was time to extubation. Secondary endpoints included the proportion of patients extubated at 6 h and indices of lung mechanics and gas exchange as well as patient clinical outcomes.

Results.—Median ventilation time was not significantly different in the low tidal volume group; a median (interquartile range) of 450 (264–1,044) min was achieved compared with 643 (417–1,032) min in the control group ($P = 0.10$). However, a higher proportion of patients in the low tidal volume group was free of any ventilation at 6 h: 37.3% compared with 20.3% in the control group ($P = 0.02$). In addition, fewer patients in the low tidal volume group required reintubation (1.3 *vs.* 9.5%; $P = 0.03$).

Conclusions.—Although reduction of tidal volume in mechanically ventilated patients undergoing elective cardiac surgery did not significantly shorten time to extubation, several improvements were observed in secondary outcomes. When these data are combined with a lack of observed complications, a strategy of reduced tidal volume could still be beneficial in this patient population (Table 4).

▶ Prolonged respiratory failure is a recognized quality indicator following cardiac surgery.[1] Many cardiac surgical centers have implemented rapid weaning protocols to address prolonged ventilations times, but there remains a significant number of patients who meet the criteria of prolonged ventilation, defined as more than 24 hours on the ventilator after cardiac surgery. Sundar and colleagues propose a novel approach to improving ventilation duration by focusing on the intraoperative, rather than postoperative, period.

Low tidal volume ventilation is a widely accepted method of managing patients with acute respiratory distress syndrome (ARDS). Many postoperative cardiac surgical patients fulfill the criteria for acute lung injury (ALI) or ARDS. The international consensus criteria include a $PaO2/FiO2$ greater than 200 mm Hg for ARDS, greater than 300 mm Hg for ALI regardless of the level of positive end-expiratory pressure, and pulmonary artery occlusion pressure

TABLE 4.—Clinical Outcomes

Outcomes	Control (n = 74)	Low Tidal Volume (n = 75)	*P* Value
Total ventilation time, min, median (IQR)	643 (417–1,032)	450 (264–1,044)	0.10
Ventilation, No. (%)	—	—	—
<6 h	15 (20.3)	28 (37.3)	0.02
<12 h	40 (54.1)	48 (64.0)	0.22
<24 h	66 (89.2)	66 (88.1)	0.82
Length of stay, median (IQR)	—	—	—
Intensive care unit, h	34.5 (26.0–94.6)	31.3 (26.0–68.0)	0.35
Postoperative hospital, days	5.5 (4.0–7.0)	5.0 (4.0–6.0)	0.16
Reintubation, No. (%)	7 (9.5)	1 (1.3)	0.03
Reason for reintubation, No. (%)	—	—	—
Arrhythmia	2	1	—
Respiratory failure	3	0	—
Pancreatitis	1	0	—
Bleeding	1	0	—
28-day mortality, No. (%)	2 (1.7)	1 (1.3)	0.62

Chi-square testing was used to analyze categorical variables appearing as No. (%). The Mann–Whitney U test was used for continuous variables with not normal distribution appearing as median (interquartile range [IQR]).

18 mm Hg or less or no clinical evidence of left atrial hypertension.[2] Furthermore, there is evidence that high tidal volumes are an independent risk factor for developing ALI in patients who did not have ALI when ventilation was initiated.[3] It is not infrequent that postoperative cardiac surgical patients meet the ALI criteria, and one of the accepted contributors to this is the systemic inflammatory response and capillary leak secondary to cardiopulmonary bypass. In addition, large tidal volume ventilation may contribute to meeting these criteria as well.

In this study, 150 patients undergoing elective cardiac surgery were randomized to two tidal volumes: 6 ml/kg (intervention) and 10 ml/kg (control). Tidal volume restriction was initiated in the operating room beginning with intubation and maintained postoperatively in the intensive care unit until extubation. Ventilator management for both arms was protocolized. Care was otherwise similar between the 2 groups. The groups were similar at baseline, with no statistically significant differences across multiple risk factors. The investigators report that more patients in the intervention (low tidal volume) arm were extubated less than hours postoperatively (37.3% vs 20.3%, $P = .02$) and fewer patients were reintubated (1.3% vs 9.5%, $P = .03$). Although their primary endpoint of time to extubation was not statistically different between the 2 groups, importantly, the trend was in the same direction (Table 4).

Although this study has important limitations such as a small sample size in a single institution in addition to caregivers being unblinded to the randomization arm, it brings to light the important consideration that something as simple as intraoperative tidal volume limitation may reduce ventilation time and, potentially, consequent respiratory complications for cardiac surgical patients. This study calls for a larger, multicenter randomized trial.

E. A. Martinez, MD, MHS

References

1. Shahian DM, Edwards FH, Jacobs JP, et al. Public reporting of cardiac surgery performance: part 2—implementation. *Ann Thorac Surg.* 2011;92:S12-S23.
2. Bernard GR, Artigas A, Brigham KL, et al. The American-European Consensus Conference on ARDS. Definitions, mechanisms, relevant outcomes, and clinical trial coordination. *Am J Respir Crit Care Med.* 1994;149:818-824.
3. Gajic O, Dara SI, Mendez JL, et al. Ventilator-associated lung injury in patients without acute lung injury at the onset of mechanical ventilation. *Crit Care Med.* 2004;32:1817-1824.

Improving Patient Care in Cardiac Surgery Using Toyota Production System Based Methodology

Culig MH, Kunkle RF, Frndak DC, et al (Forbes Regional Hosp, Monroeville, PA; Gerald McGinnis Cardiovascular Inst, Pittsburgh, PA)
Ann Thorac Surg 91:394-400, 2011

Background.—A new cardiac surgery program was developed in a community hospital setting using the operational excellence (OE) method, which is based on the principles of the Toyota production system. The initial results of the first 409 heart operations, performed over the 28 months between March 1, 2008, and June 30, 2010, are presented.

Methods.—Operational excellence methodology was taught to the cardiac surgery team. Coaching started 2 months before the opening of the program and continued for 24 months.

Results.—Of the 409 cases presented, 253 were isolated coronary artery bypass graft operations. One operative death occurred. According to the database maintained by The Society of Thoracic Surgeons, the risk-adjusted operative mortality rate was 61% lower than the regional rate. Likewise, the risk-adjusted rate of major complications was 57% lower than The Society of Thoracic Surgeons regional rate. Daily solution to determine cause was attempted on 923 distinct perioperative problems by all team members. Using the cost of complications as described by Speir and coworkers, avoiding predicted complications resulted in a savings of at least $884,900 as compared with the regional average.

Conclusions.—By the systematic use of a real time, highly formatted problem-solving methodology, processes of care improved daily. Using carefully disciplined teamwork, reliable implementation of evidence-based protocols was realized by empowering the front line to make improvements. Low rates of complications were observed, and a cost savings of $3,497 per each case of isolated coronary artery bypass graft was realized (Table 4).

▶ Culig and colleagues present their experience in establishing a new heart and vascular center. The methods that they adopted were those of the Toyota production system,[1] which "focuses on the relentless identification of defects in processes and the ongoing study of these defects while implementing trials toward their elimination." They describe how they made the Toyota system

TABLE 4.—Cost Analysis According to Speir et al [7], Forbes Ed Dardanell Heart and Vascular Center (HVC) Isolated Coronary Artery Bypass Graft Surgery (CABG), March 2008 to June 2010, 253 Cases

Complication	HVC Actual No. of Patients	STS Like Group Rate (2009) Predicted No. Patients	HVC Risk-Adjusted No. of Patients[a] (Risk-Adjusted Rate)[b]	Complications Prevented[c] × Complication Cost	Total Savings
Operative mortality	1	2.1% × 253 = 5	2 (0.63%)	3 × $49,200	$147,600
Atrial fibrillation	25	21.1% × 253 = 53	25 (NA)	28 × $2,700	$75,600
Prolonged ventilation	8	11.5% × 253 = 29	10 (3.7%)	19 × $25,700	$488,300
Renal failure	1	3.9% × 253 = 10	2 (0.74%)	8 × $22,900	$183,200
Permanent stroke	3	1.2% × 253 = 3	4 (1.58%)	−1 × $9,800	−$9,800
Total complications prevented				57	
Total savings					$884,900
Savings per CABG					$3,497

NA = not available; OE = Observed/Expected; STS = The Society of Thoracic Surgeons.
Editor's Note: Please refer to original journal article for full references.
[a]Risk-adjusted number of patients is risk-adjusted rate × 253, then rounded up.
[b]Risk-adjusted rate is OE × STS overall rate [6]; OE is reported by the Clinical Automated Office Solutions system.
[c]Complications prevented is difference of STS predicted number of patients and HVC risk-adjusted number of patients.

the norm by starting with this approach during the hiring process; each new hire was told that he or she would "be developing a new way of doing work" in the new center. They discuss how they educated the team members on the Toyota system and implemented the program. Some of the key steps were the development of a balanced scorecard with clear goals and metrics, the implementation of a daily meeting to address safety concerns from the previous 24 hours, and establishing the norm that, in order for issues to be brought to the group, the person bringing the concern forward had to think about why the event happened and what type of intervention he or she might propose. The goal for resolution of the issues is within 24 hours for all safety concerns and 48 hours for other problems.

They describe many important factors that made this successful. They highlight that this was an ongoing process with education and coaching of frontline staff for 24 months. They also emphasize the importance of the active role of leadership in being visible supporters and active participants in addressing staff safety concerns. They report that with this new program, they had better outcomes than the regional and national comparison groups. They also performed a cost analysis, using the cost estimates of Speir and colleagues.[2] They report an estimated cost savings per coronary artery bypass graft of $3497 and overall savings of $884 900 compared to the Society of Thoracic Surgeons like group (Table 4).

Although this study has limitations, including that it is observational in nature, it offers important insight into how care can be designed to reduce variation and improve outcomes in a cardiac surgical center. The opportunity to design a new surgical heart center from the ground up is somewhat unique, and it would be interesting (although difficult to study) to understand the impact of this specific intervention compared with any other method to establish processes of care in a new heart center. However, this experience provides a rare opportunity to understand the impact that a comprehensive quality improvement initiative can have on outcomes and performance. Although these findings may not be generalizable to other established centers and the patient population may have a different risk profile than at your institution, the lessons remain important. Emphasizing continuous quality improvement and giving frontline providers a safe atmosphere to bring up safety concerns are important drivers of improving outcomes.

E. A. Martinez, MD, MHS

References

1. Ono T. *Toyota production system: beyond large-scale production.* London, England: Productivity Press; 1988.
2. Speir AM, Kasirajan V, Barnett SD, Fonner E Jr. Additive costs of postoperative complications for isolated coronary artery bypass grafting patients in Virginia. *Ann Thorac Surg.* 2009;88:40-45.

Miscellaneous

Atelectasis as a Cause of Postoperative Fever: Where Is the Clinical Evidence?

Mavros MN, Velmahos GC, Falagas ME (Alfa Inst of Biomedical Sciences, Athens, Greece; Massachusetts General Hosp and Harvard Med School, Boston)

Chest 140:418-424, 2011

Background.—Atelectasis is considered to be the most common cause of early postoperative fever (EPF) but the existing evidence is contradictory. We sought to determine if atelectasis is associated with EPF by analyzing the relevant published evidence.

Methods.—We performed a systematic search in PubMed and Scopus databases to identify studies examining the association between atelectasis and EPF.

Results.—A total of eight studies, including 998 cardiac, abdominal, and maxillofacial surgery patients, were eligible for analysis. Only two studies specifically examined our question, and six additional articles reported sufficient data to be included. Only one study reported a significant association between postoperative atelectasis and fever, whereas the remaining studies indicated no such association. The performance of EPF as a diagnostic test for atelectasis was also assessed, and EPF performed poorly (pooled diagnostic OR, 1.40; 95% CI, 0.92-2.12). The significant heterogeneity among the studies precluded a formal metaanalysis.

Conclusion.—The available evidence regarding the association of atelectasis and fever is scarce. We found no clinical evidence supporting the concept that atelectasis is associated with EPF. More so, there is no clear evidence that atelectasis causes fever at all. Large studies are needed to precisely evaluate the contribution of atelectasis in EPF.

▶ The common notion for decades has been that atelectasis in the early postoperative period is the cause of early postoperative fever. The evidence to support this association has been lacking, but nonetheless, this concept has remained an "urban legend." These authors used a systematic search of PubMed and Scopus to assess the data in support of atelectasis as a cause of early postoperative fever after cardiac, abdominal, or maxillofacial surgery. Although the available studies that could validate the presence or absence of a causal relationship are few, there was no direct association between the presence of early postoperative atelectasis and fever in the first 48 hours after surgical procedures. The prevailing explanation for early postoperative fever is the release of inflammatory molecules, such as tumor necrosis factor, interleukin (IL)-1, and IL-6, as a consequence of the tissue injury and inflammation associated with the surgical procedure and tissue manipulation. To adequately answer the question concerning the relationship, if any, of postoperative atelectasis to the development of early postoperative fever, we will need large, prospective, well-designed clinical studies.

R. A. Balk, MD

Renal Dysfunction Associated with Intra-abdominal Hypertension and the Abdominal Compartment Syndrome

Mohmand H, Goldfarb S (Univ of Pennsylvania School of Medicine, Philadelphia)

J Am Soc Nephrol 22:615-621, 2011

Once considered mostly a postsurgical condition, intra-abdominal hypertension (IAH) and the abdominal compartment syndrome (ACS) are now thought to increase morbidity and mortality in many patients receiving medical or surgical intensive care. Animal data and human observational studies indicate that oliguria and acute kidney injury are early and frequent consequences of IAH/ACS and can be present at relatively low levels of intra-abdominal pressure (IAP). Among medical patients at particular risk are those with septic shock and severe acute pancreatitis, but the adverse effects of IAH may also be seen in cardiorenal and hepatorenal syndromes. Factors predisposing to IAH/ACS include sepsis, large volume fluid resuscitation, polytransfusion, mechanical ventilation with high intrathoracic pressure, and acidosis, among others. Transduction of bladder pressure is the gold standard for measuring intra-abdominal pressure, and several nonsurgical methods can help reduce IAP. The role of renal replacement therapy for volume management is not well defined but may be beneficial in some cases. IAH/ACS is an important possible cause of

TABLE 1.—Medical Treatment Options to Reduce IAP

1. Improve abdominal wall compliance
    - Sedation and analgesia
    - Neuromuscular blockade
    - Avoid head of bed >30°
2. Evacuate abdominal fluid collections
    - Paracentesis
    - Percutaneous drainage
3. Evacuate intraluminal contents
    - Nasogastric decompression
    - Rectal decompression
    - Prokinetic agents
4. Correct positive fluid balance
    - Avoid excessive fluid resuscitation
    - Diuretics
    - Colloids/hypertonic fluids (in patients with severe burns)
    - Hemodialysis/ultrafiltration
5. Organ support and reducing capillary leak
    - Maintain APP >60 mmHg with vasopressors
    - Optimize ventilation, alveolar recruitment
    - Antibiotic therapy in septic patients

Adapted with permission of WSACS from Cheetham ML: Abdominal compartment syndrome. *Curr Opin Crit Care* 15: 154–162, 2009

acute renal failure in critically ill patients and screening may benefit those at increased risk (Table 1).

▶ These authors review the background of abdominal hypertension and abdominal compartment syndrome and the adverse impact of these effects on outcome in both medical and surgical patients.[1]

The most important contribution in this report from a leading renal unit is the discussion of intrarenal vascular congestion associated with elevated renal venous pressure as a factor favoring oliguria and ultimate renal failure in the setting of increased intra-abdominal pressure. The low-pressure renal vasculature shows resistance increases beyond 500% with intra-abdominal pressure of 20 mm Hg. Finally, the authors review cardiorenal and hepatorenal syndromes and argue that control of even minor elevation in intra-abdominal pressure is essential to successful management.[2,3]

Surgical therapy is the most aggressive approach to intra-abdominal pressure elevation, but a number of medical strategies are summarized in the table reproduced here.

D. J. Dries, MSE, MD

References

1. Cheatham ML. Abdominal compartment syndrome: pathophysiology and definitions. *Scand J Trauma Resusc Emerg Med.* 2009;17:10.
2. Tang WH, Mullens W. Cardiorenal syndrome in decompensated heart failure. *Heart.* 2010;96:255-260.
3. Umgelter A, Reindl W, Franzen M, Lenhardt C, Huber W, Schmid RM. Renal resistive index and renal function before and after paracentesis in patients with hepatorenal syndrome and tense ascites. *Intensive Care Med.* 2009;35:152-156.

Preoperative Frailty and Quality of Life as Predictors of Postoperative Complications

Saxton A, Velanovich V (Henry Ford Hosp, Detroit, MI)

Ann Surg 253:1223-1229, 2011

Background.—Prediction of postoperative complications has been based on assessing comorbidities. However, the evaluation of these comorbidities has not consistently identified those at higher risk of complications, primarily due to the inability to assess how these comorbidities affect functional status. We hypothesized that preoperative functional measures of patients' health status can predict postoperative complications.

Methods.—A sample of patients undergoing general surgical operations were reviewed for age, gender, diagnosis (for severity), operations (for complexity), number of comorbidities, preoperative frailty (as determined by the Canadian Study of Health and Ageing Frailty Index), preoperative quality of life (as determined by the SF-36), occurrence of postoperative complications, number of postoperative complications, and severity of complications. Data were analyzed by linear and multiple logistic regression analyses, and the Mann-Whitney *U* test.

Results.—Two hundred and twenty-six patients were evaluated, average age 61 ± 13 years, 47% male patients. Frailty Index (FI) correlated with number of comorbidities ($r = 0.61$, $P < 0.001$), and all of the domains of the SF-36. Patients who had postoperative complications had higher median preoperative FI than those would did not [0.075 (IQR 0.046–0.118) vs. 0.059 (IQR 0.045–0.089), $P = 0.007$]. Multiple logistic regression analysis demonstrated that operation complexity, FI, and the role-emotional domain were associated with an increased risk of postoperative complications, whereas the bodily pain domain was associated with a lower risk of postoperative complications.

Conclusions.—This study demonstrates that preoperative functional status as measured by FI and SF-36 may help identify patients at higher risk of postoperative complications. In our ageing population, use of such measures may help in better patient selection.

▶ This study is remarkable in that all patients included took the 36-item Short Form Health Survey (SF-36) and were treated by one surgeon, the senior author. Defining frailty as scores on individual components of the SF-36 greater than 1 standard deviation from the mean, these authors show that lower scores on the SF-36 as well as a retrospectively calculated Canadian Study of Health and Aging 70-item Frailty Index (FI) were effective in identifying individuals at increased risk for complications. Physical stress associated with operative procedures was rigorously categorized, as was the distribution and type of postoperative complications. When multiple logistic regression to assess the likelihood of any complication occurring was applied, a Frailty Index score above the level seen in "robust" individuals was the strongest predictor of adverse outcomes. The 2 strongest predictors from the SF-36 assessment were patient assessment of health (improvement or decline over the last year) and emotional state. Preoperative quality of life, as measured by the SF-36, was correlated with preoperative frailty as measured by the FI.

The authors propose, and I agree, that an understanding of frailty may help in preoperative decision making.[1,2] As more frail patients have lower 5-year survival rates, decisions regarding operations with significant risk may be affected in the frail individual. Another vital question, which this study is not designed to answer, is whether improvement in patient conditioning in the preoperative period is associated with improvement in outcomes. Or, put another way, can the frail patient be optimized to reduce operative risk?

Another challenge faced by these and other authors doing similar work is development of a rapid bedside tool to facilitate conversations among surgeons, anesthesiologists, and patients. For example, the American Society of Anesthesiologists score, a simple 5-point criterion, can be used in this way. Particularly in emergency procedures, which are not studied here, a readily applied score could contribute significantly to perioperative decision making.

D. J. Dries, MSE, MD

References

1. Makary MA, Segev DL, Pronovost PJ, et al. Frailty as a predictor of surgical outcomes in older patients. *J Am Coll Surg*. 2010;210:901-908.
2. Malani PN. Functional status assessment in the preoperative evaluation of older adults. *JAMA*. 2009;302:1582-1583.

Evaluation of Prophylactic Anticoagulation, Deep Venous Thrombosis, and Heparin-Induced Thrombocytopenia in 21 Burn Centers in Germany, Austria, and Switzerland

Busche MN, Herold C, Krämer R, et al (Hannover Med School, Germany)
Ann Plast Surg 67:17-24, 2011

Heparin-induced thrombocytopenia (HIT) is a life-threatening complication in intensive care settings. The timely diagnosis and management of HIT are challenging, and the incidences of HIT and deep venous thrombosis (DVT) may be related to prophylactic anticoagulation standards in burn units. We therefore evaluated, using a questionnaire, prophylactic anticoagulation, HIT management, and incidences of DVT and HIT in burn centers located in the German-speaking part of Europe. In the 21 responding burn centers, 1611 patients were treated and the overall incidences for clinically overt DVT and HIT in 2008 were 1.1% and 1.4%, respectively. Burn centers using low molecular weight heparin (LMWH) subcutaneous for all patients had a low rate of DVT (0.9%) and significantly lower rates of HIT (0.2%) relative to all other centers ($P < 0.05$). The highest rates of HIT (2.7%) and DVT (3.8%) were found in burn centers administering unfractionated heparin intravenous. While current HIT guidelines do not specify the administration of unfractionated heparin or LMWH for burn patients, these data warrant controlled prospective studies to confirm the advantage of LMWH administration in burn patients.

▶ The authors have done a very nice job defining the evolution of the diagnosis of heparin-induced thrombocytopenia (HIT) and relating it to patients with thermal injury. This study compared adult burn patients from 21 burn centers in German-speaking Switzerland, Austria, and Germany. Several interesting findings emerged from this survey, which had an astounding 78% response rate:

1. The lowest rates of HIT and deep venous thrombosis (DVT) were found in centers using subcutaneous low-molecular-weight heparin (LMWH) as a prophylactic anticoagulation standard for all patients, and this was statistically lower HIT than all other burn centers ($P < .05$).
2. The highest rates of HIT and DVT were found in burn centers using intravenous unfractionated heparin (UFH) as a prophylactic anticoagulation standard for all patients ($P < .05$).
3. Burn centers using intravenous UFH had a significantly higher rate of DVT than a burn center using LMWH only ($P < .05$).

Although the DVT and pulmonary embolism rates seem low in burn centers, the occurrence of HIT is associated with significant complications or death; therefore, any steps that will either decrease the incidence or prevent altogether the occurrence of HIT should be undertaken. Bushwitz et al[1] also reported in their burn center over a 10-year period that all DVT events occurred in patients receiving UFH as prophylaxis. In their study, patients were not randomized, and the prophylactic measures used in their burn center changed during the 10-year study period.

Although both studies are retrospective, and the Bushwitz study does not represent a randomized group of patients, it does seem like the evidence is growing that LMWH is superior to UHF in preventing DVTs in burn patients. There are no good data about which patients should undergo DVT chemoprophylaxis, but the Busche article findings suggest that all burn patients who receive subcutaneous LMWH chemoprophylaxis have the lowest DVT and HIT rates. LMWH is standard of care in my burn center, as part of the electronic order set, for all burn patients. I recommend the practice to you.

B. A. Latenser, MD, FACS

Reference

1. Bushwitz J, LeClaire A, He J, Mozingo D. Clinically significant venous thromboembolic complications in burn patients receiving unfractionated heparin or enoxaparin as prophylaxis. *J Burn Care Res.* 2011;32:578-582.

Other

Variation in Quality of Care after Emergency General Surgery Procedures in the Elderly

Ingraham AM, Cohen ME, Raval MV, et al (American College of Surgeons, Chicago, IL; et al)

J Am Coll Surg 212:1039-1048, 2011

Background.—The elderly (age ≥65 years) comprise an increasing proportion of patients undergoing emergency general surgery (EGS) procedures and have distinct needs compared with the young. We postulated that the needs of the elderly require different processes of care than those required for the young to assure optimal outcomes. To explore this hypothesis, we evaluated 30-day outcomes following EGS procedures in the young and the elderly and determined whether hospital performance was consistent across these 2 age strata.

Study Design.—With data from the American College of Surgeons National Surgical Quality Improvement Program (2005 to 2008), regression models were constructed for serious morbidity and mortality for all patients undergoing EGS procedures and separately for young and elderly patients. These models allowed for estimation of the risk of adverse outcomes associated with advanced age and the generation of hospital-level observed to expected (O/E) ratios. We evaluated the correlation between hospital O/E ratios for the young and the elderly and the concordance of outlier status (hospitals with CIs of O/E ratios excluding 1) with weighted κ across these 2 age groups.

Results.—Among 68,003 procedures at 186 hospitals, elderly patients had a higher crude and adjusted risk for serious morbidity (27.9% versus 9.7%, $p < 0.0001$; odds ratio 1.17, 95% CI 1.10 to 1.24) and mortality (15.2% versus 2.5%, $p < 0.0001$; odds ratio 2.29, 95% CI 2.09 to 2.51). When outcomes for elderly versus younger patients were compared, there was fair to moderate agreement on hospital performance for serious morbidity ($r = 0.43$; $\kappa = 0.30$) but not for mortality ($r = 0.10$; $\kappa = 0.17$).

Conclusions.—Elderly patients are at substantially greater risk for adverse events following EGS procedures. Hospitals had only slight agreement in mortality outcomes in the elderly compared with those in young patients. Processes of care that may account for this disparity should be further investigated.

► The authors used the massive American College of Surgeons National Surgical Quality Improvement Program (NSQIP) database, with data provided by participating hospitals between January 1, 2005 and December 31, 2008. Several arbitrary definitions were used. The transition from young to elderly was at 65 years of age. In addition, emergency general surgery was based on NSQIP definitions. The most common procedure was appendectomy. I argue that of emergency procedures performed, appendectomy is relatively benign, although common. The outcome discrepancy between young and old patients may be far greater if only higher-acuity procedures, such as for acute diverticular disease or frank gastrointestinal tract perforation, are considered.

Variability in outcomes tended to be greater in young as opposed to elderly patients. I suspect that this is because the burden of disease varied to a greater degree in the young as opposed to the old.

I agree with several summary comments made by the authors. The NSQIP dataset does not collect information regarding the process of care. Thus, the reasons for discrepancies identified (patient- or hospital-related) remain unclear.[1,2] Second, many of the bundles and performance-improvement measures identified for surgical procedures in the elective setting have not been translated into the emergency surgical population. Emergency surgical patients offer limited opportunity for optimization of comorbidities in light of the immediacy of operative intervention. The discrepancy in outcomes between the young and elderly has been identified in a large trauma outcomes study as well.[3] Datasets available for trauma outcome evaluation have far greater maturity than those of the NSQIP dataset. In fact, a recent study argues that trauma centers did not fair as well as nontrauma hospitals in the provision of emergency general surgical care. One reason proposed for this outcome is the lack of mature process measures in emergency general surgery in comparison with those in place for trauma systems.[4]

To summarize, we continue to have significant opportunities to improve acute surgical care of the elderly, but the next steps to improve these outcomes remain unclear.

D. J. Dries, MSE, MD

References

1. Ghaferi AA, Birkmeyer JD, Dimick JB. Variation in hospital mortality associated with inpatient surgery. *N Engl J Med.* 2009;361:1368-1375.
2. McGory ML, Kao KK, Shekelle PG, et al. Developing quality indicators for elderly surgical patients. *Ann Surg.* 2009;250:338-347.
3. Haas B, Gomez D, Xiong W, Ahmed N, Nathens AB. External benchmarking of trauma center performance: have we forgotten our elders? *Ann Surg.* 2011;253: 144-150.
4. Ingraham AM, Cohen ME, Raval MV, Ko CY, Nathens AB. Effect of trauma center status on 30-day outcomes after emergency general surgery. *J Am Coll Surg.* 2011;212:277-286.

Intra-abdominal Hypertension and Abdominal Compartment Syndrome after Endovascular Repair of Ruptured Abdominal Aortic Aneurysm

Djavani Gidlund K, Wanhainen A, Björck M (Uppsala Univ, Sweden)

Eur J Vasc Endovasc Surg 41:742-747, 2011

Objectives.—To investigate the frequency of intra-abdominal hypertension (IAH) and abdominal compartment syndrome (ACS) after endovascular repair (EVAR) of ruptured abdominal aortic aneurysm (rAAA).

Methods.—This was a prospective clinical study. Patients with endovascular repair of rAAA between April 2004 and May 2010 were included. Intra-abdominal pressure (IAP) was measured in the bladder every 4 h.

IAH and ACS were defined according to the World Society of the Abdominal Compartment Syndrome consensus document. Early conservative treatments (diuretics, colloids and neuromuscular blockade) were given to patients with IAP > 12 mmHg.

Results.—Twenty-nine patients, who underwent endovascular repair of a rAAA, had their IAP monitored. Twenty-five percent of them were in shock at arrival. Postoperatively, 10/29 (34%) patients had an IAP > 15 mmHg and six (21%) had an IAP > 20 mmHg. Three (3/29, 10%) patients developed ACS that necessitated abdominal decompression in two. Five out of six patients with IAP > 20 mmHg presented with preoperative shock. All patients except one with preoperative shock developed some degree of IAH.

Conclusion.—IAH and ACS are common and potential serious complications after EVAR for rAAA. Successful outcome depends on early recognition, early conservative treatment to reduce IAH and decompression laparotomy if ACS develops (Fig 2).

▶ The authors demonstrate that although abdominal compartment syndrome and intra-abdominal hypertension are more common after open aneurysm repair, this complication may appear in patients receiving endograft management of aneurysm rupture as well.[1] Thus, bladder pressure should be monitored to avoid unnecessary end organ injury.

An important marker for intra-abdominal hypertension is shock at the time of presentation. Patients presenting in shock must be considered at high risk for intra-abdominal hypertension and its sequelae.

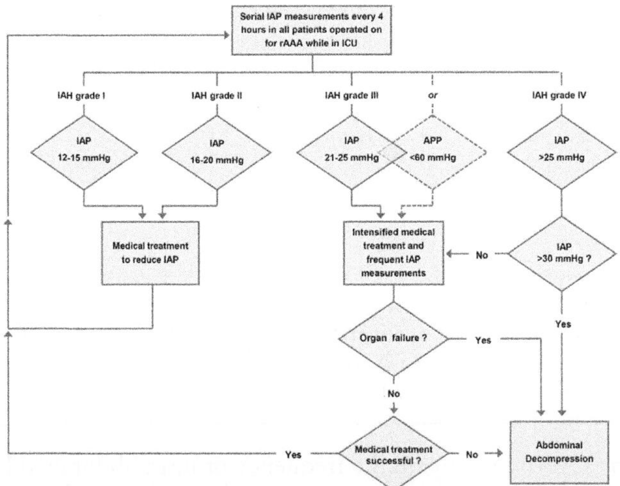

FIGURE 2.—Management algorithm for patients operated on for ruptured AAA. IAP = intra-abdominal pressure, IAH = intra-abdominal hypertension, APP = abdominal perfusion pressure (MAP – IAP), MAP = mean arterial pressure. (Reprinted from Djavani Gidlund K, Wanhainen A, Björck M. Intra-abdominal hypertension and abdominal compartment syndrome after endovascular repair of ruptured abdominal aortic aneurysm. *Eur J Vasc Endovasc Surg*. 2011;41:742-747, Copyright 2011, with permission from European Society for Vascular Surgery.)

Although abdominal decompression has been lifesaving even in patients with vascular grafts placed with open procedures, this therapy can also be safely extended to patients receiving endograft therapy.

The authors aggressively manage patients with intra-abdominal hypertension. Details of nonoperative management were not described, but the authors indicate compliance with recommendations of the World Society of the Abdominal Compartment Syndrome and early implementation of nonsurgical treatment, including aggressive provision of analgesia, diuresis, colloid administration, and neuromuscular blockade[2] (Fig 2). This carefully monitored series has an incidence of abdominal compartment syndrome of 9% to 10% with endograft placement, whereas open procedures are complicated by abdominal compartment syndrome in roughly twice the number of patients (19%).

D. J. Dries, MSE, MD

References

1. Björck M, Steuer J, Wanhainen A. Delayed abdominal closure for ruptured abdominal aortic aneurysm repair. *J Vasc Endovasc Surg.* 2010;17:107-115.
2. Cheatham ML, Malbrain ML, Kirkpatrick A, et al. Results from the International Conference of Experts on Intra-abdominal Hypertension and Abdominal Compartment Syndrome. II. Recommendations. *Intensive Care Med.* 2007;33:951-962.

Emergency surgery in the elderly patient: a quality improvement approach

Peden CJ (Royal United Hosp, Bath, UK)

Anaesthesia 66:440-445, 2011

Background.—Elderly patients with comorbidity, disability, and frailty who undergo emergency surgery are at higher risk for poor outcomes than similar patients having elective surgery. The most common operations performed in these older patients are hemiarthroplasty/sliding hip screw, laparotomy, and amputation. Emergency general and vascular surgery in elderly patients has the highest mortality of any common surgical procedure. With the aging of the population, elderly patients are increasingly the most likely group to be admitted for emergency procedures. Often these operations become a cataclysmic life event, with many patients unable to return home or to previous levels of independence. Costs are high for the patient and in terms of care for complications and increased dependency.

Identifying Problems.—It is unlikely that a new drug or surgical technique will by itself improve care for these complex patients. In addition, research is challenging, complicated by the patient's age, comorbidities, confusion or dementia, and presentation at the emergency room at non-routine working hours. The bottom line is a need to understand the size and nature of the problems and obtain high-quality risk-adjusted outcome data to support decision-making activities and counsel patient and family. Data indicate that the anesthetic management of emergency abdominal surgery varies highly, so efforts are needed to identify what high-performing centers do well and apply the same principles to poorly performing centers so they will do better. Delivery of quality care involves structure, process, and outcome components. Driver diagrams help define outcome aims and identify the primary drivers that produce those results. Secondary drivers can be addressed to improve desired outcomes. The structure to support quality care is essential, including having enough operating theaters, sufficient critical care beds available, and senior personnel handling these patients' complex care.

Management Principles.—Segmentation is dividing postoperative care into its two components: ward care and critical care. First, the focus is on ensuring the patient is delivered to the correct area of care, which requires a scoring process for patient and surgical factors. Each segment is evaluated for the process involved, which may mean focusing on more effective early detection efforts and response to complications and targeting interventions to higher-risk patients. Postoperative monitoring is often intensified to provide needed interventions in a timely fashion. Areas of concern are also identified, such as sufficient medical input and screening for psychological status.

Evidence-based care is foundational for all high-quality programs, with reliability of delivery an essential component. Key areas for evidence-based care include venous thromboembolism assessment and prophylaxis, management of sepsis using care bundles, good perioperative fluid management, dynamic cardiac output monitoring, appropriate and timely antibiotic use, and good communication and follow-through. Checklists are specifically designed to provide reliable delivery of health care in these areas.

Good communication and teamwork are also essential. Teams must be trained to perform in standardized communication methods and use briefings and checklists to facilitate the transfer of information.

More than half of surgical errors occur outside the operating theater, so the entire surgical pathway must be targeted to improve outcomes. A checklist system for the entire surgical pathway provides a comprehensive framework that reduces mortality and complications. Information loss is minimized during transfers and interdisciplinary communication is fostered. Improving one area in the pathway can trigger wider improvements. Dynamic guidelines that are constantly reviewed and revised by physicians directly involved in patient care along with regular feedback concerning outcomes to teams help in designing improvement targets.

The impact and implications of major emergency surgery on elderly patients and their families must be understood in the context of good long-term risk-adjusted data and patient-reported outcomes. The patient pathway and process must be analyzed, including nutritional assessment, medication review, management of dementia and delirium, and rehabilitation facilitated by pain management efforts. Recognizing the high mortality attending emergency procedures in elderly patients is also essential. Many of these patients do not survive the surgery. Sometimes quality of care is facilitated by allowing the patient to die with dignity.

Conclusions.—Efforts at improving patient care for elderly patients having emergency surgery should be focused on the patient and the pathway of care. Patient-centered designs improve outcomes, and protocol-driven pathways produce enhanced recovery programs. Examples of areas improved for elective surgery that may transfer well to emergency care include the design of an evidence-based pathway of care, the use of goal-directed therapy, multidisciplinary involvement in pathway design, and frequent results audits. Anesthetists serve as part of a multidisciplinary team that consider all ways to improve perioperative care for high-risk elderly patients having emergency procedures (Fig 1).

▶ This report from the United Kingdom echoes results recently published from analysis of the massive National Surgical Quality Improvement Program database in the United States.[1] Elderly patients are more likely to suffer complications and mortality in the setting of emergent abdominal procedures. Despite this, multiple lapses of the care process have been identified in patients least likely to survive mistakes. A number of glaring abnormalities were identified. Perhaps most important is the lack of a true team approach. Geriatric input was present in less than half of patients dying after femur fractures. Less than 10% of patients aged over 80 years undergoing acute abdominal operations

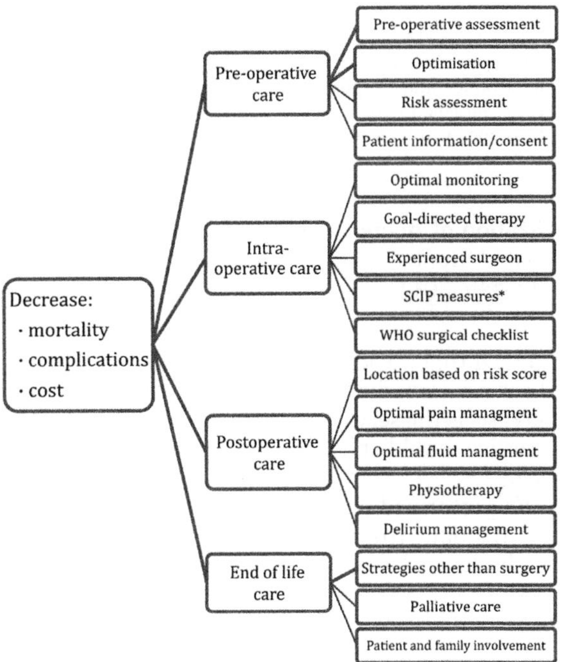

FIGURE 1.—Drivers for improving outcomes for elderly emergency surgical patients. The outcome is on the left of the diagram, then shown are the primary drivers followed by the secondary drivers. This is not an exhaustive list but serves to provide a structure to consider areas to target for quality improvement. *SCIP, Surgical Care Improvement Project [27]. *Editor's Note*: Please refer to original journal article for full references. (Reprinted from Peden CJ. Emergency surgery in the elderly patient: a quality improvement approach. *Anaesthesia*. 2011;66:440-445, with permission of John Wiley & Sons, Inc.)

received geriatric input. Management of these high-risk individuals requires a team approach. The attached figure identifies segments of care that can be studied and optimized (Fig 1).

The elderly frequently see deficits in the key areas of evidence-based practice identified in studies on both sides of the Atlantic.[2] These include careful management of venous thromboembolism prophylaxis, use of sepsis care bundles, judicious perioperative fluid management, timely antibiotic administration, and optimal communication and handoffs.

Teamwork and communication are particularly important and more difficult in the emergency setting.[3] Many of the careful methods of preoperative planning are less likely to be employed in the emergency patient. Unfortunately, these individuals may have the greatest risk. Just as a pathway of care has been identified for patients receiving elective surgery, a related group of measures with perioperative risk stratification may be invaluable in the elderly patient facing emergency surgery.

D. J. Dries, MSE, MD

References

1. Ingraham AM, Cohen ME, Raval MV, et al. Variation in quality of care after emergency general surgery procedures in the elderly. *J Am Coll Surg.* 2011;212: 1039-1048.
2. de Vries EN, Prins HA, Crolla RM, et al. Effect of a comprehensive surgical safety system on patient outcomes. *N Engl J Med.* 2010;363:1928-1937.
3. National Confidential Enquiry into Patient Outcome and Death. *Elective and Emergency Surgery in the Elderly: An Age Old Problem.* London: NCEPOD; 2010, http://www.ncepod.org.uk/2010eese.htm. Accessed 04/03/2011.

Does Regionalization of Acute Care Surgery Decrease Mortality?

Diaz JJ Jr, Norris PR, Gunter OL, et al (Vanderbilt Univ Med Ctr, Nashville, TN)
J Trauma 71:442-446, 2011

Background.—During the initial development of an Emergency General Surgery (EGS) service, severity of illness (SOI) can be expected to be high and should decrease as the service matures. We hypothesize that a matured regional EGS service would show decreasing mortality and length of stay (LOS) over time.

Methods.—We performed a retrospective study of a prospectively collected EGS registry data from 2004 to 2009. Patients were included if they had been discharged from the EGS service and were stratified by year of discharge. Systemic inflammatory response syndrome, sepsis, shock, peritonitis, perforation, and acute renal failure were used as markers of SOI. Patients were defined as high acuity if they had one or more of these SOI markers. Differences in mortality, LOS, intensive care unit admissions, SOI, charges, and distance were compared across and between years using nonparametric statistical tests (Fisher's exact, Wilcoxon rank-sum, and Kruskal-Wallis tests).

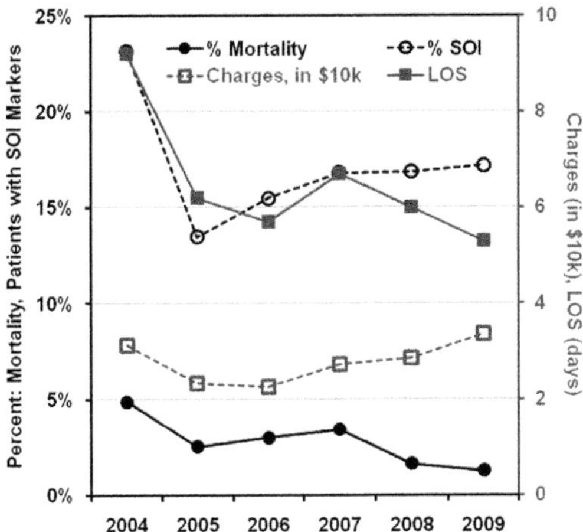

FIGURE 1.—Trends in EGS mortality, severity of illness (SOI), charges, and length of stay (LOS). (Reprinted from Diaz JJ Jr, Norris PR, Gunter OL, et al. Does regionalization of acute care surgery decrease mortality? *J Trauma*. 2011;71:442-446, with permission from Lippincott Williams & Wilkins.)

Results.—A total of 3,439 patients met study criteria. The mean age was 47 years ± 17.5 years. The majority of the patients were female (1,813, 47.3%). The overall LOS was 6.4 days ± 9.4 days (median, 4 days). In all, 2,331 (67.8%) of the patients underwent operation. Over the course of the study period, the SOI indicators stabilized at between 13% and 17% of the patient population with at least one indicator. During that time period, mortality steadily decreased from 4.9% to 1.3% ($p < 0.5$).

Conclusion.—Despite consistently high SOI, a dedicated and matured EGS service demonstrated a decrease in mortality and LOS (Fig 1).

▶ These results represent the present state of the art for implementation of acute care surgery. This medical center has made a defined commitment to development of this service independent of critical care and trauma programs.[1,2] In fact, acute care surgery is probably best separated from trauma programs, because in combination programs, including trauma, improved outcomes may not be demonstrated. A review of details in the article finds that significant resources are committed to this service. Nearly 70% of hospitalized patients receive surgical procedures.

Standardized severity-of-injury scores such as APACHE II are not available. However, the authors consistently follow a set of severity-of-injury indicators, which they have used in previous studies. Examination of the figure included with this summary finds that benefits obtained with development of an acute general surgery service should be rapidly seen (Fig 1).

This article argues effectively for the power of regionalization of acute care surgery. Not only does an acute care surgery service require significant resources to run effectively, but, without an adequate volume of clinical material, I believe that the benefits obtained from developing such a program may be harder to demonstrate.

D. J. Dries, MSE, MD

References

1. Davis KA, Rozycki GS. Acute care surgery in evolution. *Crit Care Med.* 2010;38: S405-S410.
2. Committee on Acute Care Surgery American Association for the Surgery of Trauma. The acute care surgery curriculum. *J Trauma.* 2007;62:553-556.

Infectious Complications and Soft Tissue Injury Contribute to Late Amputation After Severe Lower Extremity Trauma

Huh J, Late Amputation Study Team (Brooke Army Med Ctr, Fort Sam Houston, TX; et al)

J Trauma 71:S47-S51, 2011

Background.—Although most combat-related amputations occur early for unsalvageable injuries, >15% occur late after reconstructive attempts. Predicting which patients will abandon limb salvage in favor of definitive amputation has not been explored. The purpose of this study was to identify factors contributing to late amputation for type III open tibia fractures sustained in combat.

Methods.—Operative databases were reviewed to identify all combat-related type III open diaphyseal tibia fractures from March 2003 to September 2007. Patients were categorized based on their definitive treatment: group I, limb salvage; group II, early amputation (<12 weeks postinjury); group III, late amputation (≥12 weeks postinjury). Injury, treatment, and complication data were extracted from medical records and compared across groups.

Results.—We identified 213 consecutive fractures, including 166 (77.9%) treated definitively with limb salvage, 36 (16.9%) with early amputation, and 11 (5.2%) with late amputation. There was no difference in fracture severity among the three groups. Before amputation, group III was more likely to use autograft and bone morphogenic protein (27.3%), compared with group I (4.8%) and group II (0%), and was more likely to undergo rotational flap coverage (45.5%), compared with group II (0%). Group III patients had the highest average number of revision surgeries and rate of deep soft tissue infection and were more likely to have osteomyelitis (54.5%) before amputation compared with group I (13.9%) and group II (16.7%).

Conclusion.—Patients definitively managed with late amputation were more likely to have soft tissue injury requiring flap coverage and have their limb salvage course complicated by infection (Table 2).

► Current military practice limits early amputation to afford patients the greatest number of reconstructive opportunities. This decision is supported by aggressive provision of early care in forward battlefield medical facilities. Patients

TABLE 2.—Distribution of Injury Characteristics

	Group I, Limb Salvage (N = 166)	Group II, Early Amputees (N = 36)	Group III, Late Amputees (N = 11)	*p*
Fracture classification				
OTA type A	18.1% (30)	8.3% (3)	9.1% (1)	0.2928
OTA type B	30.1% (50)	16.7% (6)	36.4% (4)	0.2197
OTA type C	51.8% (86)	75.0% (27)	54.5% (6)	0.0395
Soft tissue classification				
G/A type IIIA	60.8% (101)	16.7% (6)	45.5% (5)	<0.0001
G/A type IIIB	34.9% (58)	36.1% (13)	45.5% (5)	0.7786
G/A type IIIC	4.2% (7)	47.2% (17)	9% (1)	<0.0001
Associated injuries				
Nerve injury	16.9% (28)	22.2% (8)	36.3% (4)	0.2171

G/A, Gustilo-Anderson; OTA, Orthopaedic Trauma Association.

are initially stabilized and transferred to the United States for ultimate reconstruction. This approach to aggressive limb salvage allows the opportunity to identify patterns of late failure. The authors note that a standard guideline is a 3.9% late amputation rate after 2 years.[1]

The authors follow tibial fractures with varying degrees of soft tissue trauma. Initial care involves external fixation with wound debridement in the theater of operations. Patients with more complex repairs (flap coverage and bone substitutes) experienced a greater incidence of late amputation. A standard indication for late amputation, nerve injury, was not present to a statistically greater degree in the late-amputation group.[2,3]

Infectious complications including soft tissue infection, presumably involving flaps and osteomyelitis, were predictors of amputation. What this study does not tell us is the morbidity associated with the increased number of reconstructive procedures these patients required and the obvious question of cost.

Regardless of the answer to the questions of cost, along with physical and emotional suffering associated with prolonged attempts at rehabilitation, these data clearly argue for better methods of infection control with complex reconstructive extremity procedures. A second lesson to note is that although fracture severity is comparable in the 3 study groups, severity of soft tissue injury appears to be a stronger determinant of both early and late amputation[4] (Table 2).

D. J. Dries, MSE, MD

References

1. Harris AM, Althausen PL, Kellam J, Bosse MJ, Castillo R. Complications following limb-threatening lower extremity trauma. *J Orthop Trauma.* 2009;23:1-6.
2. Gustilo RB, Gruninger RP, Davis T. Classification of type III (severe) open fractures relative to treatment and results. *Orthopedics.* 1987;10:1781-1788.
3. Busse JW, Jacobs CL, Swiontkowski MF, Bosse MJ, Bhandari M. Complex limb salvage or early amputation for severe lower-limb injury: a meta-analysis of observational studies. *J Orthop Trauma.* 2007;21:70-76.
4. Bosse MJ, MacKenzie EJ, Kellam JF, et al. An analysis of outcomes of reconstruction or amputation after leg-threatening injuries. *N Engl J Med.* 2002;347:1924-1931.

Are Targeted Preoperative Risk Prediction Tools More Powerful? A Test of Models for Emergency Colon Surgery in the Very Elderly

Kwok AC, Lipsitz SR, Bader AM, et al (Brigham and Women's Hosp, Boston, MA)

J Am Coll Surg 213:220-225, 2011

Background.—Whether preoperative risk prediction improves with the use of more patient- and procedure-targeted models is unclear. We created a customized preoperative mortality risk prediction score for patients 80 years or older needing an emergency colectomy and compare it with existing, more generic risk assessment methods.

Study Design.—A targeted mortality prediction model was created using 2007 to 2008 American College of Surgeons National Surgical Quality Improvement Program (ACS NSQIP) data and was validated using 2005 to 2006 data. We constructed a scoring system from the significant predictors identified. The model fit of our targeted score was compared with the American Society of Anesthesiologist's (ASA) score, the Surgical Risk Scale, and the ACS Colorectal Surgery Risk Calculator.

Results.—Analyses identified 1,358 and 372 emergency colectomies in the training and validation samples, respectively. Our targeted risk prediction score had a goodness-of-fit p value greater than 0.05 (indicating a good fit) and a c-statistic of 0.77, which represents a significantly better fit compared with the ASA score, the Surgical Risk Scale, and the ACS Colorectal Surgery Risk Calculator c-statistics (0.66, 0.66, and 0.71, respectively). When using the scores to predict mortality with 80% specificity, our targeted risk prediction score was 25% more likely to predict correctly than the ACS Colorectal Surgery Risk Calculator and 33% more likely to predict correctly compared with the ASA score and Surgical Risk Scale.

Conclusions.—Our study presents a validated preoperative mortality score for very elderly patients needing an emergency colectomy. The greater discriminating power of this targeted score indicates that preoperative risk assessment may need to be customized to specific procedures and patient circumstances (Fig 1).

▶ This article is presented by authors recently associated with the Surgical Apgar Score.[1] Now they identify risk factors for specific poor outcomes with colonic surgery and apply multivariate analysis to develop a better predictive model (Fig 1). There is logic in this approach in that it is patient and disease specific. I note, however, that the authors do not distinguish between types of colonic procedure. Clearly, a localized resection may have different physiologic implications than a total abdominal colectomy or a proctectomy.

This population should be better characterized to understand the context of this work. First, the majority of these procedures are performed using open technique. Laparoscopy is common in many settings but is not featured prominently here.

Along with age, functional status, including various predictors of function, is very important. This coincides with previous work, which identifies preoperative disability as a significant predictor of postoperative outcome.[2,3]

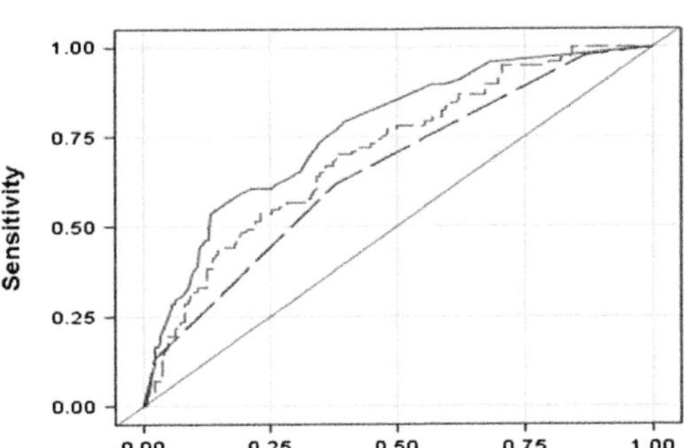

FIGURE 1.—Comparison of receiver operating characteristic (ROC) curves using the validation sample. Blue line, targeted risk prediction score (0.77); red dashed line, American College of Surgeons (ACS) Colorectal Surgery Risk Calculator (0.71); black dashed line, Surgical Risk Scale, and American Society of Anesthesiologists (ASA) score (0.66). For interpretation of the references to color in this figure legend, the reader is referred to web version of this article. (Reprinted from Kwok AC, Lipsitz SR, Bader AM, et al. Are targeted preoperative risk prediction tools more powerful? A test of models for emergency colon surgery in the very elderly. *J Am Coll Surg*. 2011;213:220-225, Copyright 2011, with permission from the American College of Surgeons.)

This study clearly demonstrates sophisticated application of our growing statistical capability with management of large datasets generated from segments of the surgical patient population. Where will these various studies lead us? Perhaps a greater sophistication regarding preoperative stratification will come. Much of this work, nevertheless, does not yet supplant but rather supports good clinical judgment.

D. J. Dries, MSE, MD

References

1. Gawande AA, Kwaan MR, Regenbogen SE, Lipsitz SA, Zinner MJ. An Apgar score for surgery. *J Am Coll Surg*. 2007;204:201-208.
2. Malani PN. Functional status assessment in the preoperative evaluation of older adults. *JAMA*. 2009;302:1582-1583.
3. Makary MA, Segev DL, Pronovost PJ, et al. Frailty as a predictor of surgical outcomes in older patients. *J Am Coll Surg*. 2010;210:901-908.

Clinical and economic burden of postoperative pulmonary complications: Patient safety summit on definition, risk-reducing interventions, and preventive strategies

Shander A, Fleisher LA, Barie PS, et al (Englewood Hosp and Med Ctr, NJ; the Univ of Pennsylvania, Philadelphia; Weill Cornell Med College, NY; et al)
Crit Care Med 39:2163-2172, 2011

Objective.—Postoperative pulmonary complications are a major contributor to the overall risk of surgery. We convened a patient safety summit to discuss ways to enhance physician awareness of postoperative pulmonary complications, advance postoperative pulmonary complications as a substantive public health concern demanding national attention, recommend strategies to reduce the deleterious impact of postoperative pulmonary complications on clinical outcomes and healthcare costs, and establish an algorithm that will help identify patients who are at increased risk for postoperative pulmonary complications.

Data Sources.—We conducted PubMed searches for relevant literature on postoperative pulmonary complications in addition to using the summit participants' experience in the management of patients with postoperative pulmonary complications.

Data Synthesis.—Postoperative pulmonary complications are common, are associated with increased morbidity and mortality, and adversely affect financial outcomes in health care. A multifaceted approach is necessary to reduce the incidence of postoperative pulmonary complications. Identifying a measurable marker of risk will facilitate the targeted implementation of risk-reduction strategies.

Conclusions.—The most practicable marker that identifies patients at highest risk for postoperative pulmonary complications is the need for postoperative mechanical ventilation of a cumulative duration >48 hrs (Table 2).

▶ This article by Shander and colleagues highlights the incidence, impact, and cost of postoperative pulmonary complications (PPCs) and proposes a metric for tracking progress along this front. They convened a group of 15 experts from the fields of surgery, anesthesiology/critical care, internal and hospital medicine, health services research, and patient safety and government health care organizations. They performed a targeted literature review of postoperative pulmonary complications and shine a spotlight on the frequency and importance of postoperative pulmonary complications. PPCs have been shown to occur twice as frequently as cardiac complications and result in longer lengths of stay and increased rates of readmission, morbidity, and mortality (Table 2). Furthermore, the cost of PPCs is estimated to contribute an additional $3.42 billion dollars to health care costs annually.[1]

TABLE 2.—Postoperative Pulmonary Complications After Elective Surgery in Adults

Bronchospasm
1 additional ICU admission for every 14 cases
1 additional ICU day for every 5 cases
1 additional hospital day and $1563 added cost per case
Other postoperative pulmonary complications (excluding bronchospasm and respiratory failure)
1 additional ICU admission for every 6 cases
0.66 additional ICU days, 3 additional hospital days, and $5771 added cost per case
Respiratory failure
1 additional ICU admission for every 2 cases
5 additional ICU days, 8 additional hospital days, and $24,000 added cost per case

ICU, intensive care unit.

Based on an analysis of a large U.S. database by Linde-Zwirble et al (72).

Editor's Note: Please refer to original journal article for full references.

This article discusses the challenges of defining PPCs, as the literature has used multiple different definitions, and the authors appropriately propose that we need to adopt a standard definition as a first step in enabling us to track this outcome and our quality of care. To that end, they propose that PPC be defined as postoperative mechanical ventilation greater than 48 hours. While adopting a standard metric is important, and adopting a metric that can be easily abstracted from administrative data is appealing, we need to be cautious about adopting this too quickly. In the accompanying editorial, Drs. Romig and Dorman[2] point out that we must be vigilant in validating this metric, prior to it being used broadly for reporting purposes. We know from experience that metrics that are drawn from administrative data have limitations[3,4] and thus need to proceed cautiously while we continue to push the quality envelope.

E. A. Martinez, MD, MHS

References

1. Linde-Zwurble WL, Bloom JD, Mecca RS, Hansell DM. Postoperative pulmonary complications in adult elective surgery patients in the US: severity, outcomes and resources use. *Crit Care.* 2010;14:210.
2. Romig MC, Dorman T. Opening our eyes to postoperative pulmonary complications. *Crit Care Med.* 2011;39:2198-2199.
3. Borzecki AM, Kaafarani HM, Utter GH, et al. How valid is the AHRQ Patient Safety Indicator "postoperative respiratory failure"? *J Am Coll Surg.* 2011;212: 935-945.
4. Rosen AK, Itani KM, Cevasco M, et al. Validating the patient safety indicators in the Veterans Health Administration: do they accurately identify true safety events? *Med Care.* 2012;50:74-85.

Development and Validation of a Risk Calculator Predicting Postoperative Respiratory Failure

Gupta H, Gupta PK, Fang X, et al (Creighton Univ, Omaha, NE; et al)
Chest 140:1207-1215, 2011

Background.—Postoperative respiratory failure (PRF) (requiring mechanical ventilation >48 h after surgery or unplanned intubation within 30 days of surgery) is associated with significant morbidity and mortality. The objective of this study was to identify preoperative factors associated with an increased risk of PRF and subsequently develop and validate a risk calculator.

Methods.—The American College of Surgeons National Surgical Quality Improvement Program (NSQIP), a multicenter, prospective data set (2007-2008), was used. The 2007 data set (n = 211,410) served as the training set and the 2008 data set (n = 257,385) as the validation set.

Results.—In the training set, 6,531 patients (3.1%) developed PRF. Patients who developed PRF had a significantly higher 30-day mortality (25.62% vs 0.98%, $P < .0001$). On multivariate logistic regression analysis, five preoperative predictors of PRF were identified: type of surgery, emergency case, dependent functional status, preoperative sepsis, and higher

American Society of Anesthesiologists (ASA) class. The risk model based on the training data set was subsequently validated on the validation data set. The model performance was very similar between the training and the validation data sets (c-statistic, 0.894 and 0.897, respectively). The high c-statistics (area under the receiver operating characteristic curve) indicate excellent predictive performance. The risk model was used to develop an interactive risk calculator.

Conclusions.—Preoperative variables associated with increased risk of PRF include type of surgery, emergency case, dependent functional status, sepsis, and higher ASA class. The validated risk calculator provides a risk estimate of PRF and is anticipated to aid in surgical decision making and informed patient consent.

▶ This study uses 2 cuts through the National Surgical Quality Improvement Program (NSQIP) data set. Data from 2007 were used to develop the model, and 2008 data were used to validate. Postoperative respiratory failure (PRF) is broadly defined. PRF occurs if patients have unplanned intubation during operation or postoperatively, were reintubated postoperatively after being extubated, or required mechanical ventilation for more than 48 hours postoperatively. Patients returned to the operating room were not counted against the PRF measure. The most powerful predictors are degree of dependency during the preoperative state and the presence of sepsis or septic shock. Consistent with traditional teaching, foregut and upper abdomen procedures also are associated with an increased risk of respiratory failure.

This study confirms another major study of preoperative frailty as a predictor of postoperative complications.[1] The authors support the power of preoperative preparation and clear risk estimation before surgery.[2] PRF incidence is similar across the spectrum of hospitals contributing to the NSQIP database. These include academic, Veterans Affairs hospitals, and private community-based facilities.

Why is this important? The 30-day mortality in this study as well as other large data sets is between 25% and 30% with PRF described in this general manner.

D. J. Dries, MSE, MD

References

1. Saxton A, Velanovich V. Preoperative frailty and quality of life as predictors of postoperative complications. *Ann Surg*. 2011;253:1223-1229.
2. Ravikumar TS, Sharma C, Marini C, et al. A validated value-based model to improve hospital-wide perioperative outcomes: adaptability to combined medical/surgical inpatient cohorts. *Ann Surg*. 2010;252:486-498.

7 Sepsis/Septic Shock

It takes an intensivist

Silverman LZ, Hoesel LM, Desai A, et al (St Joseph Mercy Hosp, Ann Arbor, MI)

Am J Surg 201:320-323, 2011

Background.—Our institution initiated the implementation of the Surviving Sepsis Campaign guidelines in 2006. We hypothesize that the addition of a surgical intensivist improved results more than the implementation of the guidelines alone.

Methods.—We collected data on 273 patients who were admitted to the surgical intensive care unit for sepsis. The groups were divided into pre-bundle, n = 19; bundle, n = 186; and bundle-plus, n = 68, to denote the method by which the patients were treated for sepsis.

Results.—There was no difference in age or sex between groups. There was a statistically significant decrease in length of stay (LOS) between the 3 groups, and in mortality between the bundle and bundle-plus treatment groups ($P < .01$). In addition, there was an average cost savings between each group.

Conclusions.—Implementation of evidence-based guidelines decreased LOS and decreased cost in our surgical intensive care unit. By adding the expertise of a surgical intensivist, we reduced LOS, cost, and relative risk of death even further than using the guidelines alone.

▶ The delivery of critical care is a complex and evolving enterprise. Models for critical care delivery are still being defined and are not uniform across hospitals in the United States. Two relevant aspects of this delivery include the use of protocolized care and the staffing of intensive care units. Protocolized care in the form of protocols, bundles, or checklists aims to decrease variability in clinical care from patient to patient. In severe sepsis, the application of "sepsis bundles" based on recommendations from the Surviving Sepsis Campaign has been associated with improved outcomes in numerous publications. Studies have also suggested that care led by a trained intensivist is associated with improved outcomes. In this study, the authors evaluated the impact on outcomes in a surgical intensive care unit of the introduction of sepsis bundles. They compared outcomes before and after the introduction of sepsis bundles and also included a third group of patients that included sepsis bundles plus care by a surgical critical care physician-led team. Not surprisingly, mortality and length of stay improved with implementation of the sepsis bundles when compared with the historical control group. Furthermore, the addition of the surgical critical care physician was associated with further decreases in mortality and length of stay. The addition of the surgical intensivist was associated with a significant increase in compliance with the sepsis bundles (10%–70%). The increase in bundle compliance by itself could easily explain the improvement in mortality. It is not possible to fully dissect the impact of the surgical intensivist. However, this study does bring to our attention the value of minimizing variability when caring for patients with severe sepsis. It further supports the use of sepsis bundles and specifically addresses their impact in a surgical intensive care unit.

S. L. Zanotti-Cavazzoni, MD

Renal effects of synthetic colloids and crystalloids in patients with severe sepsis: A prospective sequential comparison

Bayer O, Reinhart K, Sakr Y, et al (Jena Univ Hosp, Germany)
Crit Care Med 39:1335-1342, 2011

Objectives.—Hydroxyethyl starch 200 is associated with renal impairment in sepsis, but hydroxyethyl starch 130/0.4 and gelatin are considered to be less harmful. We hypothesized that fluid therapy with only crystalloids would decrease the incidence of acute kidney injury.

Design.—Prospective sequential comparison during intensive care unit stay.

Setting.—Surgical intensive care unit.

Patients.—Patients with severe sepsis.

Interventions.—Changes in standard fluid therapy, with predominantly 6% hydroxyethyl starch from January 2005 to June 2005, 4% gelatin from January 2006 to June 2006, and only crystalloids from September 2008 to June 2009.

Measurements and Main Results.—Acute kidney injury was defined by the presence of at least one RIFLE class; 118 patients received hydroxyethyl starch, 87 patients received gelatin, 141 patients received only crystalloids. Baseline serum creatinine values were similar. Patients received median cumulative doses of 46 (interquartile range, 18–92) mL/kg hydroxyethyl starch and 43 (interquartile range, 18–76) mL/kg gelatin. Total median fluid amounts were 649 (interquartile range, 275–1098) mL/kg in the hydroxyethyl starch group, 525 (237–868) mL/kg in the gelatin group, and 355 (173–911) mL/kg in the crystalloid group. The difference was statistically significant for hydroxyethyl starch after adjustment for multiple testing. Mean daily fluid intake and fluid balance were higher on days 0 and 1 in the crystalloid group. Acute kidney injury occurred in 70% of patients receiving hydroxyethyl starch (adjusted $p = .002$) and in 68% of patients receiving gelatin (adjusted $p = .025$) vs. 47% patients receiving crystalloids. Need for renal replacement therapy tended to be higher in the hydroxyethyl starch group (34%; adjusted $p = .086$) and in the gelatin group (34%; adjusted $p = .162$) in comparison to the crystalloid group (20%). Intensive care unit and hospital mortality were similar in each group (hydroxyethyl starch: 35% and 43%; gelatin: 26% and 31%; crystalloids: 30% and 37%).

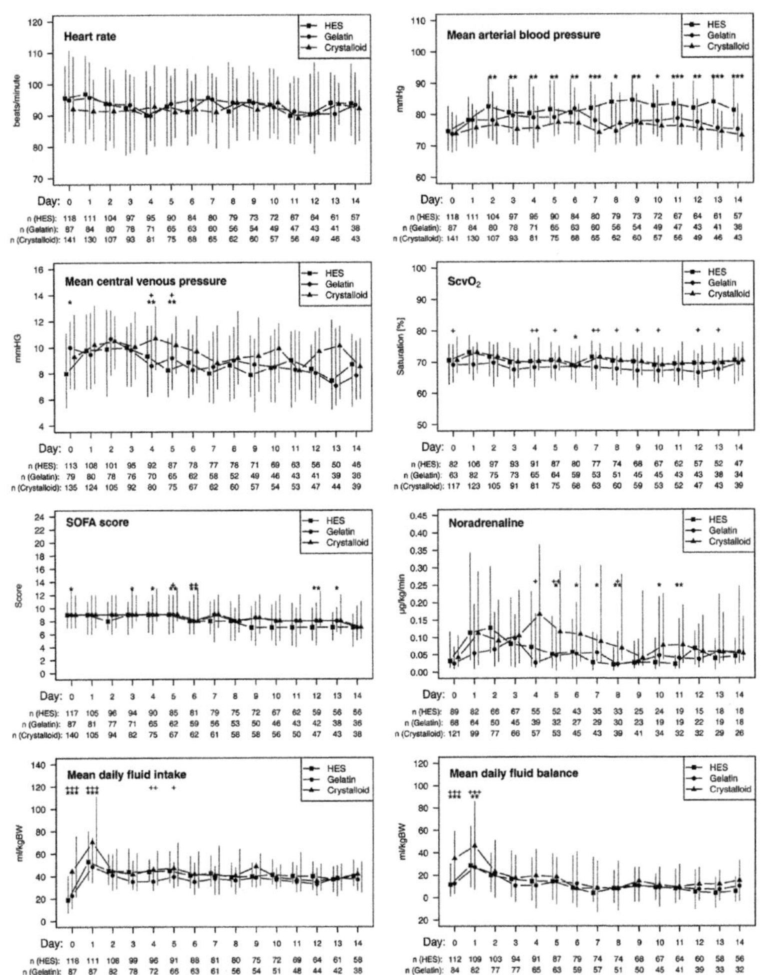

FIGURE 1.—Means of daily heart rate, daily arterial pressure, daily central venous pressure, daily central venous saturation concentrations, daily Sequential Organ Failure Assessment scores, cumulative daily dose of noradrenaline, daily fluid intake, and daily fluid balance for days 0–14. Median and interquartile range are presented. ***/+++ $p < .001$, **/++ $p < .01$, */+ $p < .05$ (*comparisons between hydroxyethyl starch [*HES*] and crystalloids groups; + comparisons between gelatin and crystalloid groups). *ScvO*$_2$, central venous oxygen saturation. (Reprinted from Bayer O, Reinhart K, Sakr Y, et al. Renal effects of synthetic colloids and crystalloids in patients with severe sepsis: a prospective sequential comparison. *Crit Care Med*. 2011;39:1335-1342, with permission from the Society of Critical Care Medicine and Lippincott Williams & Wilkins.)

Conclusion.—Fluid resuscitation with only crystalloids was equally effective, resulted in a more positive fluid balance only on the first 2 days, and was associated with a lesser incidence of acute kidney injury (Fig 1).

▶ The debate over the best type of fluid for resuscitation in critically ill patients with septic shock has gone on for years. Proponents of colloids (starches, gelatins, and albumin) have often referred to potential advantages such as less volume or increased intravascular volume expansion. On the other hand, proponents of crystalloids (saline, Ringer's lactate) have often pointed out lower cost and potential safety concerns with colloids. The largest randomized study to date, the SAFE study, compared normal saline to albumin and found no difference in the primary outcome of 28-day all-cause mortality.[1] However, questions regarding the impact of specific types of fluids on organ failure (specifically renal failure) and on overall fluid requirements still remain unanswered. One concern raised by several small studies was the potential increase in renal failure with high-molecular-weight starches. Development of newer starches with lower molecular weights seemed to resolve this issue. However, more recent systematic reviews failed to confirm that lower-molecular-weight starches had improved safety profiles when compared with older starches.

In this cohort study, the authors evaluated the effects of 3 different types of fluids in patients with severe sepsis. The primary outcome of this analysis was the development of acute kidney injury (AKI). Need for new renal replacement therapy (RRT) was a coprimary outcome. Secondary outcomes included cumulative fluid doses, fluid balance, and mortality. In a sequential design, the investigators evaluated 3 different fluid resuscitation strategies; the first group was predominantly treated with 6% hydroxyethyl starch (6% HES), the second group predominantly received 4% gelatin, and the final group was treated exclusively with crystalloids. The authors reported increased AKI in the patients treated with 6% HES and 4% gelatin when compared with the group treated with crystalloids. There was also increased need for RRT in patients in the 6% HES and 4% gelatin groups when compared with the group receiving crystalloids. Mortality was similar in all groups. Of interest, higher positive fluid balance was seen in the crystalloid group only on day 0 and day 1 of treatment, and overall the total dose of fluids was highest in the 6% HES. Additional hemodynamic outcomes are shown in Fig 1. This was not a randomized study, which is an important limitation precluding definitive conclusions from the results. However, of great interest are the findings suggesting that colloids such as 6% HES and 4% gelatin may increase the risk of AKI and need for RRT. Furthermore, it does not seem that the results of this study support a commonly held belief that resuscitation with colloids leads to less positive fluid balance. Ongoing randomized studies will hopefully help further elucidate some of these important questions.

S. L. Zanotti-Cavazzoni, MD

Reference

1. Finfer S, Bellomo R, Boyce N, et al. A comparison of albumin and saline for fluid resuscitation in the intensive care unit. *N Engl J Med.* 2004;350:2247-2256.

Successful Treatment of Severe Sepsis With Recombinant Activated Protein C During the Third Trimester of Pregnancy

Gupta R, Strickland KM, Mertz HL (Wake Forest School of Medicine, Winston Salem, NC)

Obstet Gynecol 118:492-494, 2011

Background.—Severe sepsis in pregnancy is associated with multiorgan failure and a high risk of death for the mother and fetus.

Case.—We present the case of a pregnant patient at 26 weeks of gestation with severe sepsis secondary to pneumonia. She was admitted to the intensive care unit and started on combination antibiotics and bilevel positive airway pressure. Her condition continued to deteriorate, and she was treated with recombinant activated protein C (drotrecogin alfa). She improved and delivered at 28 weeks of gestation after preterm labor; neither the patient nor the neonate had evidence of drug-related complications.

Conclusion.—This report describes a case of severe sepsis at 26 weeks of gestation secondary to pneumonia, with successful maternal and fetal outcome after use of drotrecogin alfa (activated).

▶ Sepsis remains an important cause of morbidity and mortality in pregnancy. Because of the inherent limitation of conducting scientific research during pregnancy, a great deal of clinical decision making is based on case reports, understanding of the physiologic changes associated with pregnancy, and consideration with risk to the fetus. Drotrecogin alpha (activated) was a novel therapy proposed for the treatment of severe sepsis and septic shock based on the results of 1 seminal study. In this study, no pregnant patients were included, so the experience with the use of this drug during pregnancy was very limited. These 2 case reports discuss the use of drotrecogin alpha (activated) in pregnant patients with severe sepsis. The first report describes a 20-year-old pregnant woman at 20 weeks of gestation with severe sepsis caused by a urinary tract infection. This patient completed 96 uninterrupted hours of therapy with drotrecogin alpha activated and was discharged home in good health. The second case describes a pregnant patient at 26 weeks of gestation with a diagnosis of pneumonia. Despite aggressive treatment her condition clinically deteriorated, and a decision to start drotrecogin alpha (activated) was made. Again, in this case, the patient's condition improved with therapy and she eventually delivered at 28 weeks. In both reports there was no evidence of patient or neonate drug-related complications. With the recent withdrawal of drotrecogin alpha (activated) from the market by the manufacturer, these reports mostly hold only historical interest. However, they illustrate a common problem in caring for pregnant critically ill patients. With a paucity of studies in this population, the clinician often needs to rely on case reports and very individualized risk/benefit analysis to support clinical decision making.

S. L. Zanotti-Cavazzoni, MD

Procalcitonin as a Marker for the Detection of Bacteremia and Sepsis in the Emergency Department

Riedel S, Melendez JH, An AT, et al (The Johns Hopkins Univ, Baltimore, MD)
Am J Clin Pathol 135:182-189, 2011

Rapid diagnosis of bloodstream infections (BSIs) in the emergency department (ED) is challenging, with turnaround times exceeding the timeline for rapid diagnosis. We studied the usefulness of procalcitonin as a marker of BSI in 367 adults admitted to our ED with symptoms of systemic infection. Serum samples obtained at the same time as blood cultures were available from 295 patients. Procalcitonin levels were compared with blood culture results and other clinical data obtained during the ED visit. Procalcitonin levels of less than 0.1 ng/mL were considered negative; all other levels were considered positive. In 16 patients, there was evidence of BSI by blood culture, and 12 (75%) of 16 patients had a procalcitonin level of more than 0.1 ng/mL. In 186 (63.1%) of 295 samples, procalcitonin values were less than 0.1 ng/mL, and all were culture negative. With a calculated threshold of 0.1475 ng/mL for procalcitonin, sensitivity and specificity for the procalcitonin assay were 75% and 79%, respectively. The positive predictive value was 17% and the negative predictive value 98% compared with blood cultures. Procalcitonin is a useful marker to rule out sepsis and systemic inflammation in the ED.

▶ Prompt recognition of bacteremia and sepsis is imperative to the timely initiation of antimicrobials and early goal-directed therapy in the emergency department (ED). Riedel et al utilized blood cultures positive for pathogens as the reference standard to retrospectively examine the accuracy of procalcitonin in the diagnosis of sepsis in patients presenting to the ED with signs of systemic infection. The authors established a threshold procalcitonin level of 0.1 ng/mL to exclude sepsis with a negative predictive value (NPV) of 96.3% and sensitivity of 75%. While the cutoff procalcitonin level in this study is lower than previously published reports, the high NPV value is similar, suggesting a procalcitonin <0.1 ng/mL may help rule out bacteremia in the ED population. The authors also proposed a role for procalcitonin as a prognostic marker in sepsis given that higher procalcitonin levels in this study were associated with greater sepsis severity and quantity of positive blood cultures. Prior data suggest that incorporation of procalcitonin in the algorithm for managing sepsis in the intensive care unit limits overexposure to antibiotics in the critically ill. The current study supports the use of procalcitonin as a screening tool to improve the diagnostic accuracy and risk stratification of sepsis in the undifferentiated ED patient whose management is unaided by culture data.

E. Damuth, MD
S. L. Zanotti-Cvazzoni, MD

Base excess is an accurate predictor of elevated lactate in ED septic patients

Montassier E, Batard E, Segard J, et al (Hôtel Dieu Teaching Hosp, Nantes, France; et al)

Am J Emerg Med 30:184-187, 2012

Background.—Prior studies showed that lactate is a useful marker in sepsis. However, lactate is often not routinely drawn or rapidly available in the emergency department (ED).

Objective.—The study aimed to determine if base excess (BE), widely and rapidly available in the ED, could be used as a surrogate marker for elevated lactate in ED septic patients.

Methods.—This was a prospective and observational cohort study. From March 2009 to March 2010, consecutive patients 18 years or older who presented to the ED with a suspected severe sepsis were enrolled in the study. Lactate and BE measurements were performed. We defined, a priori, a clinically significant lactate to be greater than 3 mmol/L and BE less than −4 mmol/L.

Results.—A total of 224 patients were enrolled in the study. The average BE was −4.5 mmol/L (SD, 4.9) and the average lactate was 3.5 mmol/L (SD, 2.9). The sensitivity of a BE less than −4 mmol/L in predicting elevated lactate greater than 3 mmol/L was 91.1% (95% confidence interval, 85.5%-96.6%) and the specificity was 88.6% (95% confidence interval, 83.0%-94.2%). The area under the curve was 0.95.

Conclusion.—Base excess is an accurate marker for the prediction of elevated lactate in the ED. The measurement of BE, obtained in a few minutes in the ED, provides a secure and quick method, similar to the electrocardiogram at triage for patients with chest pain, to determine the patients with sepsis who need an early aggressive resuscitation (Fig 1).

▶ The implementation of the Surviving Sepsis Campaign (SSC) guidelines through the use of sepsis bundles has been associated in with improved patient outcomes. An essential concept pushed forward by the SSC is the early identification of patients at risk for sepsis-induced hypoperfusion and the implementation of early goal-directed therapy for hemodynamic support. Among the key elements of the sepsis resuscitation bundle is the measurement of serum lactate as soon as a diagnosis of sepsis is considered. Increased lactate in patients with severe sepsis is strongly associated with increased risk of death. Increased lactate (usually >4 mmol/L) has been used as a trigger for aggressive early goal-directed hemodynamic protocols. Considering these points, it becomes important for patients presenting to the emergency department (ED) with suspected infections to have a serum lactate checked. Elevated serum lactates could improve early identification of high-risk patients with sepsis and accelerate the implementation of appropriate aggressive therapeutic strategies. A potential downside to the widespread implementation of this element of the sepsis bundles may relate to potential difficulties in obtaining serum lactates in the emergency department. Although many EDs in the United States have

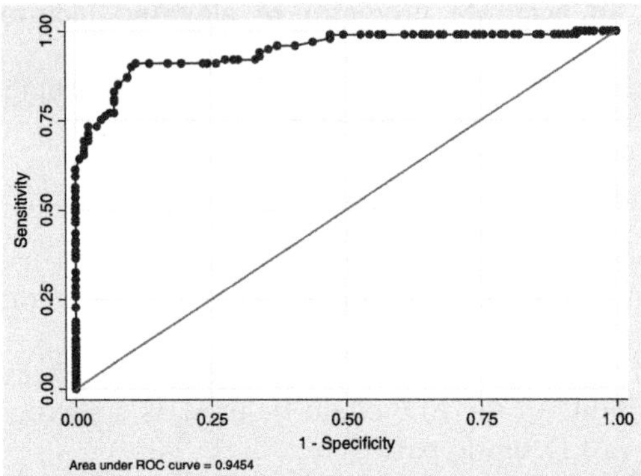

FIGURE 1.—The ROC curve for BE less than −4 mmol/L as a predictor of lactate greater than 3 mmol/L. (Reprinted from Montassier E, Batard E, Segard J, et al. Base excess is an accurate predictor of elevated lactate in ED septic patients. *Am J Emerg Med.* 2012;30:184-187, with permission from Elsevier.)

this capability, there are still multiple EDs that have limitations in quickly obtaining serum lactates. With this premise in mind, Montassier and collaborators explored the potential value of base excess (BE) in identifying patients with sepsis and an elevated lactate. They argued that BE is readily available throughout most EDs. The authors defined a clinically significant lactate to be >3.5 mmol/L and BE <−4 mmol/L. The authors reported that a BE <−4 mmol/L performed extremely well in predicting a lactate >3.5 mmol/L (sensitivity 95% and specificity 88.6%). A BE of <−4 had an excellent receiver operating curve for predicting a lactate >3.5 mmol/L (Fig 1). The results of this study suggest that BE could be used to predict elevated lactates in patients with sepsis and could be a helpful tool in triage decisions and risk stratification. However, based on the larger body of literature supporting the use of lactate in sepsis, BE should not replace lactate but more likely complement or be used as an alternative when measuring lactate is not possible.

S. L. Zanotti-Cavazzoni, MD

Initial fluid resuscitation of patients with septic shock in the intensive care unit

Carlsen S, for the East Danish Septic Shock Cohort Investigators (Copenhagen Univ Hosp, Denmark)

Acta Anaesthesiol Scand 55:394-400, 2011

Background.—Fluid is the mainstay of resuscitation of patients with septic shock, but the optimal composition and volume are unknown. Our aim was to evaluate the current initial fluid resuscitation practice in patients with septic shock in the intensive care unit (ICU) and patient characteristics and outcome associated with fluid volume.

Methods.—This was a prospective, cohort study of all patients with septic shock ($n = 132$) admitted in six ICUs during a 3-month period. Patients were divided into two groups according to the overall median volume of resuscitation fluid administered during the first 24 h after the diagnosis. Baseline characteristics, other treatments, monitoring and outcome were compared between the groups.

Results.—The mean volume of resuscitation fluid was 4.9 l (median 4.0 l and SD 3.5). Patients in the higher volume group received more crystalloids (3.7 vs. 1.2 l, $P < 0.0001$), colloids (1.8 vs. 0.9 l, $P < 0.0001$), blood products (1.8 vs. 0.6 l, $P = 0.0004$), a higher maximum vasopressor dose (0.37 vs. 0.21 µg/kg/min, $P < 0.0001$) and had a higher initial plasma concentration of lactate (4.0 vs. 3.0 mM, $P = 0.009$) compared with the lower volume group. Simplified acute physiology score II in the lower and higher dose group were 52 and 58 ($P = 0.07$). There were no differences in 30-, 90- or 365-day mortality between the two fluid volume groups.

Conclusion.—In the ICU, patients with septic shock were resuscitated with a combination of crystalloids, colloids and blood products. Although the more severely shocked patients received higher volumes of crystalloids, colloids and blood products, mortality did not differ between the groups.

▶ Sepsis is characterized by inflammation-induced endothelial dysfunction leading to vascular leakage and vasodilatation, ultimately resulting in hypovolemia, organ hypoperfusion, and septic shock. Inadequately treated shock may lead to progressive multiple organ failure and high mortality. Current guidelines emphasize the importance of early aggressive hemodynamic support in patients with septic shock. Hemodynamic support in septic shock is based on resuscitation with fluids (crystalloids or colloids) and then, if needed, vasopressors, inotropes, or blood transfusion to optimize cardiac preload and organ perfusion.

In this observational prospective, cohort study, the authors evaluate the initial fluid resuscitation practice in patients with septic shock admitted to Danish critical care units. This was a multicenter study involving 3 university hospital intensive care units (ICUs) and 3 regional hospital ICUs. It utilized a well-defined definition of septic shock and follow-up through a national patient registry. The data obtained are representative of the current care of septic patients in Danish ICUs. This study found a direct linear correlation with administration of higher fluid resuscitation with a higher lactate on presentation, higher doses of vasopressors, and more frequent invasive hemodynamic monitoring. However, there was no difference in mortality at 30 days, 90 days, and 365 days between patients that had higher (> 4 L) or lower (< 4 L) fluid resuscitation in the initial 24 hours. The data for the type and amount of fluids and use of vasopressors, blood in the first 6 hours of septic shock, were not included for analysis because of poor documentation in the emergency department or general wards. Patients could have received more fluids in those first 6 hours; however, this was not accounted for in the total resuscitation fluid. Moreover, the type of fluids and end points for resuscitation were clinician dependent and not preset for the study.

This study provides a snapshot of current practice patterns in Danish ICUs. It dose not clarify the role of specific types of fluids. This study does highlight the need for larger randomized, controlled trials to evaluate the best fluid regimens in resuscitating patients with septic shock. Furthermore, the true impact of aggressive fluid administration remains unclear. Data suggest that early aggressive fluid administration may help. However, it is still unclear if aggressive fluid administration beyond the early phases of septic shock can be harmful.

M. Mehta, MD
S. L. Zanotti-Cavazzoni, MD

The Epidemiology of Sepsis in General Surgery Patients

Moore LJ, McKinley BA, Turner KL, et al (Methodist Hosp Res Inst/Weill Cornell Med College, Houston, TX; et al)
J Trauma 70:672-680, 2011

Background.—Sepsis is increasing in hospitalized patients. Our purpose is to describe its current epidemiology in a general surgery (GS) intensive care unit (ICU) where patients are routinely screened and aggressively treated for sepsis by an established protocol.

Methods.—Our prospective, Institutional Review Board-approved sepsis research database was queried for demographics, biomarkers reflecting organ dysfunction, and mortality. Patients were grouped as sepsis, severe sepsis, or septic shock using refined consensus criteria. Data are compared by analysis of variance, Student's t test, and χ^2 test ($p < 0.05$ significant).

Results.—During 24 months ending September 2009, 231 patients (aged 59 years ± 3 years; 43% men) were treated for sepsis. The abdomen was the source of infection in 69% of patients. Several baseline biomarkers of organ dysfunction (BOD) correlated with sepsis severity including lactate, creatinine, international normalized ratio, platelet count, and D-dimer. Direct correlation with mortality was noted with particular baseline BODs including beta natriuretic peptide, international normalized ratio, platelet count, aspartate transaminase, alanine aminotransferase, and total bilirubin. Most patients present with severe sepsis (56%) or septic shock (26%) each with increasing multiple BODs. Septic shock has prohibitive mortality rate (36%), and those who survive septic shock have prolonged ICU stays.

Conclusion.—In general surgery ICU patients, sepsis is predominantly caused by intra-abdominal infection. Multiple BODs are present in severe sepsis and septic shock but are notably advanced in septic shock. Despite aggressive sepsis screening and treatment, septic shock remains a morbid condition.

► Sepsis in surgical patients may differ from that of nonsurgical patients because of the modulation of immune functions and other significant alterations in physiology resulting from surgery itself. These populations, however, are seldom assessed separately, and the impact of sepsis in surgical patients is underappreciated. Recent National Surgical Quality Improvement Program data have shown that the incidence of sepsis and septic shock exceed pulmonary embolism and myocardial infarction 10-fold. Additionally, the development of septic shock is associated with a 30% mortality rate in elective surgical patients and a 39% mortality rate in emergent surgical patients.

In this retrospective analysis, the authors evaluated 4154 patients admitted to a general surgery intensive care unit setting during a 24-month period ending in September 2009. A total of 231 (5.1%) patients in the study population were treated for sepsis. The abdomen was the predominant source of infection (63%) followed by pulmonary/thoracic (17%), and wound/soft tissue (10%) (Table 3 in the original article). Biomarkers of organ dysfunction were also correlated with sepsis severity and mortality. Beta natriuretic peptide, international normalized ratio, platelet count, aspartate transaminase (AST), alanine transferase (ALT), and total bilirubin directly correlated with mortality.

Sepsis in the surgical patient presents unique challenges as surgical infections profound enough to trigger sepsis often require reoperation. The sequelae of sepsis also present increased risks in the surgical patient during the perioperative period: disorders of coagulopathy and bleeding, secondary infection, hypotension, and frequent changes in venue and transportation risk. Despite these challenges, the authors of this study had an overall hospital mortality rate of 18%, which is significantly lower than the quoted mortality rates from other studies. They cite their utilization of mandatory sepsis screening as well as the use of a computerized clinical decision support application to implement evidence-based treatment guidelines as the reason for their decreased mortality rates. Surgical sepsis remains a morbid condition that requires diligent sepsis screening and early identification of pertinent patient risk factors.

R. Perez, MD
S. L. Zanotti-Cavazzoni, MD

Incident Stroke and Mortality Associated With New-Onset Atrial Fibrillation in Patients Hospitalized With Severe Sepsis

Walkey AJ, Wiener RS, Ghobrial JM, et al (Boston Univ School of Medicine, MA; Univ of Washington School of Medicine, Seattle; et al)
JAMA 306:2248-2255, 2011

Context.—New-onset atrial fibrillation (AF) has been reported in 6% to 20% of patients with severe sepsis. Chronic AF is a known risk factor for stroke and death, but the clinical significance of new-onset AF in the setting of severe sepsis is uncertain.

Objective.—To determine the in-hospital stroke and in-hospital mortality risks associated with new-onset AF in patients with severe sepsis.

Design and Setting.—Retrospective population-based cohort of California State Inpatient Database administrative claims data from nonfederal acute care hospitals for January 1 through December 31, 2007.

Patients.—Data were available for 3 144 787 hospitalized adults. Severe sepsis (n=49 082 [1.56%]) was defined by validated *International Classification of Diseases, Ninth Revision, Clinical Modification* (*ICD-9-CM*) code 995.92. New-onset AF was defined as AF that occurred during the hospital stay, after excluding AF cases present at admission.

Main Outcome Measures.—A priori outcome measures were in-hospital ischemic stroke (*ICD-9-CM* codes 433, 434, or 436) and mortality.

Results.—Patients with severe sepsis were a mean age of 69 (SD, 16) years and 48% were women. New-onset AF occurred in 5.9% of patients with severe sepsis vs 0.65% of patients without severe sepsis (multivariable-adjusted odds ratio [OR], 6.82; 95% CI, 6.54-7.11; *P*<.001). Severe sepsis was present in 14% of all new-onset AF in hospitalized adults. Compared with severe sepsis patients without new-onset AF, patients with new-onset AF during severe sepsis had greater risks of in-hospital stroke (75/2896 [2.6%] vs 306/46 186 [0.6%] strokes; adjusted OR, 2.70; 95% CI, 2.05-3.57; *P*<.001) and inhospital mortality (1629 [56%] vs 18 027 [39%] deaths; adjusted relative risk, 1.07; 95% CI, 1.04-1.11; *P*<.001). Findings were robust across 2 definitions of severe sepsis, multiple methods of addressing confounding, and multiple sensitivity analyses.

Conclusion.—Among patients with severe sepsis, patients with new-onset AF were at increased risk of in-hospital stroke and death compared with patients with no AF and patients with preexisting AF.

▶ Severe sepsis is a major cause of morbidity and mortality in patients admitted to the intensive care unit. The incidence and mortality of severe sepsis increase with age and with the number of associated comorbid diseases. Arrhythmias are common in the intensive care unit; they occur in more than 10% of all patients admitted to the intensive care unit (ICU). Arrhythmias are more likely in older patients and those with severe sepsis. Despite being common, the impact of atrial fibrillation on clinical outcomes in critically ill patients is still not fully defined. Furthermore, there are even fewer data on the relationship and impact of new-onset atrial fibrillation in patients with severe sepsis.

In this study, the authors used claims from a large administrative database in 2007 to address the clinical significance of new-onset atrial fibrillation in the setting of severe sepsis. The authors report that patients with severe sepsis and new-onset atrial fibrillation had increased odds of in-hospital stroke (adjusted odds ratio, 2.70; 95% confidence interval [CI], 2.75–3.57) and increased hospital mortality (adjusted relative risk, 1.70; 95% CI, 1.04–1.11). These findings have significant implications for practicing intensivists caring for severe sepsis patients. However, because many other studies are derived from large administrative databases, the results should be evaluated with some caution. There are challenges inherent to studies that utilize large databases; central to these challenges is the understanding of the potential flaws the data contained in the database itself may possess. To overcome these limitations, the authors performed a series of sensitivity analyses, the results of which supported the primary findings of this study—that new-onset atrial fibrillation in the setting of severe sepsis is associated with an increased risk of stroke and increased mortality. Additional limitations that need further consideration regarding this study are: (1) the inability of the authors to precisely determine the relationship of sepsis, atrial fibrillation, and stroke and (2) the possibility that (due to the nature of the data) the authors were unable to control for all potential confounders. For example, the dose and type of vasopressor used to treat septic shock could predispose to atrial fibrillation. This could also be an indicator of severity of disease and is associated by itself with a high risk of death. This is specifically relevant to septic shock patients who are treated with dopamine, as recent studies have found that the incidence of arrhythmias is much higher with dopamine than with other vasopressors such as norepinephrine.

The limitations notwithstanding, the findings of this study are still very relevant, and this area should be investigated further. If additional studies support the findings of this study, that new-onset atrial fibrillation in the setting of severe sepsis is associated with an increased risk of stroke and increased mortality, it would seem logical for the next step to be the critical evaluation of potential therapies to best prevent and treat new-onset atrial fibrillation in patients with severe sepsis and septic shock.

S. L. Zanotti-Cavazzoni, MD

Nursing considerations to complement the Surviving Sepsis Campaign guidelines

Aitken LM, Williams G, Harvey M, et al (Griffith Univ, Nathan, Queensland, Australia; Gold Coast Health Services District, Queensland; Consultants in Critical Care, Glenbrook, NV; et al)

Crit Care Med 39:1800-1818, 2011

Objectives.—To provide a series of recommendations based on the best available evidence to guide clinicians providing nursing care to patients with severe sepsis.

Design.—Modified Delphi method involving international experts and key individuals in subgroup work and electronic-based discussion among the entire group to achieve consensus.

Methods.—We used the Surviving Sepsis Campaign guidelines as a framework to inform the structure and content of these guidelines. We used the Grades of Recommendation, Assessment, Development, and Evaluation (GRADE) system to rate the quality of evidence from high (A) to very low (D) and to determine the strength of recommendations, with grade 1 indicating clear benefit in the septic population and grade 2 indicating less confidence in the benefits in the septic population. In areas without complete agreement between all authors, a process of electronic discussion of all evidence was undertaken until consensus was reached. This process was conducted independently of any funding.

Results.—Sixty-three recommendations relating to the nursing care of severe sepsis patients are made. Prevention recommendations relate to education, accountability, surveillance of nosocomial infections, hand hygiene, and prevention of respiratory, central line-related, surgical site, and urinary tract infections, whereas infection management recommendations related to both control of the infection source and transmission-based precautions. Recommendations related to initial resuscitation include improved recognition of the deteriorating patient, diagnosis of severe sepsis, seeking further assistance, and initiating early resuscitation measures. Important elements of hemodynamic support relate to improving both tissue oxygenation and macrocirculation. Recommendations related to supportive nursing care incorporate aspects of nutrition, mouth and eye care, and pressure ulcer prevention and management. Pediatric recommendations relate to the use of antibiotics, steroids, vasopressors and inotropes, fluid resuscitation, sedation and analgesia, and the role of therapeutic end points.

Conclusion.—Consensus was reached regarding many aspects of nursing care of the severe sepsis patient. Despite this, there is an urgent need for further evidence to better inform this area of critical care.

▶ Severe sepsis and septic shock are a major cause of morbidity and mortality. With increasing incidence, severe sepsis continues to be an important health care problem worldwide. Significant improvements in the care of patients afflicted with this complex disease have materialized with the implementation of the Surviving Sepsis Campaign guidelines and sepsis bundles. These evidence-based guidelines and quality assurance programs have guided physicians caring for severe sepsis patients. However, the care of critically ill patients with severe sepsis in the intensive care unit requires a true multidisciplinary team approach to be successful. In that respect, guidelines and research specifically aimed at interventions related to nursing care are lacking.

In this important and opportune article, a group of thought leaders from the field of critical care nursing provide a series of recommendations based on best available evidence to guide nursing care of patients with severe sepsis. The authors used the Surviving Sepsis Campaign guidelines as a framework to inform the structure and content of their document. Available evidence was reviewed and systematically appraised using the GRADE system. Based on the strength of the available evidence, sixty-three recommendations relating to the nursing care of patients with severe sepsis were made. Consensus was reached on many aspects of nursing care in severe sepsis. However, it was also evident from this document that many areas are lacking in data, and future research in sepsis should also target various aspects of nursing care.

This is an extremely relevant article. It is always important to remind physicians that care in the intensive care unit is a team effort. Medical knowledge and therapies do not translate to patients at the bedside based solely on the efforts of physicians. Ultimately, the level of nursing care in the intensive care unit is often the main difference maker in our patients. This document should be read by all intensivists and shared with nursing staff in their intensive care units.

S. L. Zanotti-Cavazzoni, MD

Nationwide Trends of Severe Sepsis in the 21st Century (2000-2007)

Kumar G, from the Milwaukee Initiative in Critical Care Outcomes Research (MICCOR) Group of Investigators (Med College of Wisconsin, Milwaukee; et al)

Chest 140:1223-1231, 2011

Background.—Severe sepsis is common and often fatal. The expanding armamentarium of evidence-based therapies has improved the outcomes of persons with this disease. However, the existing national estimates of the frequency and outcomes of severe sepsis were made before many of the recent therapeutic advances. Therefore, it is important to study the outcomes of this disease in an aging US population with rising comorbidities.

Methods.—We used the Healthcare Costs and Utilization Project's Nationwide Inpatient Sample (NIS) to estimate the frequency and outcomes of severe sepsis hospitalizations between 2000 and 2007. We identified hospitalizations for severe sepsis using *International Classification of Diseases, Ninth Revision, Clinical Modification* codes indicating the presence of sepsis and organ system failure. Using weights from NIS, we estimated the number of hospitalizations for severe sepsis in each year. We combined these with census data to determine the number of severe sepsis hospitalizations per 100,000 persons. We used discharge status to identify in-hospital mortality and compared mortality rates in 2000 with those in 2007 after adjusting for demographics, number of organ systems failing, and presence of comorbid conditions.

Results.—The number of severe sepsis hospitalizations per 100,000 persons increased from 143 in 2000 to 343 in 2007. The mean number of organ system failures during admission increased from 1.6 to 1.9 ($P < .001$). The mean length of hospital stay decreased from 17.3 to 14.9 days. The mortality rate decreased from 39% to 27%. However, more admissions ended with discharge to a long-term care facility in 2007 than in 2000 (35% vs 27%, $P < .001$).

Conclusions.—An increasing number of admissions for severe sepsis combined with declining mortality rates contribute to more individuals surviving to hospital discharge. Importantly, this leads to more survivors being discharged to skilled nursing facilities and home with in-home care. Increased attention to this phenomenon is warranted (Fig 1).

▶ Sepsis is a common and fatal disease. Two landmark studies published in early 2000 have shaped our knowledge regarding the epidemiology of severe sepsis.[1,2] Angus et al[1] published a landmark study using discharge databases from 7 states. This study calculated the incidence of severe sepsis in the United States as 750,000 cases per year. Furthermore, this study projected an increase in the incidence of sepsis of 1.5% annually, mostly because of a growing proportion of the population in the 65-year-and-older age group. Martin et al[2] published a subsequent report that showed increasing frequencies of sepsis over the last 20 years and an estimated incidence for severe sepsis of 80.8 cases per 100 000 in 2000. Since the publication of these seminal studies, treatment strategies for severe

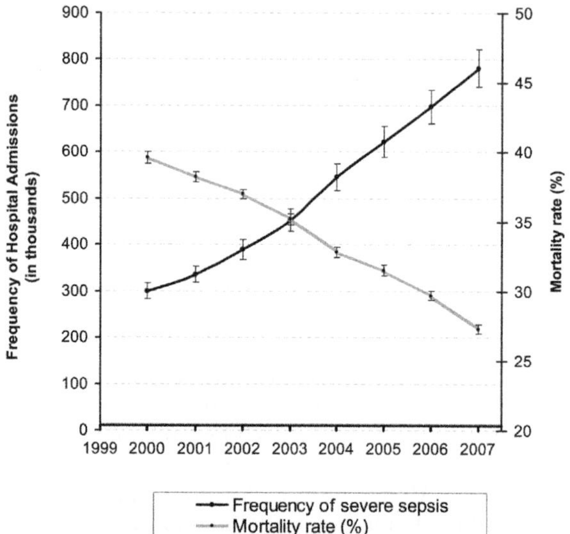

FIGURE 1.—Frequency of admission and mortality rates due to severe sepsis, 2000-2007. Bars represent SEM. (Reprinted from Kumar G, from the Milwaukee Initiative in Critical Care Outcomes Research (MICCOR) Group of Investigators. Nationwide trends of severe sepsis in the 21st century (2000-2007). *Chest.* 2011;140:1223-1231, with permission from American College of Chest Physicians.)

sepsis and septic shock have evolved. Understanding how the epidemiology of this disease evolves over time remains a critical piece in our efforts to provide the best care for critically ill patients with sepsis.

In this study, the authors reexamine this important topic. They used the Healthcare Costs and Utilization Project's Nationwide Inpatient Sample (NIS) to estimate trends in the frequency and outcomes of hospitalizations for severe sepsis in the United States between 2000 and 2007. The principal finding of this study was that the incidence of sepsis increased over this time period and this was associated with a decrease in mortality (Fig 1). The frequency of hospitalizations for severe sepsis increased from 143 per 100 000 US adults in 2000 to 343 per 100 000 in 2007. This represents an annual increase of approximately 16.5%, an increase that is significantly higher than previous projections. In-hospital mortality for severe sepsis decreased from 39.6% in 2000 to 27.3% in 2007. During this time period, mortality for septic shock also decreased by more than 10%. This is remarkable if one considers that during this time, the number of organ failures increased. With regard to organ failures, a shift in the most frequent organ failure from respiratory to renal occurred during this time period. Another important outcome measure that improved was length of hospital stay (this includes survivors and nonsurvivors). Finally, this study also showed an increase in the number of patients being discharged to skilled nursing facilities (SNFs). This finding has important health care implications because it probably represents a rapidly increasing need for SNF beds in the future. This is an extremely valuable study that builds on previous work and provides clinicians an updated snapshot of severe sepsis.

The increasing frequency is concerning because it will likely continue to represent a significant burden to our ability to provide critical care. However, the decrease in mortality is reassuring because it correlates with new strategies in treating this disease earlier and more aggressively.

S. L. Zanotti-Cavazzoni, MD

References

1. Angus DC, Linde-Zwirble WT, Lidicker J, Clermont G, Carcillo J, Pinsky MR. Epidemiology of severe sepsis in the United States: analysis of incidence, outcome, and associated costs of care. *Crit Care Med.* 2001;29:1303-1310.
2. Martin GS, Mannino DM, Eaton S, Moss M. The epidemiology of sepsis in the United States from 1979 through 2000. *N Engl J Med.* 2003;348:1546-1554.

Successful Treatment with Drotrecogin alfa (activated) in a Pregnant Patient with Severe Sepsis

Eppert HD, Goddard KB, King CL (Blount Memorial Hosp, Maryville, TN; Grady Health System, Atlanta, GA)

Pharmacotherapy 31:50e-55e, 2011

Sepsis remains one of the leading causes of mortality during pregnancy. Because of the inherent limitations of conducting scientific investigations during pregnancy, a great deal of clinical decision making is based on observational reports, an understanding of the physiologic changes of pregnancy, and consideration for risk to the fetus. We describe a 20-year-old pregnant woman at 20 weeks' gestation who was admitted to an obstetric ward for dehydration and a urinary tract infection. Approximately 36 hours later, the patient's clinical status deteriorated, with the development of mental status changes, acute respiratory failure, and renal failure. Drotrecogin alfa (activated) was started, as the patient's Acute Physiology and Chronic Health Evaluation II score was 27 (> 25 is the typical score required for drotrecogin alfa [activated] therapy); within 48 hours the patient's clinical status dramatically improved. The patient completed 96 uninterrupted hours of therapy and was subsequently discharged after a 15-day hospitalization, with no apparent sequelae. Approximately 17 weeks later, the patient gave birth to a 3.42-kg female infant with no congenital abnormalities. To our knowledge, this represents the second case report to describe the use of drotrecogin alfa (activated) along with the status of the mother and fetus both after completion of therapy and after subsequent delivery. Because of the threat of mortality from sepsis during pregnancy, combined with the inherent limitations associated with clinical research during pregnancy, further reports and investigation into the treatment of sepsis in the pregnant patient are warranted.

▶ Sepsis remains an important cause of morbidity and mortality in pregnancy. Because of the inherent limitation of conducting scientific research during pregnancy, a great deal of clinical decision making is based on case reports, understanding of the physiological changes associated with pregnancy, and consideration of risk to the fetus. Drotrecogin alpha (activated) was a novel therapy proposed for the treatment of severe sepsis and septic shock based on the results of one seminal study. In this study, no pregnant patients were included, so the experience with the use of this drug during pregnancy was very limited. There have been 2 case reports discussing the use of drotrecogin alpha (activated) in pregnant patients with severe sepsis. The current report describes a 20-year-old pregnant woman at 20 weeks' gestation with severe sepsis caused by a urinary tract infection. This patient completed 96 uninterrupted hours of therapy with drotrecogin alpha (activated) and was discharged home in good health. The second case report describes a pregnant patient at 26 weeks' gestation with a diagnosis of pneumonia. Despite aggressive treatment, she clinically deteriorated, and a decision to start drotrecogin alpha (activated) was made. Again, in this case, the patient improved with therapy and eventually delivered at 28 weeks. In both reports there was no evidence of patient or neonate drug-related complications. With the recent withdrawal of drotrecogin alpha (activated) from the market by the manufacturer, these reports mostly hold only historical interest. However, they illustrate a common problem in caring for pregnant critically ill patients. With a paucity of studies in this population, the clinician often needs to rely on case reports and very individualized risk/benefit analysis to support clinical decision making.

S. L. Zanotti-Cavazzoni, MD

Short-term effects of terlipressin bolus infusion on sublingual microcirculatory blood flow during septic shock

Morelli A, Donati A, Ertmer C, et al (Univ of Rome, Italy; Marche Polytechnique Univ, Ancona, Italy; Univ Hosp of Muenster, Münster, Germany)
Intensive Care Med 37:963-969, 2011

Purpose.—Terlipressin bolus infusion may contribute to overshooting increases in systemic vascular resistance with concomitant reductions in systemic blood flow and oxygen delivery. Whether these effects negatively impact on microcirculatory perfusion is still not known. The objective of the present study was, therefore, to elucidate the effects of a single terlipressin bolus dose of 0.5 mg on microcirculatory perfusion in patients with catecholamine-dependent septic shock.

Methods.—This prospective clinical cohort study was performed in a multidisciplinary intensive care unit at a university hospital. We enrolled 20 patients suffering from catecholamine-dependent septic shock. After restoring normovolaemia, norepinephrine (NE) was titrated to maintain mean arterial pressure (MAP) between 65 and 75 mmHg. Thereafter, all patients received a bolus infusion of 0.5 mg terlipressin, and NE was adjusted to maintain MAP between the threshold values. Sublingual microcirculatory blood flow of small vessels was assessed by sidestream dark-field imaging. All measurements, including data from right heart catheterization and NE requirements, were obtained at baseline and 6 h after terlipressin administration.

Results.—Terlipressin stabilized haemodynamics and, at the same time, decreased NE requirements (0.42 ± 0.67 vs. 0.74 ± 0.73 μg/kg per minute, $p < 0.05$). Whereas the pH and arterial lactate concentrations remained unchanged, microcirculatory flow index of small vessels had increased at the end of the 6-h study period (2.6 ± 0.6 vs. 2.0 ± 0.5 units, $p < 0.05$).

Conclusion.—In fluid-resuscitated patients with septic shock (with a MAP between 65 and 75 mmHg), a bolus infusion of 0.5 mg terlipressin was effective in reducing NE requirements without worsening microcirculatory blood flow. Randomized clinical trials are now warranted to verify these preliminary results.

▶ The pathogenesis of septic shock is complex and poorly understood, and significant morbidity and mortality occurs despite achieving target blood pressure, central venous pressure (CVP), and measured venous oxygen saturation as per the current Surviving Sepsis guidelines.[1] New technologies (Orthogonal Polarizing Spectrum and side stream dark-field [SDF] imaging) emerged in the past decade as tools for imaging the microcirculation, which is arguably one of the central pieces to the pathophysiological abnormalities in septic shock. Many have proposed that nitric oxide (NO) overproduction and/or vasopressin deficiency play a chief role in the unresponsiveness of the vasculature to vasoconstrictors, resulting in vasodilatory shock. Vasopressin analogs (VA)—namely, vasopressin and terlipressin—act on V1 and V2 receptors to cause dose-dependent vasoconstriction in myocardial, splanchnic, digital, and skin circulation. Terlipressin, a long-acting V1 agonist, is currently used in Europe in managing patients with catecholamine refractory septic shock. It is a pro-drug and capable of releasing sustained amount of metabolite lysine vasopressin. Clinically it is given as an intermittent infusion bolus of dose ranging from 0.5 to 2 mg.

Morelli et al looked at short-term effects of terlipressin bolus on microcirculatory blood flow in patients with septic shock using SDF technology. A bolus of 0.5 mg of terlipressin was given to 20 patients who fulfilled international criteria for septic shock and required norepinephrine (NE) to keep mean arterial pressure (MAP) between 65 and 75 mm Hg despite adequate volume resuscitation (CVP 8–12, pulmonary artery occlusion pressure [PAOP] 12–15). Sublingual microcirculation was assessed using Microscan (an SDF imaging device) at 0 hours and 6 hours after infusion of terlipressin. All images were analyzed and scored by an automated software and an independent investigator who was not aware of study protocol. Microcirculation was scored based on index of vascular density (total and perfused), 2 assessments of capillary perfusion (proportion of perfused vessels [PPV] and microcirculatory flow index), and the heterogeneity index, based on an international round table consensus. The primary endpoint of the study was change in microcirculatory flow index (MFI) of small vessels in response to terlipressin administration.

Following terlipressin bolus administration, NE requirements in patients were significantly lower at 6 hours. Other clinical and lab parameters remained unchanged (heart rate, MAP, POAP, CVP, lactate, mixed venous oxygen saturation, oxygenation) except for a lower arterial carbon dioxide tension. There was a significant change in the microcirculatory variables. MFI of small vessels, total vessel density, perfused vessel density, and PPVs significantly increased. Conversely, the heterogeneity index significantly decreased (all $P < .05$). In this study, a bolus of 0.5-mg infused terlipressin showed a reduction in NE requirements in adequately resuscitated patients with septic shock. However, this reduction in NE requirement did not come at a cost of impaired microcirculatory flow, as evidenced by increased MFI of small vessels and decreased heterogeneity index at the level of microcirculation, as well as no change in arterial pH or lactate level at end of study.

Morelli et al's study has certain limitations. It had an open-label design without a control group. Thus, it cannot be concluded that the observed effects were from terlipressin or improvement of patients over time. The study population was small in number, and patients were enrolled in the study at different times during the evolution of septic shock. Therefore, varying severities in cardiovascular dysfunction among study patients would have affected results. Furthermore, SDF imaging provides a semiquantitative assessment of microcirculatory variables and is subject to interobserver bias and technical expertise. Lastly, microcirculation of sublingual mucosa may not be representative of circulation in other areas of the body. Despite these limitations, this study showed that in fluid-resuscitated patients with septic shock, a bolus dose of 0.5 mg terlipressin is effective in reducing NE requirements, and this occurs without worsening microcirculatory blood flow. Additional studies are needed to better understand the impact of different vasopressors in septic shock and the microcirculation.

U. Patel, MD
S. L. Zanotti-Cavazzoni, MD

Reference

1. Dellinger RP, Levy MM, Carlet JM, et al. Surviving sepsis campaign: international guidelines for management of severe sepsis and septic shock: 2008. *Intensive Care Med.* 2008;34:17-60.

Prolonged methylene blue infusion in refractory septic shock: a case report

Dumbarton TC, Minor S, Yeung CK, et al (Dalhousie Univ, Halifax, Nova Scotia, Canada)

Can J Anesth 58:401-405, 2011

Purpose.—Methylene blue (MB) has been advocated for the treatment of refractory hemodynamic instability in patients with septic shock. However, the use of MB infusions in septic shock is not considered standard treatment, and the available literature describes infusions of short duration, typically less than six hours.

Clinical Features.—We report a case of septic shock in a 67-yr-old male who required maximal vasopressor support with norepinephrine, epinephrine, and vasopressin. Despite standard protocols for the treatment of septic shock, the patient's hemodynamic status was refractory 80 hr post admission. However, initiation of a MB infusion resulted in the rapid restoration of hemodynamic stability and a subsequent decrease in vasopressor requirements. Multiple attempts to discontinue the MB infusion resulted in immediate and repeated increases in vasopressor requirements, necessitating a continuous infusion with a slow taper of MB for 120 hr. Ultimately, the patient survived the illness and was discharged home. We observed no adverse events that could be attributed to the use of MB.

Conclusion.—In our patient, the use of MB resulted in hemodynamic stability unattained with standard vasopressor support. Further research is warranted on the use of MB in patients with septic shock.

▶ Current treatment for patients with septic shock is based on early antibiotic administration and aggressive hemodynamic support. Hemodynamic support includes the use of fluids and, if needed, vasopressors to maintain a mean arterial pressure > 65 mm Hg. Based on current guidelines, norepinephrine constitutes the first-line vasopressor therapy for patients with septic shock. Other options that are utilized commonly in patients not responding to norepinephrine include epinephrine, dopamine, phenylephrine, and noncatecholamines, such as vasopressin. There are a few reports of the use of methylamine blue (MB) in patients with refractory septic shock. However, little is known about the clinical utility and optimal dosing/duration for MB in septic shock. The few published reports describe relatively short infusion times, usually less than 6 hours. In this case report, the authors describe a patient with septic shock who, despite maximum vasopressor support with norepinephrine, epinephrine, and vasopressin, remained hypotensive. The patient was started on an infusion of MB, which was associated with restoration of hemodynamic stability and the subsequent decrease of vasopressin requirements. The case reports that multiple attempts to discontinue the MB infusion resulted in hemodynamic instability and repeat increases of vasopressor requirements. This resulted in a prolonged MB total infusion time (approximately 120 hours). This patient ultimately survived his septic shock episode and was discharged home. The authors did not observe any adverse events attributable to the MB despite the prolonged infusion time. A case report such as this one does not constitute a high level of evidence and should not support the widespread of use of therapy such as MB for septic shock. However, this case report does suggest that in selected cases of refractory septic shock, the clinician may consider starting an MB infusion. Perhaps, this case even more strongly supports the need for trials to determine the proper role of MB in the treatment of sepsis-induced vasodilatory shock.

S. L. Zanotti-Cavazzoni, MD

Corticosteroid therapy for patients in septic shock: Some progress in a difficult decision

Sprung CL, Brezis M, Goodman S, et al (Hadassah Hebrew Univ Med Ctr, Jerusalem, Israel)

Crit Care Med 39:571-574, 2011

Objectives.—Reversible adrenal insufficiency has been frequently diagnosed in critically ill patients with sepsis who have either low basal cortisol levels or low cortisol responses to adrenocorticotrophic hormone (ACTH) stimulation. It is generally accepted that a phenomenon called "endotoxin tolerance" contributes to immunosuppression during sepsis. The present study was to investigate whether endotoxin tolerance occurs in the adrenal gland, leading to hyporesponsiveness of adrenal gland during sepsis.

Design.—Controlled laboratory experiment.

Setting.—University research laboratory.

Subjects.—Sprague-Dawley male rats 200–250 g, and primary isolated adrenal fasciculata-reticularis cells.

Interventions.—Rats received intra-arterial injection of purified lipopolysaccharide (LPS, 0.5 mg/kg) through indwelling femoral arterial catheters, and 24 h later the adrenocortical sensitivity to exogenous ACTH (10 ng/kg) was detected. Primary F/R cells were pretreated with LPS at 0.1–100 ng/mL or with ACTH at 0.01–10 ng/mL, and then challenged, in fresh media, with 1 μg/mL LPS or 10 ng/mL ACTH.

Measurements and Main Results.—Toll-like receptor 4 were expressed in adrenal gland and primary fasciculata-reticularis cells. Plasma corticosterone response to ACTH was decreased in rats receiving preinjection of LPS. LPS pretreatment caused a significant decrease in corticosterone production in response to subsequent ACTH and LPS stimulation in primary fasciculata-reticularis cells. LPS pretreatment inhibited ACTH- and LPS-induced expression of steroid metabolizing enzymes. LPS significantly decreased toll-like receptor 4 and ACTH receptor expression.

Conclusions.—Pre-exposure to LPS resulted in hyporesponsiveness to ACTH stimulation in rats. *In vitro*, LPS pretreatment impaired corticosterone production of F/R cells in response to ACTH and LPS, which was associated with decreased expression of synthetic enzymes required for corticosterone production. Our results indicate that endotoxin tolerance of adrenal gland is one of mechanisms for adrenocortical insufficiency during sepsis.

▶ The use of corticosteroids in patients with severe sepsis and septic shock has been a topic of debate for several decades. Initial use of corticosteroids at high doses to modulate the inflammatory response of sepsis was stopped after several randomized trials showed no benefit and even potential harms. After some time, the concept of relative adrenal insufficiency in sepsis emerged. An initial study suggested that corticosteroids at lower physiologic doses for 7 days could improve outcomes in patients with relative adrenal insufficiency. However, a subsequent larger, multicenter study (the CORTICUS study) did not show improved survival with corticosteroids. Furthermore, more recent data have challenged the validity of testing the adrenal axis in patients with septic shock.

In this special article, the authors evaluate in a rat model the effects of endotoxin on adrenal function. The authors report that preexposure to endotoxin resulted in hyporesponsiveness to adrenocorticotrophic hormone stimulation. They also reported that in vitro, pretreatment with endotoxin decreased cortisol production. The results of this study support endotoxin tolerance of the adrenal gland as one potential mechanism for adrenal dysfunction in sepsis. The article also includes an extensive discussion of the most relevant clinical trials and meta-analyses on this topic. Ultimately, the authors make some recommendations based on their evaluation of the available data and expertise.

M. Charrion, MD
S. L. Zanotti-Cavazzoni, MD

Impact of previous antibiotic therapy on outcome of Gram-negative severe sepsis

Johnson MT, Reichley R, Hoppe-Bauer J, et al (UIC-College of Pharmacy, Chicago, IL; BJC Healthcare, St Louis, MO; Barnes-Jewish Hosp, St Louis, MO; et al)

Crit Care Med 39:1859-1865, 2011

Objective.—To determine whether exposure to antimicrobial agents in the previous 90 days resulted in decreased bacterial susceptibility and increased hospital mortality in patients with severe sepsis or septic shock attributed to Gram-negative bacteremia.

Design.—A retrospective cohort study of hospitalized patients (January 2002 to December 2007).

Setting.—Barnes-Jewish Hospital, a 1200-bed urban teaching hospital.

Patients.—Seven hundred fifty-four consecutive patients with Gram-negative bacteremia complicated by severe sepsis or septic shock.

Interventions.—Data abstraction from computerized medical records.

Measurements and Main Results.—*Escherichia coli* (30.8%), *Klebsiella pneumoniae* (23.2%), and *Pseudomonas aeruginosa* (17.6%) were the most common isolates from blood cultures. Three hundred ten patients (41.1%) had recent antibiotic exposure. Cefepime was the most common agent with previous exposure (50.0%) followed by ciprofloxacin (32.6%) and imipenem or meropenem (28.7%). Patients with prior antibiotic exposure had significantly higher rates of resistance to cefepime (29.0% vs. 7.0%), piperacillin/tazobactam (31.9% vs. 11.5%), carbapenems (20.0% vs. 2.5%), ciprofloxacin (39.7% vs. 17.6%), and gentamicin (26.1% vs. 7.9%) ($p < .001$ for all comparisons). Patients with recent antibiotic exposure had greater inappropriate initial antimicrobial therapy (45.4% vs. 21.2%; $p < .001$) and hospital mortality (51.3% vs. 34.0%; $p < .001$) compared with patients without recent antibiotic exposure. Multivariate logistic regression analysis demonstrated that recent antibiotic exposure was independently associated with hospital mortality (adjusted odds ratio, 1.70; 95% confidence interval, 1.41–2.06; $p = .005$). Other variables independently associated with hospital mortality included use of vasopressors, infection resulting from *P. aeruginosa*, inappropriate initial antimicrobial therapy, increasing Acute Physiology and Chronic Health Evaluation II scores, and the number of acquired organ failures.

Conclusions.—Recent antibiotic exposure is associated with increased hospital mortality in Gram-negative bacteremia complicated by severe sepsis or septic shock. Clinicians caring for patients with severe sepsis or septic shock should consider recent antibiotic exposure when formulating empiric antimicrobial regimens for suspected Gram-negative bacterial infection.

▶ Prior antibiotic exposure is often cited as a risk factor for the development of resistant infections. The potential mechanism relates to shifts to colonization with subsequent infection by bacteria resistant to the prior antibiotics. In addition, prior antibiotic therapy has been shown to be associated with inadequate empirical initial antibiotics regimes, which in turn increases mortality in critically ill patients.

In this retrospective cohort study, Johnson et al evaluated the impact of previous antibiotic exposure on outcomes in patients with gram-negative sepsis. The authors found that recent antibiotic exposure was associated with increased hospital mortality in gram-negative bacteremia complicated by severe sepsis or septic shock. This was most likely explained by the significantly higher frequency of resistance to multiple antibiotics found in patients with previous antibiotic exposure. Patients with previous antibiotic exposure also had significantly higher chances of receiving inadequate initial empirical antibiotic therapy.

This study builds on a existing body of literature showing a strong link between previous antibiotic treatment and increased resistant infections with increased morbidity and mortality. This study is particular in describing this phenomenon in patients with gram-negative sepsis. Furthermore, the results of this study should serve as a strong reminder to clinicians with regard to the value of identifying and understanding recent history of previous antibiotic use in patients with severe sepsis and septic shock. A good clinical history could help guide appropriate empiric antibiotics and ultimately have a positive impact on outcomes in this critically ill patient population.

M. Charron, MD
S. L. Zanotti-Cavazzoni, MD

Epidemiology and risk factors of sepsis after multiple trauma: An analysis of 29,829 patients from the Trauma Registry of the German Society for Trauma Surgery

Wafaisade A, Trauma Registry of the German Society for Trauma Surgery (Univ of Witten/Herdecke, Cologne, Germany; et al)

Crit Care Med 39:621-628, 2011

Objectives.—The objectives of this study were 1) to assess potential changes in the incidence and outcome of sepsis after multiple trauma in Germany between 1993 and 2008 and 2) to evaluate independent risk factors for posttraumatic sepsis.

Design.—Retrospective analysis of a nationwide, population-based prospective database, the Trauma Registry of the German Society for Trauma Surgery.

Setting.—A total of 166 voluntarily participating trauma centers (levels I–III).

Patients.—Patients registered in the Trauma Registry of the German Society for Trauma Surgery between 1993 and 2008 with complete data sets who presented with a relevant trauma load (Injury Severity Score of ≥9) and were admitted to an intensive care unit (n = 29,829).

Interventions.—None.

Measurements and Main Results.—Over the 16-yr study period, 10.2% (3,042 of 29,829) of multiply injured patients developed sepsis during their hospital course. Annual data were summarized into four subperiods: 1993–1996, 1997–2000, 2001–2004, and 2005–2008. The incidences of sepsis for the four subperiods were 14.8%, 12.5%, 9.4%, and 9.7% ($p < .0001$), respectively. In-hospital mortality for all trauma patients decreased for the respective subperiods (16.9%, 16.0%, 13.7%, and 11.9%; $p < .0001$). For the subgroup of patients with sepsis, the mortality rates were 16.2%, 21.5%, 22.0%, and 18.2% ($p = .054$), respectively. The following independent risk factors for posttraumatic sepsis were calculated from a multivariate logistic regression analysis: male gender, age, preexisting medical condition, Glasgow Coma Scale Score of ≤8 at scene, Injury Severity Score, Abbreviated Injury Scale$_{\text{THORAX}}$ Score of ≥3, number of injuries, number of red blood cell units transfused, number of operative procedures, and laparotomy.

Conclusions.—The incidence of sepsis decreased significantly over the study period; however, in this decade the incidence remained unchanged. Although overall mortality from multiple trauma has declined significantly since 1993, there has been no significant decrease of mortality in the subgroup of septic trauma patients. Thus, sepsis has remained a challenging complication after trauma during the past 2 decades. Recognition of the identified risk factors may guide early diagnostic workup and help to reduce septic complications after multiple trauma.

▶ Over the past few decades, the mortality from multiple trauma has gradually decreased. However, the incidence of sepsis and its associated mortality in trauma patients has not been well studied. Additionally, no consensus has been reached on independent risk factors for sepsis in trauma patients to guide proper early patient management and reduce septic complications. The authors of this retrospective analysis used the Trauma Registry for the German Society of Trauma Surgery from 1993 to 2008 to identify a study population of 29 829 patients to assess incidence and outcomes of sepsis after multiple trauma in Germany and identify risk factors for posttraumatic sepsis. These patients had severe traumatic injury, defined as Injury Severity Score (ISS) of ≥9, and were admitted to an intensive care unit setting. Annual data were summarized into 4 subperiods to evaluate temporal influences: 1993–1996, 1997–2000, 2001–2004, and 2005–2008.

This analysis represents the largest study on sepsis in severely injured patients to date with a mean ISS of 26 ± 13 and an overall incidence of sepsis totaling 10.2%. The authors identified male gender, age, preexisting medical condition, Glasgow Coma Score of ≤8 at the scene, ISS, AIS_{THORAX} score of ≥3, number of injuries, number of red blood cell units transfused, number of operative procedures, and laparotomy as independent risk factors of the development of sepsis (Table 4 in the original article). Although overall mortality from multiple trauma decreased significantly in this study, there was no decrease in mortality in the subgroup of septic trauma. The authors cite an increase in multiple organ failure (MOF) in the septic subgroup as well as the emergence of fungal pathogens or microbial resistance as possible contributions to the static mortality rates. Interestingly, mortality in sepsis patients increased in each subsequent time interval, but a significant decrease was observed when the 2 most recent subperiods (2001–2004 vs 2005–2008) were compared. This decrease directly coincides with the Surviving Sepsis Campaign and the publication of their evidence-based clinical practice guidelines. Improved adherence to these guidelines and early identification of patients at risk for sepsis are needed to decrease sepsis related mortality in the trauma patient.

R. Perez, MD
S. L. Zanotti-Cavazzoni, MD

Identification of Cardiac Dysfunction in Sepsis with B-Type Natriuretic Peptide

Turner KL, Moore LJ, Todd SR, et al (The Methodist Hosp Res Inst, Houston, TX)

J Am Coll Surg 213:139-147, 2011

Background.—B-type natriuretic peptide (BNP) is secreted in response to myocardial stretch and has been used clinically to assess volume overload and predict death in congestive heart failure. More recently, BNP elevation has been demonstrated with septic shock and is predictive of death. How BNP levels relate to cardiac function in sepsis remains to be established.

Study Design.—Retrospective review of prospectively gathered sepsis database from a surgical ICU in a tertiary academic hospital. Initial BNP levels, patient demographics, baseline central venous pressure levels, and in-hospital mortality were obtained. Transthoracic echocardiography was performed during initial resuscitation per protocol.

Results.—During 24 months ending in September 2009, two hundred and thirty-one patients (59 ± 3 years of age, 43% male) were treated for sepsis. Baseline BNP increased with initial sepsis severity (ie, sepsis vs severe sepsis vs septic shock, by ANOVA; $p < 0.05$) and was higher in those who died vs those who lived (by Fisher's exact test; $p < 0.05$). Of these patients, 153 (66%) had early echocardiography. Low ejection fraction (<50%) was associated with higher BNP (by Fisher's exact test; $p < 0.05$) and patients with low ejection fraction had a higher mortality (39% vs 20%; odds ratio = 3.03). We found no correlation between baseline central venous pressure (12.7 ± 6.10 mmHg) and BNP (526.5 ± 82.10 pg/mL) (by Spearman's ρ, $R_s = .001$) for the entire sepsis population.

Conclusions.—In surgical sepsis patients, BNP increases with sepsis severity and is associated with early systolic dysfunction, which in turn is associated with death. Monitoring BNP in early sepsis to identify occult systolic dysfunction might prompt earlier use of inotropic agents.

▶ This is a retrospective review of a surgical sepsis database. The hypothesis of the authors was that B-type natriuretic peptide (BNP) could be used as a predictor of mortality and early myocardial dysfunction in sepsis patients. In the 231 patients entered into the database, higher baseline levels of BNP did correlate both with sepsis severity and mortality. Sixty-six of the patients had a transthoracic echocardiography within 24 hours of presentation. There was a significant correlation between systolic dysfunction identified on echo and higher BNP levels. Notably, there was no correlation between BNP and the presence of diastolic dysfunction.

Identifying which septic patients have a component of cardiac dysfunction is important for both clinical decision making and prognosis. This article shows once again the potential use of BNP as a marker for mortality in sepsis. In this study, BNP levels correlated with severity as measured by the presence of sepsis, severe sepsis, or septic shock. Another important finding is the correlation with BNP and low ejection fraction. Both systolic and diastolic dysfunction have been observed in patients with sepsis. Use of a biomarker to help identify these patients would potentially be helpful. The results of this article do not support the use of BNP to identify diastolic dysfunction. They do seem to support the use of BNP to identify systolic dysfunction.

There are important limitations to this article and its conclusions. Not knowing the prior ejection fraction of the patients' baseline functional status could profoundly alter the conclusions of the study. Also, not knowing the trend of the BNP during the patients' admission and instead having an isolated BNP level on presentation may limit the conclusions we can make on its association with cardiac dysfunction. The authors acknowledged all of this in their discussion. Furthermore, because of the multiple etiologies for elevated BNP, we are left with the same question as in the use of BNP to identify decompensated heart failure. More specifically, is the cause of the elevated BNP a reflection of cardiac dysfunction? For this reason, the authors reached a conclusion that the main strength of BNP levels in sepsis may be as negative predictors of volume overload. Interestingly, there was no correlation between BNP levels and central venous pressure. This may indicate a problem with using central venous pressure as a measure of intravascular volume status rather than BNP not holding up as a predictor of volume overload.

B. Goodgame, MD
S. L. Zanotti-Cavazzoni, MD

Use of procalcitonin for the detection of sepsis in the critically ill burn patient: A systematic review of the literature

Mann EA, Wood GL, Wade CE (Univ of Texas Health Sciences Ctr, Houston; US Army Inst of Surgical Res, San Antonio, TX)
Burns 37:549-558, 2011

The purpose of this systematic review was to assess the evidence for use of routine procalcitonin testing to diagnose the presence of sepsis in the burn patient. The electronic databases MEDLINE, Cochrane, CINAHL, ProQuest, and SCOPUS were searched for relevant studies using the MeSH terms burn, infection, procalcitonin, and meta-analysis. The focus of the review was the adult burn population, but other relevant studies of critically ill patients were included as data specific to the patient with burns are limited. Studies were compiled in tabular form and critically appraised for quality and level of evidence. Four meta-analyses, one review of the literature, one randomized controlled trial, nine prospective observational, and three retrospective studies were retrieved. Six of these studies were specific to the burn population, with one specific to burned children. Only one meta-analysis, one adult burn and one pediatric burn study reported no benefit of procalcitonin testing to improve diagnosis of sepsis or differentiate sepsis from non-infectious systemic inflammatory response. The collective findings of the included studies demonstrated benefit of incorporating procalcitonin assay into clinical sepsis determination. Evaluation of the burn specific studies is limited by the use of guidelines to define sepsis and inconsistent results from the burn studies. Utility of the procalcitonin assay is limited due to the lack of availability of rapid, inexpensive tests. However, it appears procalcitonin assay is a safe and beneficial addition to the clinical diagnosis of sepsis in the burn intensive care unit.

▶ Burn patients with sepsis represent a complex challenge. Early identification at the bedside is difficult. In this group of patients, signs of sepsis are nonspecific, because many burn patients carry the criteria for systemic inflammatory response. Delaying antibiotic therapy in patients with sepsis, including patients with burns, is always a concern because it carries the risk of increased mortality. This is even more true in burn patients in whom significant difficulty in differentiating severe sepsis from systemic inflammatory response syndrome is noted.

In this article, Mann et al conducted a systematic overview of the literature to evaluate whether procalcitonin (PCT) can be used as a marker of sepsis in burn patients. The review included 4 meta-analyses: 1 randomized controlled trial, a prospective observational, and 3 retrospective studies. Six of the 18 studies were burn-specific. Given that the diagnostic odds ratio of all studies combined was 7.79, the authors concluded the PCT could be a beneficial addition to the clinical diagnosis of sepsis in the burn intensive care unit (ICU).

The possible role of PCT in a burn ICU setting seems interesting, because PCT level is easy, fast, and relatively inexpensive, which makes the use of this test in this setting very compelling. However, it is not clear from this article that we can draw a clear-cut conclusion.

A closer look at the burn-specific studies in this article shows that the number is limited to 5 observational and 1 retrospective study. The burn patients are relatively heterogeneous with total body surface area (TBSA) of burns ranging between 32% and 62%. Given the reports of PCT values correlating with the severity of TBSA, this heterogeneity adds further limitation to the use of PCT in burn patients, something not commented on in this article. In addition, the cutoff value of PCT between septic and nonseptic patients is still to be determined. This number was clearly different among the studies, raising significant discrepancies in sensitivity and specificity of the test (sensitivity: 46% to 100%; specificity: 67% to 89%). Moreover, most of the studies used the LUMItest for PCT detection. A more sensitive second-generation assay using time-resolved amplified cryptate emission (Kryptor assay, BRAHMS) has recently been developed. Knowing that nonseptic patients with severe burns can have elevated PCT, a more sensitive assay could help detect minimal changes, especially in the group of patients in whom PCT levels are indeterminate.

To conclude, this review seems in agreement with previous studies that support the use of PCT as a diagnostic marker of sepsis. However, it still does not resolve the current limitations of the test, nor does it answer how to incorporate such information into clinical decision making.

Z. Kobeissi, MD

Norepinephrine increases cardiac preload and reduces preload dependency assessed by passive leg raising in septic shock patients

Monnet X, Jabot J, Maizel J, et al (Hôpital de Bicêtre, Service de Réanimation Médicale, France)

Crit Care Med 39:689-694, 2011

Objective.—To assess the effects of norepinephrine on cardiac preload, cardiac index, and preload dependency during septic shock.

Design.—Prospective interventional study.

Setting.—Medical Intensive Care Unit.

Patients.—We included 25 septic shock patients (62 ± 13 yrs old, Simplified Acute Physiology Score II 53 ± 12, lactate 3.5 ± 2.1 mmol/L, all receiving norepinephrine at baseline at 0.24 [25%–75% interquartile range: 0.12–0.48] μg/kg/min) with a positive passive leg raising test (defined by an increase in cardiac index ≥10%) and a diastolic arterial pressure ≤40 mm Hg.

Interventions.—We performed a passive leg raising test (during 1 min) at baseline. Immediately after, we increased the dose of norepinephrine (to 0.48 [0.36–0.71] μg/kg/min) and, when the hemodynamic status was stabilized, we performed a second passive leg raising test (during 1 min). We finally infused 500 mL saline.

Measurements and Main Results.—Increasing the dose of norepinephrine significantly increased central venous pressure (+23% ± 12%), left ventricular end-diastolic area (+9% ± 6%), E mitral wave (+19% ± 23%), and global end-diastolic volume (+9% ± 6%). Simultaneously, cardiac index significantly increased by 11% ± 7%, suggesting that norepinephrine had recruited some cardiac preload reserve. The second passive leg raising test increased cardiac index to a lesser extent than the baseline test (13% ± 8% vs. ± 19% ± 6%, $p < .05$), suggesting that norepinephrine had decreased the degree of preload dependency. Volume infusion significantly increased cardiac index by 26% ± 15%. However, cardiac index increased by <15% in four patients (fluid unresponsive patients) while the baseline passive leg raising test was positive in these patients. In three of these four patients, the second passive leg raising test was also negative, i.e., the second passive leg raising test (after norepinephrine increase) predicted fluid responsiveness with a sensitivity of 95 [76–99]% and a specificity of 100 [30–100]%.

Conclusions.—In septic patients with a positive passive leg raising test at baseline suggesting the presence of preload dependency, norepinephrine increased cardiac preload and cardiac index and reduced the degree of preload dependency.

▶ Volume resuscitation and vasopressor therapy remains a cornerstone in the management of critically ill patients with shock and hypotension. Accumulating evidence over the last few years, both experimental and clinical, shows the limitation of static measures, such as central venous pressure and pulmonary artery occlusion pressure, in determining cardiac preload in critically ill patients.

Dynamic indices, such as pulse pressure variation (PPV) and stroke volume variation (SVV), have been shown to be superior in the assessment of fluid responsiveness. Despite the growing variety of techniques to assess preload or responsiveness to volume challenges, none have been shown to be completely reliable in all patient groups. The limitations have been attributed, among other causes (eg, variations in intrathoracic pressure, myocardial dysfunction), to the concomitant use of vasopressor therapy with fluid resuscitation.

In this study, Monnet et al studied the effect of norepinephrine (NE) on cardiac preload and cardiac index (CI) using passive leg raising (PLR) in septic shock patients. Twenty-five patients were included. All patients were receiving NE at baseline, were intubated, were sedated, and showed a positive response to PLR. Patients were monitored by the PiCCO2 device, invasive arterial pressure, central venous pressure, and transesophageal echocardiography. Several hemodynamic studies were taken, at baseline level, after 1 minute of PLR, after NE increase, after second PLR, and after 500 mL of saline bolus.

The authors noted that NE caused a significant increase in the cardiac preload parameters such as central venous pressure, left ventricular end-diastolic area (LVEDA), global end-diastolic volume, and CI that was in comparison with similar effects caused by increased preload induced by the first PLR. On the other hand, NE caused a lesser increase in cardiac index during the second PLR. The authors concluded the NE exerts part of its hemodynamic effect through increasing cardiac preload with subsequent decrease in cardiac preload reserve in addition to its known effect of restoring arterial tone.

The authors concluded that NE exerted its effect through mobilizing unstressed volume in the venous reservoir through increase in vascular tone acting like an endogenous fluid challenge and thus may decrease the amount of fluid administration. It should be noted that this study did not address the component of organ perfusion or the issue of mortality.

Although this study was not powered to address mortality or to detect tissue perfusion, a few observations are worth discussing:

1. The study was performed with patients in septic shock without adequate fluid resuscitation, as noted from the significant increase in preload parameters and cardiac index after both PLR and the saline challenge. The authors reported that their recruited patients were in their early stages of sepsis. If so, this should be considered a major deviation from early goal-directed therapy and Surviving Sepsis Campaign guidelines.
2. More importantly, the increase in mean arterial pressure after the first PLR (before NE increase) decreased significantly during the second PLR and after the saline bolus (from 36% to ~6%), whereas similar augmentation in CI and LVEDA were noted in both groups (before and after NE increase). Despite the fact that NE increased preload parameters and CI, further significant increases were noted after the second PLR and the saline bolus. This reflects that the vasoconstrictive effect of NE in enhancing preload is limited. It also highlights the importance of the need of continued early adequate volume resuscitation in the group studied.
3. No information was provided on subsequent lactic acid and SVO2 results. Given the fact that NE could induce venous blood shift from the unstressed to the stressed vascular bed, advocating the use of NE as a first-line therapy could entail the risk of increasing cardiac work and vasoconstriction in an already compromised region of microcirculation.

This shows that PLR remains a good predictor of fluid responsiveness even while patients are on NE. This article highlights some of the hemodynamic effects of NE, namely, its effect on cardiac preload. It also shows that NE does not preclude using the PLR to determine fluid responsiveness at the bedside in septic shock patients. However, it is important to note that the NE effect on cardiac function was not studied as to guide volume resuscitation. Further studies looking at peripheral tissue perfusion and outcome are needed before advising such a clinical approach.

Z. Kobeissi, MD

Cost-effectiveness of an emergency department-based early sepsis resuscitation protocol

Jones AE, Troyer JL, Kline JA (Carolinas Med Ctr, Charlotte, NC; Univ of North Carolina at Charlotte)

Crit Care Med 39:1306-1312, 2011

Objectives.—Guidelines recommend that sepsis be treated with an early resuscitation protocol such as early goal-directed therapy. Our objective was to assess the cost-effectiveness of implementing early goal-directed therapy as a routine protocol.

Design.—Prospective before and after study.

Setting.—Large urban hospital emergency department with >110,000 visits/yr.

Patients.—The target population was patients with consensus criteria for septic shock. We excluded those with age <18 yrs, no aggressive care desired, or need for immediate surgery.

Interventions.—Clinical and cost data were prospectively collected on two groups: 1) patients from 1 yr before; and 2) 2 yrs after implementing early goal-directed therapy as standard of care. Before phase patients received nonprotocolized care at attending discretion. The primary outcomes were 1-yr mortality, discounted life expectancy, and quality-adjusted life-years. Using costs and quality-adjusted life-years, we constructed an incremental cost-effectiveness ratio and performed a net monetary benefit analysis, producing the probability that the intervention was cost-effective given different values for the willingness to pay for a quality-adjusted life-year.

Results.—Two hundred eighty-five subjects, 79 in the before and 206 in the after phases, were enrolled. Treatment with early goal-directed therapy was associated with an increased hospital cost of $7,028 and an increase in both discounted sepsis-adjusted life expectancy and quality-adjusted life years of 1.5 and 1.3 yrs, respectively. Early goal-directed therapy use was associated with a cost of $5,397 per quality-adjusted life-years gained and the net monetary benefit analysis indicates a 98% probability ($p = .038$) that early goal-directed therapy is cost-effective at a willingness to pay of $50,000 per quality-adjusted life-years.

Conclusion.—Implementation of early goal-directed therapy in the emergency department care of patients with severe sepsis is cost-effective.

▶ Introduction of new therapies is often associated with perceived increase in costs and resource utilization. However, understanding the true cost-effectiveness impact of a specific therapeutic intervention requires consideration of multiple factors. In this article, the authors aim to identify whether an early goal-directed therapy for sepsis resuscitation is cost effective. When comparing total cost per patient before and after implementation of this protocol, there is increased cost of $7028 in the protocol-treated patients. Evaluating cost effectiveness must take into account survivors' life expectancy and quality of life. The authors use a sepsis-adjusted life expectancy, which allows the comparison to take into account the fact that survivors of sepsis have an overall decreased life expectancy compared with their counterparts in the general population with the same age, sex, and race. Quality of life is also measured by assigning a utility to each year or partial year of gained life. The utility is adjusted for the postsepsis population by taking the average utility level of a person in the general population with the same sepsis-adjusted life expectancy rather than the same actual age. Patients treated with the protocol had an increase sepsis-adjusted life expectancy of 1.5 years and increase in quality-adjusted life-years (QALY) of 1.3 years.

The main determinant of cost effectiveness seems to be what the general population is willing to pay for an additional year of life. Although there is no clear cutoff, the authors cite a $50 000 per QALY to be a frequently used value in the literature. The authors identify the Incremental Cost Effectiveness Ratio, which is basically the added cost per QALY gained. Additionally, they calculate a net monetary benefit analysis (NMB), which allows a comparison while taking into account varying willingness to pay for an additional year of life. Using the cutoff of $50 000 and a NMB analysis, the authors conclude that early goal-directed therapy is cost effective. The authors make the point that some of the barriers to implementing a sepsis resuscitation protocol may certainly be cost effectiveness. To this end, it seems reasonable to perform a cost-effectiveness evaluation. I think the concern that cost is a barrier is well founded. This solid analysis of cost effectiveness for a sepsis protocol may be well used to persuade hospital administration to invest in the training, education, and equipment that is needed for this type of protocol implementation.

B. Goodgame, MD
S. L. Zanotti-Cavazzoni, MD

Understanding the potential role of statins in pneumonia and sepsis

Yende S, Milbrandt EB, Kellum JA, et al (Univ of Pittsburgh School of Medicine, PA; et al)

Crit Care Med 39:1871-1878, 2011

Objective.—To examine the association of statin use with clinical outcomes and circulating biomarkers in community-acquired pneumonia and sepsis.

Design.—Multicenter inception cohort study.

Setting.—Emergency departments of 28 U.S. hospitals.

Patients.—A total of 1895 subjects hospitalized with community-acquired pneumonia.

Interventions.—None.

Measurements and Main Results.—Our approach consisted of two different comparison cohorts, each reflecting methods used in prior publications in this area. We first compared subjects with prior statin use (prior use cohort), defined as a history of statin use in the week before admission, with those with no prior use. We then compared prior statin users whose statins were continued inhospital (continued use cohort) with those with either no prior use or no inhospital use. We adjusted for patient characteristics, including demographics, comorbid conditions, and illness severity, and accounted for healthy user effect and indication bias using propensity analysis. We determined risk of severe sepsis and 90-day mortality. We measured markers of inflammation (tumor necrosis factor, interleukin-6, interleukin-10), coagulation (antithrombin, factor IX, plasminogen activator inhibitor, D-dimer, thrombin antithrombin complex), and lymphocyte cell surface protein expression during the first week of hospitalization. There were no differences in severe sepsis risk between statin users and nonusers for prior (30.8% vs. 30.7%, $p = .98$) or continued statin use (30.2% vs. 30.8%, $p = .85$) in univariate analyses and after adjusting for patient characteristics and propensity for statin use. Ninety-day mortality was similar in prior statin users (9.2% vs. 12.0%, $p = .11$) and lower in continued statin users (7.9% vs. 12.1%, $p = .02$). After adjusting for patient characteristics and propensity for statin use, there was no mortality benefit for prior (odds ratio, 0.90 [0.63–1.29]; $p = .57$) or continued statin use (odds ratio, 0.73 [0.47–1.13]; $p = .15$). Only antithrombin activity over time was higher in statin subjects, yet the magnitude of the difference was modest. There were no differences in other coagulation, inflammatory, or lymphocyte cell surface markers.

Conclusions.—We found no evidence of a protective effect for statin use on clinical outcomes and only modest differences in circulating biomarkers in community-acquired pneumonia, perhaps as a result of healthy user effects and indication bias.

▶ Community-acquired pneumonia (CAP) is a potentially life-threatening disease and a frequent reason for hospitalization in the United States. When associated with severe sepsis, the morbidity and mortality of CAP increases significantly. HMG CoA inhibitors , more popularly known as statins, are widely utilized for their low-density lipoprotein–lowering properties. However, statins have also been shown to have many direct and indirect anti-inflammatory and immunomodulatory effects in animal and human studies. Furthermore, studies have found a potential role for statins in improving endothelial function and modulating the coagulation cascade in a favorable way. These non–lipid-lowering effects have led many investigators to propose a potential role for statins in treating sepsis.

The study by Yende et al is a large multicenter prospective cohort study that looks at statin use in a cohort of patients older than 18 years with CAP and sepsis. They compared patients within two groups: (1) group 1 compared subjects with prior statin use with subjects with no statin use, (2) the second group compared subjects with prior statin use who continued statins while in the hospital with those who either never took statins or did not continue them during their hospital stay.

The authors did not find evidence of any protective effect of statins in the patients with CAP and sepsis. However, this study also raises a few important questions. Firstly, was the dose of statins used by patients in this study sufficient to exert their immunomodulatory effects? Moreover, are all the classes of statins equally efficacious in exerting their immunomodulatory effects?

Another area for debate might relate to the fact that in this study most severely ill intubated intensive care unit patients were not included. Did the mild/moderate nature of the illness in the patients studied affect the visible change (delta) in the levels of markers of inflammation between the cases and controls leading to discrepancy in the results? Although the results of this study do not point to a significant clinical benefit of statin use in sepsis, they are unlikely to settle this fascinating debate.

V. Punjabi, MD
S. L. Zanotti-Cavazzoni, MD

8 Metabolism/ Gastrointestinal/ Nutrition/ Hematology-Oncology

Aprotinin Versus Tranexamic Acid During Liver Transplantation: Impact on Blood Product Requirements and Survival

Massicotte L, Denault AY, Beaulieu D, et al (Centre hospitalier de l'Université de Montréal, Quebec, Canada; et al)

Transplantation 91:1273-1278, 2011

Background.—Historically, orthotopic liver transplantation (OLT) has been associated with major blood loss and the need for blood product transfusions. Activation of the fibrinolytic system can contribute significantly to bleeding. Prophylactic administration of antifibrinolytic agents was found to reduce blood loss.

Methods.—The efficacy of two antifibrinolytic compounds—aprotinin (AP) and tranexamic acid (TA)—was compared in OLT. Four hundred consecutive OLTs were studied: 300 patients received AP and 100 received TA. Multivariate logistic regression analysis was used to identify independent predictors of intraoperative transfusion requirement and 1-year patient mortality.

Results.—There was no intergroup difference in intraoperative blood loss (1082 ± 1056 vs. 1007 ± 790 mL), red blood cell transfusion per patient (0.5 ± 1.4 vs. 0.5 ± 1.0), final hemoglobin (Hb) concentration (93 ± 20 g/L vs. 95 ± 22 g/L), the percentage of OLT cases requiring no blood product administration (80% vs. 82%), and 1-year survival (85.1% vs. 87.4%). Serum creatinine concentrations were also the same (116 ± 55 vs. 119 ± 36 μmol/L) 1 year after surgery. Two variables, starting Hb and phlebotomy, correlated with the two primary outcome measures (transfusion and 1-year survival).

Conclusions.—In our experience, administration of AP was not superior to TA with regards to blood loss and blood product transfusion requirement during OLT. In addition, we found no difference between the groups in the 1-year survival rate and renal function. Furthermore, we suggest that starting Hb concentration should be considered when prioritizing patients on the waiting list and planning perioperative care for OLT recipients.

▶ Although effective at controlling bleeding both as an inhibitor of the conversion of plasminogen to plasmin as well as a protease inhibitor, aprotinin (AP) has been widely unavailable outside the research environment since 2007, when it was shown to increase renal failure and mortality in cardiac surgical patients receiving this medication for hemostasis.[1] Other antifibrinolytic agents remain available, including tranexamic acid (TA) and epsilon-amino caproic acid. While the efficacy of these agents has been relatively well studied in cardiac surgery, their effectiveness in orthotopic liver transplant (OLT) is less well documented. These investigators undertook to determine whether AP was different than TA in controlling bleeding in this high-risk population. Using AP under an investigational protocol, they prospectively compared 300 patients on AP with 100 receiving TA. No advantage was demonstrated for AP in that outcomes were identical between the groups: blood loss, transfusion requirements, and final hemoglobins were similar in the 2 groups. Interestingly, unlike the data from the cardiac surgical population, however, no detrimental effects were identified with the use of AP. One-year survival was similar in both groups, as was renal function. In patients undergoing OLT, this initial data indicate that AP appears to offer a safe alternative to other antifibrinolytic agents. However, as it also appears to offer no advantages, confirmatory data would be useful before drawing final conclusions; even if these results are confirmed, the use of this agent should probably be reserved for patients unresponsive to or unable to receive other antifibrinolytic agents.

D. R. Gerber, DO, FCCP

Reference

1. Mangano DT, Tudor IC, Dietzel C. The risk associated with aprotinin in cardiac surgery. *N Engl J Med.* 2006;354:353-365.

Furosemide for Packed Red Cell Transfusion in Preterm Infants: A Randomized Controlled Trial

Balegar V KK, Kluckow M (Royal North Shore Hosp, Sydney, Australia)
J Pediatr 159:913-918, 2011

Objective.—To assess the effect of furosemide administered with packed red blood cell transfusion on cardiopulmonary variables of hemodynamically stable, electively transfused preterm infants beyond the first week of life.

Study Design.—A randomized, stratified, double-blind, placebo-controlled trial of intravenous furosemide (1 mg/kg) versus placebo (normal saline) just before "top-up" packed red blood cell transfusion (20 mL/kg over 4 hours) in a tertiary neonatal intensive care unit.

Results.—The primary outcome was a change in fraction of inspired oxygen (FiO_2) during the 24 hours posttransfusion compared with the 6-hour pretransfusion period. Secondary outcomes were functional echocardiographic and clinical/biochemical variables. Of 51 consecutive preterm infants with mean (± SD) birth weights of 900 g (± 28); enrollment weights of 1342 g (± 432); birth gestation of 27 weeks (± 1); and postmenstrual age of 32 weeks (± 4), 40 completed the study. Pretransfusion variables were comparable between the furosemide (n = 21) and placebo (n = 19) groups. There was a small but significant increase ($P < .05$) in posttransfusion FiO_2 in placebo (relative increase of 7%, equivalent to an absolute increase from 0.27 to 0.29) compared with the furosemide group. Other variables were similar. No infant received open-label furosemide.

Conclusions.—Routine furosemide in electively transfused preterm infants confers minimal clinical benefits. Prevention of a clinically insignificant FiO_2 rise needs to be balanced against potential adverse effects.

▶ It is common practice in critically ill patients and in adult patients in general to use a so-called "loop diuretic," such as furosemide, especially when multiple units of packed red blood cells (PRBC) are being transfused, with the intent of preventing circulatory overload and hypoxemic respiratory failure. The literature supporting this practice is sketchy at best, however, and a significant proportion of patients likely have no need for this intervention. This practice is also undertaken by neonatologists when transfusing premature infants, with similar goals in mind. In an effort to determine whether this intervention has clinical merit, these investigators performed a double-blind prospective trial in which they gave preterm infants either furosemide or placebo before PRBC transfusion and assessed the impact on oxygen requirements in the 24 hours after transfusion as well as echocardiographic and other clinical and biochemical parameters. While the infants receiving diuretic had a slightly lower oxygen requirement that was statistically significant, the investigators felt the difference was of no clinical significance. Echocardiographic, biochemical, and other clinical parameters were similar in the 2 groups. Overall, the investigators felt that diuresis conveyed no benefit in transfused premature infants, and carried potential risks, such as induction of fluid and electrolyte disturbances. While it is uncertain whether these findings can be extrapolated to a critically ill adult population, they should raise the question of whether the routine use of diuresis before or in between units of PRBC is necessary or appropriate as it is commonly applied. While there is certainly a population of patients at risk for transfusion-associated circulatory overload, most specifically those patients with preexisting poor myocardial contractility or otherwise compromised hemodynamics, it is most likely unnecessary and potentially harmful to routinely perform diuresis on otherwise stable patients receiving PRBC. Prospective evaluation of this issue in adults would seem warranted.

D. R. Gerber, DO, FCCP

Transfusion-related acute lung injury: reports to the French Hemovigilance Network 2007 through 2008

Ozier Y, Muller J-Y, Mertes P-M, et al (Université Paris Descartes, France; CHU de Nantes, France; CHU Nancy, France; et al)
Transfusion 51:2102-2110, 2011

Background.—Transfusion-related acute lung injury (TRALI) is a major cause of transfusion-related mortality and morbidity. Epidemiologic studies using data from national transfusion schemes can help achieve a better understanding of TRALI incidence.

Study Design and Methods.—A multidisciplinary working group analyzed TRALI cases extracted from the French Hemovigilance Network Database (2007-2008). All notified cases were reviewed for diagnosis. Those meeting the Canadian Consensus Conference criteria for TRALI were classified according to imputability to transfusion and clinical severity. Patient data (clinical characteristics, number and types of products transfused, and serology results) were obtained.

Results.—There were 62 TRALI cases and 23 possible TRALI cases during the 2-year period. An immune-mediated mechanism was identified in 30 of 50 TRALI cases with complete serology. TRALI was considered to be the cause of death in 7.1% of patients and might have contributed to death in an additional 9.4% of TRALI or possible TRALI patients. Occurrence ranked high in obstetrics (15%), after surgery (34%), and in hematologic malignancies (21%). Single-donor high-plasma-volume components were involved in half of the cases where the implicated blood product could be determined and carried the highest risk per component (1:31,000 for single-donor fresh-frozen plasma units and apheresis platelet [PLT] concentrates, and 1:173,000 for red blood cells). No incident could be definitively related to the transfusion of solvent/detergent-treated pooled plasma (>200,000 units transfused), nor to pooled PLT concentrates.

Conclusion.—The proportion of TRALI cases related to plasma-rich components was lower than previously described.

▶ Transfusion-related acute lung injury (TRALI) is a significant cause of morbidity and mortality associated with the use of blood products. Its true incidence is difficult to determine, with variably reported rates and widely estimated incidences by clinicians. In this study, the investigators used data reported to the French Haemovigilance Network over a 2-year period and established diagnostic criteria to try to determine the incidence of this entity in France as well as the blood products most often responsible for its occurrence.

Eighty-five cases, 62 definite and 23 probable, were identified in the study period. Surgical patients were most likely to develop TRALI followed in decreasing order by patients with hematologic/oncologic disorders and then obstetric patients. The incidence was highest among recipients of single-donor, high-volume blood components, occurring at a rate of 1 in 31 000 transfusions, followed by packed red blood cell transfusions, which resulted in TRALI at a rate of 1 in 173 000.

TRALI presents an important clinical conundrum. On one hand, while relatively rare, it may still be underdiagnosed if not looked for. In addition, given the frequency with which blood products are utilized, even an entity with a low frequency of occurrence will appear from time to time. Conversely, familiarity with the diagnostic criteria is essential to make the diagnosis correctly, to avoid missing other pathologies which would, or may, require different interventions.

D. R. Gerber, DO, FCCP

High Oxygen Partial Pressure Decreases Anemia-induced Heart Rate Increase Equivalent to Transfusion

Feiner JR, Finlay-Morreale HE, Toy P, et al (Univ of California, San Francisco; et al)

Anesthesiology 115:492-498, 2011

Background.—Anemia is associated with morbidity and mortality and frequently leads to transfusion of erythrocytes. The authors sought to directly compare the effect of high inspired oxygen fraction *versus* transfusion of erythrocytes on the anemia-induced increased heart rate (HR) in humans undergoing experimental acute isovolemic anemia.

Methods.—The authors combined HR data from healthy subjects undergoing experimental isovolemic anemia in seven studies performed by the group. HR changes associated with breathing 100% oxygen by nonrebreathing facemask *versus* transfusion of erythrocytes at their nadir hemoglobin concentration of 5 g/dl were examined. Data were analyzed using a mixed-effects model.

Results.—HR had an inverse linear relationship to hemoglobin concentration with a mean increase of 3.9 beats per min per gram of hemoglobin (beats/min/g hemoglobin) decrease (95% CI, 3.7–4.1 beats/min/g hemoglobin), $P < 0.0001$. Return of autologous erythrocytes significantly decreased HR by 5.3 beats/min/g hemoglobin (95% CI, 3.8–6.8 beats/min/g hemoglobin) increase, $P < 0.0001$. HR at nadir hemoglobin of 5.6 g/dl (95% CI, 5.5–5.7 g/dl) when breathing air (91.4 beats/min; 95% CI, 87.6–95.2 beats/min) was reduced by breathing 100% oxygen (83.0 beats/min; 95% CI, 79.0–87.0 beats/min), $P < 0.0001$. The HR at hemoglobin 5.6 g/dl when breathing oxygen was equivalent to the HR at hemoglobin 8.9 g/dl when breathing air.

Conclusions.—High arterial oxygen partial pressure reverses the heart rate response to anemia, probably because of its usability rather than its effect on total oxygen content. The benefit of high arterial oxygen partial pressure has significant potential clinical implications for the acute treatment of anemia and results of transfusion trials.

▶ Packed red blood cells (PRBC) are transfused for a variety of purposes, most importantly to increase oxygen delivery to tissue. Among other goals of transfusion is the correction of symptomatic anemia, including the correction of tachycardia believed to be the result of low hemoglobin (Hgb) levels. The use of high fractional inspired oxygen (F_IO_2) levels has previously been shown to be as effective or more so than PRBC transfusion as a means of delivering oxygen to tissue in surgical patients in an article by Suttner and coworkers, although this study has recently been retracted due to lack of appropriate institutional review board approval. In the present study, Feiner et al investigated whether a high F_IO_2 could be used to control the tachycardia induced by isovolemic anemia in healthy volunteers. Data collected on subjects studied in prospective trials performed separately over several years was reviewed and demonstrated that when subjects were bled in an isovolemic fashion with albumin replacement, a high F_IO_2 (100%) was extremely effective at reducing heart rate. Application of oxygen at an F_IO_2 of 100% at isovolemic anemia to a mean Hgb of 5.9 gm/dL reduced heart rate by the equivalent of 3 g of Hgb. The authors also determined that, in these health volunteers, heart rate increased by about 3.4 beats per minute for every gram drop in Hgb in men and about 4.6 for every gram in women. The findings that heart rate appears to respond as well to oxygen as to PRBC has significant clinical implications. Oxygen is immediately available in almost any health care setting. Although not completely without complications, it carries far fewer risks and complications than blood transfusion. At the very least, the application of high-flow oxygen can be used for symptomatic anemia as a temporizing measure until PRBC are available and may help minimize the number of units of red cells transfused. It should be noted, however, that the data presented in this study are from healthy volunteers. The applicability of this approach to critically ill patients, the elderly, or others in the real-world setting has yet to be established. Nevertheless, it seems reasonable to attempt to use this approach in tachycardic, anemic patients both as a stabilizing tool and perhaps in an effort to limit the volume of transfused PRBC.

D. R. Gerber, DO, FCCP

Association of admission hematocrit with 6-month and 1-year mortality in intensive care unit patients

Mudumbai SC, Cronkite R, Hu KU, et al (VA Palo Alto HCS, CA; Stanford Univ, CA; VA San Francisco/Univ of California at San Francisco)

Transfusion 51:2148-2159, 2011

Background.—This study examined the association of hematocrit (Hct) levels measured upon intensive care unit (ICU) admission and red blood cell transfusions to long-term (1-year or 180-day) mortality for both surgical and medical patients.

Study Design and Methods.—Administrative and laboratory data were collected retrospectively on 2393 consecutive medical and surgical male patients admitted to the ICU between 2003 and 2009. We stratified patients based on their median Hct level during the first 24 hours of their ICU stay (Hct < 25.0%, 25% ≤ Hct < 30%, 30% ≤ Hct < 39%, and 39.0% and higher). An extended Cox regression analysis was conducted to identify the time period after ICU admission (0 to <180, 180 to 365 days) when low Hct (<25.0) was most strongly associated with mortality. The unadjusted and adjusted relationship between admission Hct level, receipt of a transfusion, and 180-day mortality was assessed using Cox proportional hazards regression modeling.

Results.—Patients with an Hct level of less than 25% who were not transfused had the worst mortality risk overall (hazard ratio [HR], 6.26; 95% confidence interval [CI], 3.05-12.85; $p < 0.001$) during the 6 months after ICU admission than patients with a Hct level of 39.0% or more who were not transfused. Within the subgroup of patients with a Hct level of less than 25% only, receipt of a transfusion was associated with a significant reduction in the risk of mortality (HR, 0.40; 95% CI, 0.19-0.85; $p = 0.017$).

Conclusion.—Anemia of a Hct level of less than 25% upon admission to the ICU, in the absence of a transfusion, is associated with long-term mortality. Our study suggests that there may be Hct levels below which the transfusion risk-to-benefit imbalance reverses.

▶ It is now widely, if not quite universally, accepted that a broad variety of critically ill patients can tolerate what had for many years been considered unacceptably low levels of anemia. This was first well documented by the Transfusion Requirements In Critical Care (TRICC) trial[1] and has subsequently been confirmed by numerous other studies. An extensive body of literature, essentially beginning with that study, has evolved demonstrating that packed red blood cell (PRBC) transfusion is often not only not beneficial even in critically ill patients but may be harmful in some subpopulations. As a result, the specific indications for transfusion in the absence of active bleeding and the level of anemia that should trigger a transfusion, if such a "routine" response exists, have become a matter of controversy. In this study, the authors retrospectively reviewed data on a mixed medical-surgical population of nearly 2400 male intensive care unit (ICU) patients, evaluating hematocrit (Hct) levels during the first 24 hours of their intensive care stays. Patients were stratified according to Hct (< 25%, 25%–30%, 30%–39%, and > 39%) and also assessed for transfusion history. Groups were compared for 6-month and 1-year mortality using a Cox proportion hazard method. Overall, patients in the group with Hct levels < 25% who were not transfused had the highest mortality; within that subgroup, transfusion resulted in a significant reduction in mortality. This study suggests that a Hct < 25% may be an appropriate threshold for transfusion in critically ill patients, because these patients appear to have responded with a significant reduction in mortality with this intervention. Hct of 25% of is generally accepted as correlating with a hemoglobin (Hgb) of approximately 8 g/dL. The results of the TRICC trial indicated that a broad array of critically ill patients did as well, or possibly better, if not transfused unless their Hgb levels were approximately 7 g/dL compared with those transfused at Hgb levels at 9 g/dL. It is unclear how low the Hcts actually were in the group of patients with values < 25%, because these data were not reported in the article. It would seem reasonable that if a substantial proportion had profound anemia on presentation, transfusion would likely be beneficial, regardless of any potential detrimental effects of this intervention. Other limitations in comparing the results of this study to previous studies is the difficulty in comparing the acuity of the patients. Although most ICU-based studies use APACHE, SAPS, SOFA, and other systems as indicators of acuity, the authors used the Charlson scoring system as their index. Despite these shortcomings, this retrospective study raises an interesting question: is there a reasonable transfusion trigger in the critically ill patient population? The blood supply is different now than it was when the TRICC trial was originally performed. In the United States, Canada, and most if not all of the developed world, transfused PRBC are now leukodepleted. Although not all complications and deficiencies associated with transfusion can be blamed on the presence of white blood cells (WBCs), it is likely that WBCs were at least partially responsible for past problems. These findings may be an impetus for a new prospective to confirm these results.

D. R. Gerber, DO, FCCP

Reference

1. Hébert PC, Wells G, Blajchman MA, et al. A multicenter, randomized, controlled clinical trial of transfusion requirements in critical care. Transfusion Requirements in Critical Care investigators, Canadian critical care trials group. *N Engl J Med.* 1999;340:409-417.

Effect of Single Recombinant Human Erythropoietin Injection on Transfusion Requirements in Preoperatively Anemic Patients Undergoing Valvular Heart Surgery

Yoo Y-C, Shim J-K, Kim J-C, et al (Yonsei Univ Health System, Seoul, Korea)
Anesthesiology 115:929-937, 2011

Background.—The authors investigated the effect of a single preoperative bolus of erythropoietin on perioperative transfusion requirement and erythropoiesis in patients with preoperative anemia undergoing valvular heart surgery.

Methods.—In this prospective, single-site, single-blinded, randomized, and parallel-arm controlled trial, 74 patients with preoperative anemia were randomly allocated to either the erythropoietin or the control group. The erythropoietin group received 500 IU/kg erythropoietin and 200 mg iron sucrose intravenously 1 day before the surgery. The control group received an equivalent volume of normal saline. The primary endpoint was transfusion requirement assessed during the surgery and for 4 days postoperatively. Reticulocyte count and iron profiles were measured serially and compared preoperatively and on postoperative days 1, 2, 4, and 7.

Results.—Transfusion occurred in 32 patients (86%) of the control group *versus* 22 patients (59%) of the erythropoietin group ($P = 0.009$). The mean number of units of packed erythrocytes transfused per patient during the surgery and for 4 postoperative days (mean ± SD) was also significantly decreased in the erythropoietin group compared with the control group (3.3 ± 2.2 *vs.* 1.0 ± 1.1 units/patient, $P = 0.001$). The reticulocyte count was significantly greater in the erythropoietin group at postoperative days 4 ($P = 0.001$) and 7 ($P = 0.001$).

Conclusions.—A single intravenous administration of erythropoietin and an iron supplement 1 day before surgery significantly reduced the perioperative transfusion requirement in anemic patients undergoing valvular heart surgery, implicating its potential role as a blood conservation strategy.

▶ Transfusion of packed red blood cells (PRBC) is a commonly applied intervention in patients undergoing cardiac surgical procedures. A significant body of literature exists indicating that patients undergoing coronary artery bypass graft (CABG) surgery who receive PRBC have significantly worse outcomes as measured by a variety of parameters than similar patients who do not. There are few data published on cardiac surgical patients receiving red cell transfusion who have undergone isolated valvular surgery, but it is reasonable, as with most patient populations, to try to limit the exposure to transfusions if possible in light of the extensive and growing body of literature demonstrating limited efficacy and potential complications associated with this intervention. In this small study involving 74 anemic patients undergoing isolated valve surgery, the investigators prospectively administered a single dose of recombinant erythropoietin (EPO) in a single-blind fashion to half of them preoperatively and evaluated both groups for the need for perioperative transfusion, reticulocyte count, and hemoglobin levels. EPO recipients had significantly lower postoperative transfusion requirements and higher reticulocyte counts than did the nonrecipients in this study. They also had higher hemoglobins on postoperative days 2, 3, and 4 despite similar rates of intraoperative transfusions. These findings suggest that a single dose of EPO administered in close proximity to cardiac surgery (in this case 1 day before) is effective in augmenting intrinsic red blood cell production and limiting the need for PRBC transfusion. These findings are different from those previously described in a more diverse range of critically ill patients. EPO has previously been investigated for its ability to augment hemoglobin levels in the critically ill.[1,2] Although preliminary results were initially encouraging, subsequent studies failed to validate these initial findings, although trauma patients receiving this agent were identified as having a lower mortality rate unrelated to a decreased number of transfusions. The results of the present study suggest that EPO may have benefit as adjunctive therapy in some patient populations that might otherwise require or at least receive blood transfusions on a regular basis. The small number of patients in this study make it hard to adopt this as a routine approach at this time and would suggest a larger, double-blind study. In addition, evaluation of this intervention in patients undergoing CABG surgery, who appear to be at particularly high risk of complications from PRBC transfusion, would seem reasonable.

D. R. Gerber, DO, FCCP

References

1. Corwin HL, Gettinger A, Pearl RG, et al. Efficacy of recombinant human erythropoietin in critically ill patients: a randomized controlled trial. *JAMA*. 2002;288: 2827-2835.
2. Corwin HL, Gettinger A, Fabian TC, et al; for the EPO Critical Care Trials Group. Efficacy and safety of epoetin alfa in critically ill patients. *N Engl J Med*. 2007; 357:965-976.

The impact of fresh frozen plasma vs coagulation factor concentrates on morbidity and mortality in trauma-associated haemorrhage and massive transfusion

Nienaber U, Innerhofer P, Westermann I, et al (Univ of Witten/Herdecke, Cologne, Germany; Innsbruck Med Univ, Austria)

Injury 42:697-701, 2011

Introduction.—Clinical observations together with recent research highlighted the role of coagulopathy in acute trauma care and early aggressive treatment has been shown to reduce mortality.

Methods.—Datasets from severely injured and bleeding patients with established coagulopathy upon emergency room (ER) arrival from two retrospective trauma databases, (i) TR-DGU (Germany) and (ii) Innsbruck Trauma Databank/ITB (Austria), that had received two different strategies of coagulopathy management during initial resuscitation, (i) fresh frozen plasma (FFP) without coagulation factor concentrates, and (ii) coagulation factor concentrates (fibrinogen and/or prothrombin complex concentrates) without FFP, were compared for morbidity, mortality and transfusion requirements using a matched-pair analysis approach.

Results.—There were no major differences in basic characteristics and physiological variables upon ER admission between the two cohorts that were matched. ITB patients had received substantially less packed red blood cell (pRBC) concentrates within the first 6 h after admission (median 1.0 (IQR_{25-75} 0–3) vs 7.5 (IQR_{25-75} 4–12) units; $p < 0.005$) and the first 24 h as compared to TR-DGU patients (median 3 (IQR_{25-75} 0–5) vs 12.5 (8–20) units; $p < 0.005$). Overall mortality was comparable between both groups whilst the frequency for multi organ failure was significantly lower within the group that had received coagulation factor concentrates exclusively and no FFP during initial resuscitation ($n = 3$ vs $n = 15$; $p = 0.015$). This translated into trends towards reduced days on ventilator whilst on ICU and shorter overall in-hospital length of stays (LOS).

Conclusion.—Although there was no difference in overall mortality between both groups, significant differences with regard to morbidity and need for allogenic transfusion provide a signal supporting the management of acute post-traumatic coagulopathy with coagulation factor concentrates rather than with traditional FFP transfusions. Prospective and randomised clinical trials with sufficient patient numbers based upon this strategy are advocated.

▶ Treatment of the actively bleeding patient is a common and crucial problem in critical care, and no more so than for clinicians involved in the care of trauma patients. In addition to mechanical control of bleeding and maintenance of adequate circulating blood volume with intravenous fluid and blood as indicated, correction of any underlying coagulopathy/repletion of clotting factors is recognized as an essential aspect of therapy. While historically this last piece of the picture has usually been achieved through the administration of fresh frozen plasma (FFP), in recent years, clotting factor (CF) concentrates have become more widely and readily available. Whether either approach has an advantage over the other remains an unanswered question. To try to resolve this question, these authors reviewed data from 2 retrospective trauma databases that had the merits of including patients who had been treated using distinct regimens: the German group used an approach using FFP but no CF during their initial resuscitation efforts; their Austrian counterparts conversely used only CF and no FFP in the correction of coagulopathy. Patients from these 2 registries were compared for morbidity, mortality, and transfusion requirements. Although overall mortality was the same in both groups, the Austrian group, which used CF, had significantly lower use of red cell transfusions. Patients treated by this group also had signifiacntly lower rates of organ failure. Whether the lower rates of organ failure are related to the use of CF versus FFP, the lower rate of red cell transfusion, or some other undetermined factors, would only be speculative. However, based on what is known about the deleterious effects of blood products, it is not unreasonable to hypothesize that at least some of the difference is a result of the lower rate of blood use. As with any retrospective study, prospective validation would strengthen these findings. In addition, it is uncertain whether these findings are generalizable to nontrauma patients, and more specifically, patients with major coagulopathies, such as those with advanced liver disease. Evaluation of such questions would be both interesting and clinically important.

D. R. Gerber, DO, FCCP

Changes in Cardiac Physiology After Severe Burn Injury
Williams FN, Herndon DN, Suman OE, et al (The Univ of Texas, Galveston)
J Burn Care Res 32:269-274, 2011

Cardiac stress, mediated by increased catecholamines, is the hallmark of severe burn injury typified by marked tachycardia, increased myocardial oxygen consumption, and increased cardiac output (CO). It remains one of the main determinants of survival in large burns. Currently, it is unknown for how long cardiac stress persists after a severe injury. Therefore, the aim of this study was to determine the extent and duration of cardiac stress after a severe burn. To determine persistence of cardiac alteration, the authors determined cardiac parameters of all surviving patients with burns ≥40% TBSA from 1998 to 2008. One hundred ninety-four patients were included in this study. Heart rate, mean arterial pressure, CO, stroke volume, cardiac index, and ejection fractions were measured at regular intervals from admission up to 2 years after injury. Rate pressure product was calculated as a correlate of myocardial oxygen consumption. All values were compared with normal nonburned children to validate the findings. Statistical analysis was performed using log transformed analysis of variance with Bonferroni correction and Student's *t*-test, where applicable. Heart rate, CO, cardiac index, and rate pressure product remained significantly increased in burned children for up to 2 years when compared with normal ranges ($P < .05$), indicating vastly increased cardiac stress. Ejection fraction was within normal limits for 2 years. Cardiac stress persists for at least 2 years postburn, and the authors suggest that attenuation of these detrimental responses may improve long-term morbidity.

▶ Burns represent a specialized form of trauma. The changes in cardiac physiology represent just 1 example of the differences between blunt and penetrating trauma when compared with thermal trauma. Because of the prolonged exposure to elevated catecholamine levels, a hyperdynamic state exists in the postburn period, which is associated with impaired wound healing, erosion of lean body mass, and prolonged rehabilitation. The detrimental cardiac effects of this sustained process are unknown. What this study nicely demonstrates is that pediatric burn patients remain in a hyperdynamic process for longer than we thought, with increased cardiac stress remaining at the end of the study 2 years after the burn. Beta-adrenergic blockade with propranolol has been the most efficacious anticatabolic therapy in the treatment of burns, although the underlying mechanism of action regarding catabolism reversal is still unclear. This modality is being used with increasing frequency in burn centers. What remains to be seen is the most efficacious treatment regimen for propranolol in both children and adults with severe burn injury.

B. A. Latenser, MD, FACS

Body Mass Index (BMI) and mortality in patients with severe burns: Is there a "tilt point" at which obesity influences outcome?

Ghanem AM, Sen S, Philp B, et al (Broomfield Hosp, Chelmsford, Essex, UK)
Burns 37:208-214, 2011

Background.—Obesity is a serious health hazard. Despite advances in burn care severely obese patients with large burns have higher mortality compared with normal-weight patients. The Body Mass Index is the universal measure to define and classify obesity. This study aims to evaluate the effect of Body Mass Index (BMI) on mortality of severe burn patients.

Methods.—A retrospective study of 95 patients treated over 2-year period in a dedicated burn ITU. Mortality was studied in relation to BMI as well as demographic, burn characteristics well as length of hospital stay. Logistic regression model and non-parametric comparison tests were used for analysis.

Results.—Mean age was 42 ± 22 years (mean ± SD), Total Burn Surface area (TBSA) 33 ± 16%, BMI 29 ± 7.5 (kg/m^2) and hospital stay was 37 ± 33 days. Incidence of inhalation injury was 29% and over all mortality was 19%. By logistic regression age, TBSA and inhalation injury were separately associated with mortality. Patients with BMI $\geq$ 35 (kg/m^2) had significantly higher mortality compared with patients with BMI < 25 (kg/m^2) [$p = 0.037$ (Fisher's exact test)].

Conclusions.—Body Mass Index ≥ 35 (kg/m^2) is a tilt point, which is associated with a higher than predicted mortality following burns when compared to burned patients with a normal BMI.

▶ Although the authors have concluded that a body mass index (BMI) greater than 35 is associated with increased mortality rate in burn patients and the finding makes sense to the teleologist, the study does not support the conclusion. With only 4.2% of the study patients having a BMI greater than 40, drawing the conclusion that there is a 20 times higher risk of death in this patient population is not supported. The other significant problem with this study, which the authors admit, is that patients in the BMI greater than 35 category have a disproportionate amount of inhalation injury and larger thermal burns, predisposing them to an increased mortality rate regardless of their obesity status.

However, the authors are to be commended in asking the question about obesity and its impact on burn outcomes. This study question is perfect for a multicenter evaluation. The National Burn Repository of the American Burn Center should be used as a resource by some enterprising investigator(s) to pursue this research inquiry.

B. A. Latenser, MD, FACS

Epidemiology of burns throughout the world. Part I: Distribution and risk factors

Peck MD (Arizona Burn Ctr, Phoenix)

Burns 37:1087-1100, 2011

Globally in 2004, the incidence of burns severe enough to require medical attention was nearly 11 million people and ranked fourth in all injuries, higher than the combined incidence of tuberculosis and HIV infections. Fortunately, although burns and fires account for over 300,000 deaths each year throughout the world, the vast majority of burns are not fatal. Nonetheless, fire-related burns are also among the leading causes of disability-adjusted life years (DALYs) lost in low- and middle-income countries (LMIC).

Morbidity and mortality due to fire and flames has declined worldwide in the past decades. However, 90% of burn deaths occur in LMIC, where prevention programs are uncommon and the quality of acute care is inconsistent. Even in high-income countries, burns occur disproportionately to racial and ethnic minorities such that socioeconomic status—more than cultural or educational factors—account for most of the increased burn susceptibility.

Risk factors for burns include those related to socioeconomic status, race and ethnicity, age, and gender, as well as those factors pertaining to region of residence, intent of injury, and comorbidity. Both the epidemiology and risk factors of burns injuries worldwide are reviewed in this paper.

▶ I recommend this article to those who participate in burn care in low-, middle-, or high-income countries. For those living in high-income countries but performing burn care, teaching, or other volunteering efforts in low- or middle-income countries, the data review provided by Peck in this article will come as no surprise. For those restricting their health care delivery to high-income countries, a snapshot into some of the economic and racial differences will be enlightening. For those in a position to fund burn outreach and prevention programs, this review provides a nice 10 000-foot overview of some of the drawbacks to current data and knowledge about burn care. Peck eloquently and simply points out the impact of burn care and burn prevention programs in countries of various incomes. Knowledge of epidemiology in burn care can guide prevention programs, the only sure way to lessen the impact of burns in the global community.

B. A. Latenser, MD, FACS

Gastric Feedings Effectively Prophylax Against Upper Gastrointestinal Hemorrhage in Burn Patients

Yenikomshian H, Reiss M, Nabavian R, et al (Keck School of Medicine Univ of Southern California, Los Angeles, CA)

J Burn Care Res 32:263-268, 2011

The purpose of this study was to examine the effectiveness of gastric feeding in prevention of upper gastrointestinal (GI) hemorrhage. A retrospective chart review of 50 consecutive burn intensive care unit patients with admission dates from January 1, 2005, to December 31, 2007, was conducted. Five of 50 patients (10%) developed GI hemorrhage. Three men of 36 developed a GI hemorrhage (8%) compared with 2 of 14 women (14%). Patients who developed hemorrhage had a higher abbreviated burn severity index score of 11 compared with the control group of 9 and having a higher mortality rate of 80% compared with controls of 27%. Those patients who developed abdominal compartment syndrome were more likely to develop GI hemorrhage (40% rate compared with 4% in patients who did not develop abdominal compartment syndrome). Of 13 patients who were not tolerating their tube feed at some point during treatment, 4 developed hemorrhage (31%), whereas only 1 patient who was tolerating his or her tube feed developed hemorrhage (3%). Three of 19 (16%) patients on proton pump inhibitor prophylaxis developed a GI hemorrhage compared with 2 of 31 (6%) of patients who were not undergoing prophylaxis. Because of the potential side effects of proton pump inhibitor prophylaxis, the authors believe that when tolerated, gastric feedings should be the standard prophylaxis to prevent upper gastrointestinal hemorrhage. Acid suppression therapy may only be necessary for patients who are not tolerating their tube feeds, have other abdominal pathologies, or with a previous history of peptic ulcer disease.

▶ Stress gastritis and gastrointestinal (GI) bleeding used to be frequent complications in patients with severe thermal injury. In days of yore, it was not unusual for those of us caring for burns to perform major gastric surgery in most patients with severe burns. Once H2 blockers and proton pump inhibitors (PPI) became a routine part of burn critical care, any kind of stress gastritis or upper GI bleeding became a thing of the past. Side effects of these medications, including the possibility of gastric bacterial overgrowth and possible pneumonia from aspiration, have led some to question regarding their rather ubiquitous use. One theory is that early feeding into the stomach obviates the need for H2 blockers or PPI. In this study, patients fed into the stomach developed upper GI bleeding at the same rates with or without PPI. Patients not on PPI were started on PPI if they developed an upper GI bleed. The authors conclude that enteral feeds are an effective and easy way to prevent GI bleeding without the risks associated with PPIs.

Although I think the authors may be correct in their assertion, this study does not support their claim. This study found an alarmingly high rate of upper GI bleeding (10%) in the study population, which was not prospective or randomized, and the sample size was small. The high mortality rate in the group developing upper GI bleeding is not controlled for by the authors. Another alarming finding is the unacceptably high rate of abdominal compartment syndrome (4/50 patients) in this study. The effect of abdominal compartment syndrome (ACS) on the study outcomes is unknown. The mortality rate was high in those patients with severe burn injuries, who may have succumbed to their injuries too early in their course to develop GI bleeding. In summary, early tube feedings may prophylax against upper GI bleeding in burn patients, but this study does not adequately make that case.

B. A. Latenser, MD, FACS

Early Glycemic Control in Critically Ill Patients With Burn Injury

Murphy CV, Coffey R, Cook CH, et al (The Ohio State Univ Med Ctr, Columbus)
J Burn Care Res 32:583-590, 2011

Glucose management in patients with burn injury is often difficult because of their hypermetabolic state with associated hyperglycemia, hyperinsulinemia, and insulin resistance. Recent studies suggest that time to glycemic control is associated with improved outcomes. The authors sought to determine the influence of early glycemic control on the outcomes of critically ill patients with burn injury. A retrospective analysis was performed at the Ohio State University Medical Center. Patients hospitalized with burn injury were enrolled if they were admitted to the intensive care unit between March 1, 2006, and February 28, 2009. Early glycemic control was defined as the achievement of a mean daily blood glucose of ≤150 mg/dl for at least two consecutive days by postburn day 3. Forty-six patients made up the study cohort with 26 achieving early glycemic control and 20 who did not. The two groups were similar at baseline with regard to age, pre-existing diabetes, APACHE II score and burn size and depth. There were no differences in number of surgical interventions, infectious complications, or length of stay between patients who achieved or failed early glycemic control. Failure of early glycemic control was, however, associated with significantly higher mortality both by univariate (35.0 vs 7.7%, $P = .03$) and multivariate analyses (hazard ratio 6.754 [1.16–39.24], $P = .03$) adjusting for age, TBSA, and inhalation injury. Failure to achieve early glycemic control in patients with burn injury is associated with an increased risk of mortality. However, further prospective controlled trials are needed to establish causality of this association.

▶ Hyperglycemia in critically burned patients has come under increasing scrutiny over the last decade. The landmark van den Berghe article in 2001 regarding the benefits of tight glycemic control in critically ill patients did not include burn patients, and many subsequent articles have likewise excluded burn patients. Follow-on studies focusing on burn patients rather than the intensive care unit population have examined the effect of glycemic control on many facets of burn care, including skin graft take rates, donor site healing, remote site infections, and hospital length of stays. Some articles even discussed how to implement a strict glycemic control protocol in a burn center. However, none of these studies found an effect on mortality rates related to glucose management. Although small and retrospective in nature, this study adds another bit of data that the current glucose management protocols in most burn centers are of benefit to patient outcomes. However, the question of what the optimal glucose level might be has not been answered by this study. The higher mortality rate in patients who did not achieve early glycemic control (33% vs 7.7%) when compared with patients who did achieve early control is impressive. I agree with the authors that a retrospective study cannot determine causality. This topic would be an excellent one for a prospective, multicenter, randomized study performed through the American Burn Association Burn Science Advisory Panel.

B. A. Latenser, MD, FACS

9 Trauma and Overdose

Development and Testing of Low-Volume Hyperoncotic, Hyperosmotic Spray-Dried Plasma for the Treatment of Trauma-Associated Coagulopathy

Shuja F, Finkelstein RA, Fukudome E, et al (Massachusetts General Hosp/ Harvard Med School, Boston; et al)

J Trauma 70:664-671, 2011

Background.—Trauma-associated coagulopathy carries an extremely high mortality. Fresh-frozen plasma (FFP) is the mainstay of treatment; however, its availability in the battlefield is limited. We have already shown that lyophilized, freeze-dried plasma (FDP) reconstituted in its original volume can reverse trauma-associated coagulopathy. To enhance the logistical advantage (lower volume and weight), we developed and tested a hyperoncotic, hyperosmotic spray-dried plasma (SDP) product in a multiple injuries/hemorrhagic shock swine model.

Methods.—Plasma separated from fresh porcine blood was stored as FFP or preserved as FDP and SDP. In in vitro testing, SDP was reconstituted in distilled water that was either equal (1 × SDP) or one-third (3 × SDP) the original volume of FFP. Analysis included measurements of prothrombin time (PT), partial thromboplastin time (PTT), fibrinogen levels, and activity of selected clotting factors. In in vivo testing, swine were subjected to multiple injuries (femur fracture and grade V liver injury) and hemorrhagic shock (60% arterial hemorrhage, with the "lethal triad" of acidosis, coagulopathy, and hypothermia) and were treated with FFP, FDP, or 3 × SDP ($n = 4-5$/group). Coagulation profiles (PT, PTT, and thromboelastography) were measured at baseline, post-shock, post-crystalloid, treatment (M_0), and during 4 hours of monitoring (M_{1-4}).

Results.—In vitro testing revealed that clotting factors were preserved after spray drying. The coagulation profiles of FFP and 1 × SDP were similar, with 3 × SDP showing a prolonged PT/PTT. Multiple injuries/ hemorrhagic shock produced significant coagulopathy, and 3 × SDP infusion was as effective as FFP and FDP in reversing it.

Conclusion.—Plasma can be spray dried and reconstituted to one-third of its original volume without compromising the coagulation properties in vivo. This shelf-stable, low-volume, hyperoncotic, hyperosmotic plasma is a logistically attractive option for the treatment of trauma-associated coagulopathy in austere environments, such as a battlefield.

▶ Early coagulopathy is a frequent source of morbidity and mortality in severely injured patients. The components are hemodilution, hypothermia, acidosis, and clotting factor consumption. A common denominator is soft-tissue injury.[1,2]

These authors have developed a plasma product for use in resuscitation, which can be rapidly reconstituted and stored at room temperature for extended periods of time. The volume of material is smaller than traditional fresh frozen plasma and features ABO universality and viral inactivation. They argue that protein viability is better maintained with the spray-drying process than the freezing used in blood banks today.

This work in a large animal model suggests the potential for this product. However, additional testing is clearly necessary. I note that the animal preparation used does not truly replicate the coagulopathic injured patient. The component of soft-tissue injury in this model is relatively small. Shock is secondary to bleeding as in a Wiggers preparation.

This is intriguing material. We have much more to learn.

D. J. Dries, MSE, MD

References

1. Brohi K, Singh J, Heron M, Coats T. Acute traumatic coagulopathy. *J Trauma.* 2003;54:1127-1130.
2. Dries DJ. The contemporary role of blood products and components used in trauma resuscitation. *Scand J Trauma Resusc Emerg Med.* 2010;18:63.

Does Temporary Chest Wall Closure With or Without Chest Packing Improve Survival for Trauma Patients in Shock After Emergent Thoracotomy?

Lang JL, Gonzalez RP, Aldy KN, et al (Univ of Texas-Southwestern Med Ctr, Dallas; Univ of South Alabama Med Ctr, Mobile)
J Trauma 70:705-709, 2011

Background.—Many surgeons avoid the damage-control techniques of intrathoracic packing and temporary chest wall closure after thoracotomy for trauma because of concerns about packing's effects on intrathoracic pressure and infectious risks. We hypothesized that temporary chest closure with or without intrathoracic packing (TCC-P) as a method of thoracic damage control would yield higher than expected survival rates for trauma thoracotomy patients with metabolic exhaustion, whereas traditional definitive chest closure (DEF) would exhibit predicted survival rates.

Methods.—This was a retrospective cohort study by two urban Level I trauma centers on patients who (1) underwent emergent thoracotomy for trauma, (2) received ≥10 units (U) packed red blood cells and/or sustained a cardiac arrest before starting chest closure, and (3) survived to intensive care unit arrival. Demographic/physiologic data, chest closure method, and thoracic complications were gathered. Trauma injury severity scores (TRISS) were used to calculate survival probability for TCC-P and DEF. Nonparametric statistics were used for all comparisons. All values are expressed as medians and interquartile ranges (IQR).

Results.—Sixty-one patients met inclusion criteria. Both TCC-P (n = 17) and DEF (n = 44) were severely injured (ISS = 35 [IQR, 25–42] vs. 29 [IQR 19–45] and packed red blood cells = 16.5 U [IQR, 12.3–25.5 U] vs. 15 U [IQR, 11–23 U], respectively; p = ns). Patient demographics were similar except for the findings that the TCC-P cohort had higher rates of cardiac arrest before starting chest closure (TCC-P 82% vs. DEF 48%, $p = 0.04$), significantly more severe abdominal injuries, and less severe head injuries than the DEF group. No significant differences were observed in survival of the overall samples (TCC-P = 47% vs. DEF = 57%), nor for observed: expected (O:E) survival ratio in 13 patients with TCC-P and 30 with DEF meeting criteria for TRISS calculation (TCC-P O:E, 46%:39%; DEF O:E, 53%:57%). No significant differences were found for TCC-P and DEF thoracic infectious (24% vs. 25%) or hemorrhagic (18% vs. 14%) complications. Surprisingly, peak inspiratory pressures on intensive care unit arrival were markedly better after TCC-P (20 cm H_2O [IQR, 18–31 cm H_2O]) than after DEF (32.5 cm H_2O [IQR, 28–37.5 cm H_2O], $p = 0.003$).

Conclusion.—Concerns about TCC-P are not borne out as thoracic infection rates are unaffected and peak pressures are actually lower, possibly due to greater pleural volume from an open chest wall and skin-only closure. However, no significant survival benefit was seen with TCC-P.

▶ This is a retrospective cohort of patients from 2 trauma centers sustaining shock frequently associated with thoracic trauma. We are not given specifics on injury. A nonspecific scoring system (Injury Severity Score) is presented. One remarkable difference is the greatly increased number of cardiac arrests in patients receiving chest packing. In many settings, cardiac arrest is a marker for adverse outcome. That the experimental group with a significantly greater incidence of cardiac arrest had comparable survival with standard care argues for the viability of this approach.[1-4]

Another obvious observation is the retrospective nature of this data and the lack of specified criteria for choosing packing or definitive closure. It is very encouraging to see the lack of hemorrhagic or infectious thoracic complications when packing is used.

D. J. Dries, MSE, MD

References

1. Seamon MJ, Shiroff AM, Franco M, et al. Emergency department thoracotomy for penetrating injuries of the heart and great vessels: an appraisal of 283 consecutive cases from two urban trauma centers. *J Trauma.* 2009;67:1250-1258.
2. Branney SW, Moore EE, Feldhaus KM, et al. Critical analysis of two decades of experience with postinjury emergency department thoracotomy in a regional trauma center. *J Trauma.* 1998;45:87-95.
3. Seamon MJ, Fisher CA, Gaughan JP, Kulp H, Dempsey DT, Goldberg AJ. Emergency department thoracotomy: survival of the least expected. *World J Surg.* 2008;32:604-612.
4. Seamon MJ, Pathak AS, Bradley KM, et al. Emergency department thoracotomy: still useful after abdominal exsanguination? *J Trauma.* 2008;64:1-8.

Glasgow Coma Scale and laboratory markers are superior to COHb in predicting CO intoxication severity

Grieb G, Simons D, Schmitz L, et al (Hosp of the RWTH Aachen Univ, Germany)

Burns 37:610-615, 2011

Carbon monoxide (CO) intoxications can affect several organ systems and lead to coma or death in severe cases. To date, COHb is routinely used as a marker for detecting CO intoxication. In this retrospective study, we investigated 173 patients admitted with CO intoxication to our intensive care unit (ICU) over a period of 8 years. Standardised blood tests, chest X-ray and neurological status evaluation were performed on admission and throughout the inpatient treatment. The duration of inpatient treatment was considered to be an indication of the severity of CO-related illness. Interestingly, the data did not reveal a significant correlation between initial COHb level and the duration of inpatient treatment. Instead, a significant inverse correlation was found between the initial Glasgow Coma Scale and the duration of inpatient treatment. Furthermore, significant correlations were found between the duration of inpatient treatment and the occurrence of elevated leucocyte numbers, elevated C-reactive protein (CRP) serum concentrations and the presence of lung infiltrates. In conclusion, we postulate that clinical parameters, such as the Glasgow Coma Scale and the laboratory markers CRP and leucocyte count are adequate supportive tools for evaluating the severity of CO-related illness, and further, that the measurement of COHb alone is insufficient for this purpose.

▶ The authors point out, appropriately, that we can learn more about the impact of carbon monoxide (CO) intoxication than can be determined by a simple determination of carboxyhemoglobin level.[1,2] The Glasgow Coma Scale (GCS) is a valuable, ubiquitous, clinical assessment tool, whereas C-reactive protein and leukocyte count are readily available. Ultimately, I believe that care of the patient with CO intoxication is based on clinical presentation (better understood with GCS) rather than a carboxyhemoglobin level.

There are a number of limitations to this study because of its retrospective nature, which are worthy of comment. First, most patients had only 1 day of inpatient treatment. Thus, a wide range of injury acuity is not present. Second, the duration of inpatient treatment was considered to be a surrogate for severity of carbon monoxide–related illness. Did other factors contribute to length of stay? What about comorbid conditions? Not all patients had the same degree of care. Fifty-six patients in this series were treated with hyperbaric oxygen. What if all patients had either received hyperbaric oxygen or none had been given hyperbaric oxygen? Finally, patients who did not recover to meet stated discharge criteria were excluded from this study. We are not told how many patients were excluded. Only 17 patients demonstrated "massive neurological disorder or coma." Thus, severity of disease was not great in this population.

As the authors appropriately indicate, further prospective data are needed. I commend them for suggesting additional clinical markers of injury severity and emphasizing the importance of clinical function in the triage of the patient with CO intoxication.

D. J. Dries, MSE, MD

References

1. Weaver LK. Carbon monoxide poisoning. *N Engl J Med.* 2009;360:1217-1225.
2. Kealey GP. Carbon monoxide toxicity. *J Burn Care Res.* 2009;30:146-147.

Retrospective Review of Lumbosacral Dissociations in Blast Injuries

Helgeson MD, Lehman RA Jr, Cooper P, et al (Walter Reed Natl Military Med Ctr, Washington, DC; Walter Reed Army Med Ctr, Washington, DC; et al)

Spine 36:E469-E475, 2011

Study Design.—Retrospective review of medical records and radiographs.

Objective.—We assessed the clinical outcomes of lumbosacral dissociation (LSD) after traumatic, combat-related injuries, and to review our management of these distinct injuries and report our preliminary follow-up.

Summary of Background Data.—LSD injuries are an anatomic separation of the pelvis from the spinal column, and are the result of high-energy trauma. A relative increase in these injuries has been seen in young healthy combat casualties subjected to high-energy blast trauma.

Methods.—We performed a retrospective review of inpatient/outpatient medical records and radiographs for all patients treated at our institution with combat-related lumbosacral dissociations. Twenty-three patients met inclusion criteria of combat-related lumbosacral dissociations with one-year follow-up. Patients were treated as follows: no fixation (9), sacroiliac screw fixation (8), posterior spinal fusion (5) and sacral plate (1). All patients with radiographic evidence of a zone III sacral fracture, in addition to associated lumbar fractures indicating loss of the iliolumbar ligamentous complex integrity were included.

Results.—In 15 patients, the sacral fracture were an H or U type zone III fracture, whereas in the remaining nine, the sacral fracture was severely comminuted and unable to classify (six open fractures). There was no difference in visual analog scale (VAS) between treatment modalities. Two open injuries had residual infections. One patient treated with an L4-ilium posterior spinal fusion with instrumentation required instrumentation removal for infection. At a mean follow-up of 1.71 years (range, 1–4.5), 11 patients (48%) still reported residual pain and the mean VAS at latest follow-up was 1.7 (range, 0–7).

Conclusion.—Operative stabilization promoted healing and earlier mobilization, but carries a high-postoperative risk of infection. Nonoperative

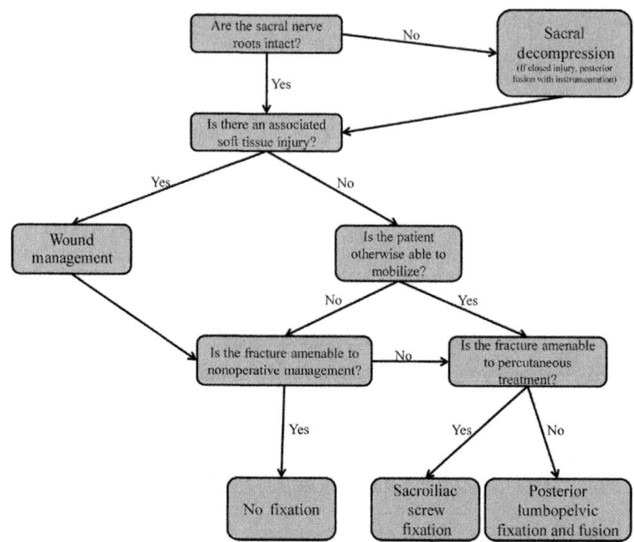

FIGURE 1.—Treatment algorithm used at our institution for lumbosacral dissociations. (Reprinted from Helgeson MD, Lehman RA Jr, Cooper P, et al. Retrospective review of lumbosacral dissociations in blast injuries. *Spine*. 2011;36:E469-E475, with permission from Lippincott Williams & Wilkins.)

management should be considered in patients whose comorbidities prevent safe stabilization (Fig 1).

▶ This is a small series of high-energy injuries.[1] There are a number of lessons to be learned from it, but the limitations of a small retrospective series cannot be ignored.

The first observation is that specific injuries did not dictate specific treatment modalities in this series. Second, open wounds bring significant infection risk. Even with repeated debridement of open wounds, operative stabilization was associated with a 3-fold increase in infectious risk compared with wounds that were closed. Third, early stabilization did not appear to confer recovery benefit. This seems counterintuitive and may be explained by a relatively small series of cases. Finally, hardware can erode through thin soft tissue and poorly healed wounds in malnourished patients. Aggressive nutrition support is vital.

The most important clinical distinctions were overall functional status (immobile patients could consolidate fractures in 3 months) and the quality of soft tissue, as the infection risk is real (Fig 1).

D. J. Dries, MSE, MD

Reference

1. Schildhauer TA, Bellabarba C, Nork SE, Barei DP, Routt ML Jr, Chapman JR. Decompression and lumbopelvic fixation for sacral fracture-dislocations with spino-pelvic dissociation. *J Orthop Trauma*. 2006;20:447-457.

Prospective Identification of Patients at Risk for Massive Transfusion: An Imprecise Endeavor

Vandromme MJ, Griffin RL, McGwin G Jr, et al (Univ of Alabama at Birmingham School of Medicine)

Am Surg 77:155-161, 2011

Most retrospective studies evaluating fresh-frozen plasma: packed red blood cell ratios in trauma patients requiring massive transfusion (MT) are limited by survival bias. As prospective resource-intensive studies are being designed to better evaluate resuscitation strategies, it is imperative that patients with a high likelihood of MT are identified early. The objective of this study was to develop a predictive model for MTin civilian trauma patients. Patients admitted to the University of Alabama at Birmingham Trauma Center from January 2005 to December 2007 were selected. Admission clinical measurements, including blood lactate 5 mMol/L or greater, heart rate greater than 105 beats/min, international normalized ratio greater than 1.5, hemoglobin 11 g/dL or less, and systolic blood pressure less than 110 mmHg, were used to create a predictive model. Sensitivity (Sens), specificity (Spec), positive predictive value (PPV), and negative predictive value (NPV) were calculated for all possible combinations of clinical measurements as well as each measure individually. A total of 6638 patients were identified, of whom 158 (2.4%) received MT. The best-fit predictive model included three or more positive clinical measures (Sens: 53%, Spec: 98%, PPV: 33%, NPV: 99%). There was increased PPV when all clinical measurements were positive (Sens: 9%, Spec: 100%, PPV: 86%, NPV: 98%). All combinations or clinical measures alone yielded lower predictive probability. Using these emergency department clinical measures, a predictive model to successfully identify civilian trauma patients at risk for MT was not able to be constructed. Given prospective identification of patients at risk for MT remains an imprecise undertaking, appropriate resources to support these efforts will need to be allocated for the completion of these studies (Tables 2 and 4).

▶ One of the hot topics in trauma care is provision of high fresh frozen plasma to red blood cell ratios in patients receiving massive transfusion, now defined as the administration of 10 units of packed red blood cells per 24 hours. Early administration of massive transfusion is associated with optimal resuscitation outcomes, although many studies suggesting this result are limited by survival bias. A large multicenter trial of massive transfusion is now underway. The prevailing dilemma is rapid identification of patients requiring this therapy.[1-3]

The University of Alabama group developed a model with retrospective data that was then tested prospectively. Criteria used, as reflected in the abstract, can readily be obtained in the emergency department.

The authors were able to identify patients who did not require massive transfusion, but rapid identification of those requiring this therapy was more difficult. An attractive analysis was also performed comparing this work to other parameters that have been proposed. Many of these parameters are flawed in that

TABLE 2.—Odds Ratios*† (ORs) and Associated 95% Confidence Intervals (95% CIs) for the Association between Admission Clinical Characteristics and the Need for 10 or More Units of Packed Red Blood Cells within 24 Hours of Admission

Variables	Development Period‡ OR (95% CI)	P	Validation Period§ OR (95% CI)	P
Blood lactate 5 mMol/L or greater	3.13 (1.96–5.00)	<0.0001	3.57 (1.89–6.67)	<0.0001
Heart rate greater than 105 beats/min	3.55 (2.22–5.66)	<0.0001	3.51 (1.81–6.80)	0.0002
Hemoglobin 11 g/dL or less	10.12 (6.01–17.04)	<0.0001	2.20 (1.21–3.99)	0.01
INR greater than 1.5	5.61 (3.28–9.61)	<0.0001	44.89 (21.44–94.00)	<0.0001
SBP less than 110 mmHg	2.08 (1.27–3.43)	0.0039	35.06 (19.06–64.47)	<0.0001

INR, international normalized ratio; SBP, systolic blood pressure.
*Based on weighted data.
†Adjusted for other variables listed.
‡Patients admitted between January 2005 and January 22, 2007.
§Patients admitted between January 23, 2007 and December 2008.

TABLE 4.—Comparison of MT Prediction Formulas, Factors Used for Prediction, and Corresponding Statistics of Predictability

	Factors Used	AUC	Other Measures of Predictability
Current study	Hb, SBP, INR, BL, HR	0.90	Sensitivity 53% Specificity 98% PPV 33% NPV 99%
Yucel et al.,[19] "TASH" Score	Hb, BE, SBP, HR, FAST, gender, and presence extremity injury	0.89	
McLaughlin et al.[13]	HR, SBP, Hct, and pH	0.86	Sensitivity 59% Specificity 77% PPV 66% NPV 72%
Nunez et al.,[18] "ABC" Score	SBP, HR, FAST, and penetrating mechanism of injury	0.87	Sensitivity 75% Specificity 86% Correctly classified 84%

MT, massive transfusion; AUC, area under the receiver operator curve; Hb, hemoglobin; SBP, systolic blood pressure; INR, international normalized ratio; BL, blood lactate; HR, heart rate; BE, base excess; FAST, Focused Assessment Sonography in Trauma; Hct, hematocrit, PPV, positive predictive value; NPV, negative predictive value.
Editor's Note: Please refer to original journal article for full references.

calculation is difficult or does not reflect parameters that are immediately available to the clinician. This study, although carefully designed, may be fatally flawed by a limited event rate. For example, in the validation cohort, only 9 patients had all 5 positive predictors.

Two other interesting observations can be made. The odds ratios as reflected in the first of the two tables retained from this article changed significantly for some variables between the development and validation periods. Second, the authors provide a comparison of massive transfusion prediction formulas in the second table retained from this article.

D. J. Dries, MSE, MD

References

1. McLaughlin DF, Niles SE, Salinas J, et al. A predictive model for massive transfusion in combat casualty patients. *J Trauma.* 2008;64:S57-S63.
2. Nunez TC, Voskresensky IV, Dossett LA, Shinall R, Dutton WD, Cotton BA. Early prediction of massive transfusion in trauma: simple as ABC (assessment of blood consumption)? *J Trauma.* 2009;66:346-352.
3. Yücel N, Lefering R, Maegele M, et al. Trauma Associated Severe Hemorrhage (TASH)-Score: probability of mass transfusion as surrogate for life threatening hemorrhage after multiple trauma. *J Trauma.* 2006;60:1228-1237.

Effect Of Trauma Center Status on 30-Day Outcomes After Emergency General Surgery

Ingraham AM, Cohen ME, Raval MV, et al (American College of Surgeons, Chicago, IL; et al)

J Am Coll Surg 212:277-286, 2011

Background.—Trauma surgeons increasingly care for emergency general surgery (EGS) patients. The extent to which trauma center (TC) performance improvement translates into improved quality for EGS is unknown. We hypothesized that EGS outcomes in TCs would be similar to outcomes in non-trauma centers (NTC); failure to support our hypothesis suggests that the effects of trauma performance improvement have extended beyond trauma patients.

Study Design.—We retrospectively studied EGS procedures at TCs versus NTCs among American College of Surgeons National Surgical Quality Improvement Program participants (2005–2008). Thirty-day outcomes were overall morbidity, serious morbidity, and mortality. TC versus NTC outcomes were compared using regression modeling, observed-to-expected (O/E) ratios (among hospitals submitting ≥20 EGS procedures), and outlier status (hospitals whose O/E confidence interval excludes 1.0).

Results.—Of 68,003 patients at 222 hospitals, 42,264 (62.2%) were treated at 121 TCs; 25,739 (37.8%) were treated at 101 NTCs. TCs had significantly higher overall morbidity (21.4% versus 17.2%; $p < 0.0001$), serious morbidity (15.8% versus 12.3%; $p < 0.0001$), and mortality (6.4% versus 4.8%; $p < 0.0001$) than NTCs. On adjusted analyses, TC status was a significant predictor of overall morbidity (odds ratio = 1.11; 95% CI, 1.01–1.21), but not serious morbidity (odds ratio = 1.08; 95% CI, 0.98–1.19) or mortality (odds ratio = 0.92; 95% CI, 0.82–1.04). Among 211 hospitals assigned O/E ratios, TCs were more likely, although not significantly so, to be high outliers for overall morbidity (7.6% versus 4.3%; $p = 0.017$), serious morbidity (5.1% versus 4.3%; $p = 0.034$), and mortality (3.4% versus 2.2%; $p > 0.099$).

Conclusions.—Although overall morbidity tended to favor NTCs, mortality was no different. This suggests that the trauma performance improvement processes have not been applied to EGS patients, despite

TABLE 3.—Comparison of 30-Day Outcomes after Emergency General Surgery Procedures at Trauma Centers versus Non-Trauma Centers Among 222 American College of Surgeons National Surgical Quality Improvement Program Hospitals

Outcomes	Trauma Centers (n = 42,264) N	%	Non-Trauma Centers (n = 25,739) n	%	p Value
Overall morbidity	9,054	21.4	4,425	17.2	<0.0001
Serious morbidity	6,694	15.8	3,160	12.3	<0.0001
Mortality	2,687	6.4	1,242	4.8	<0.0001
Individual morbidities					
Superficial SSI	1,727	4.1	900	3.5	0.0001
Deep SSI	479	1.13	244	0.95	0.02
Organ space SSI	1,283	3.0	574	2.2	<0.0001
Wound disruption	635	1.5	268	1.0	<0.0001
Pneumonia	1,896	4.5	797	3.1	<0.0001
Unplanned intubation	1,253	3.0	548	2.1	<0.0001
Pulmonary embolism	220	0.5	106	0.4	0.05
Fail to wean	2,715	6.4	1,077	4.2	<0.0001
Renal failure	692	1.6	368	1.4	0.03
Urinary tract infection	1,082	2.6	424	1.7	<0.0001
Neurological event	280	0.7	135	0.5	0.03
Deep vein thrombosis	278	0.7	120	0.5	0.002
Sepsis or septic shock	3,706	8.8	1,789	7.0	<0.0001
Bleeding requiring transfusion	518	1.2	220	0.9	<0.0001
Cardiac arrest	494	1.2	213	0.8	<0.0001
Neurologic event	280	0.7	135	0.5	0.03

A hospital was categorized as a trauma center if the hospital was verified or designated as a Level I or II center by either the American College of Surgeons or regional authorities. Level III and IV centers as well as all hospitals not designated as trauma centers were categorized as non-trauma centers. Individual morbidities reaching statistical significance between emergency general surgery patients treated at trauma centers versus non-trauma centers are presented. SSI, surgical site infection.

being cared for by similar providers. Despite having processes for trauma, there remains the opportunity for quality improvement for EGS care (Table 3).

▶ This article casts doubt on the value of using a trauma center model for management of emergency general surgery.[1] By virtually every index evaluated, nontrauma hospitals were better able to manage common emergency general surgery problems than were trauma centers.

This study is done with the extensive National Surgical Quality Improvement Program database of the American College of Surgeons.[2] Thus, I believe the data are strong. The reproduced table indicates that morbidity and mortality indices favor the nontrauma hospital for the management of general surgery emergencies.

Why is this? One possibility is the lack of structure for emergency general surgery care that exists for management of nonburn trauma or burn patients.[3] These patients are followed by strict registry data collection and quality assurance programs. Second, emergency general surgery may not receive the same emphasis as injured patients do in trauma centers. Another possibility is that trauma centers are organized to provide optimal care for the most severely injured and ill patients.[4] Patients with common problems may not receive comparable rapid attention. Trauma centers also tend to care for a higher percentage of uninsured or underinsured patients. Insurance status has been linked with outcomes.

Regardless of the reason for relatively poor trauma center performance in this study, it highlights the need for improved attention to the management of emergency general surgery. The combination of emergency general surgery with trauma care, which is increasingly nonoperative, is felt to sustain the operative skills of the trauma surgeon. Optimal quality of practice for the trauma surgeon and outcomes for the emergency general surgery patient must align.

D. J. Dries, MSE, MD

References

1. Committee to Develop the Reorganized Specialty of Trauma, Surgical Critical Care, and Emergency Surgery. Acute care surgery: trauma, critical care, and emergency surgery. *J Trauma.* 2005;58:614-616.
2. MacKenzie EJ, Rivara FP, Jurkovich GJ, et al. A national evaluation of the effect of trauma-center care on mortality. *N Engl J Med.* 2006;354:366-378.
3. Utter GH, Maier RV, Rivara FP, Nathens AB. Outcomes after ruptured abdominal aortic aneurysms: the "halo effect" of trauma center designation. *J Am Coll Surg.* 2006;203:498-505.
4. Khuri SF. The NSQIP: a new frontier in surgery. *Surgery.* 2005;138:837-843.

The Evolving Management of Venous Bullet Emboli: A case series and literature review

Miller KR, Benns MV, Sciarretta JD, et al (Univ of Louisville, KY)
Injury 42:441-446, 2011

Bullet emboli are an infrequent and unique complication of penetrating trauma. Complications of venous and arterial bullet emboli can be devastating and commonly include limb-threatening ischaemia, pulmonary embolism, cardiac valvular incompetence, and cerebrovascular accidents. Bullets from penetrating wounds can gain access to the venous circulation and embolise to nearly every large vascular bed. Venous emboli are often occult phenomenon and may remain unrecognised until migration leads to vascular injury or flow obstruction with resultant oedema. The majority of arterial emboli present early with end-organ or limb ischaemia. We describe four separate cases involving venous bullet embolism and the subsequent management of each case. Review of the literature focusing on the reported management of these injuries, comparison of techniques of management, as well as the evolving role of endovascular techniques in the management of bullet emboli is provided.

► The authors clearly demonstrate that venous bullet emboli, while infrequent, can now be addressed with endovascular techniques. Simple expectant management is no longer the standard of care.

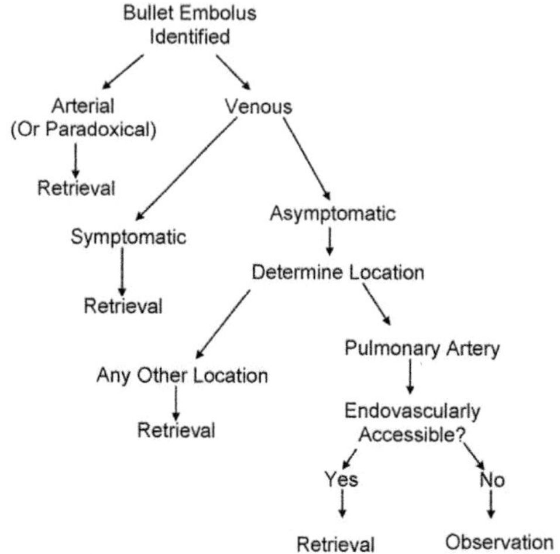

In the algorithm, the authors suggest that an endovascular approach may also be appropriate for emboli in the pulmonary arterial bed (Box 1). I doubt that many lesions in the pulmonary arteries will be accessible to endovascular technique. The authors have not shown the feasibility of this approach in this brief case series. Bullets removed here come from the great veins, atrial appendage, and right ventricle.

I also note that the missiles retrieved were obtained within days of injury. The authors have not demonstrated the effectiveness of endovascular technique when a missile has been in place for an extended period. Projectiles that have been in place over longer periods of time may be more difficult to remove using the endovascular approach. The authors do provide an extensive series of case reports in which venous emboli are addressed. In only one of these case reports was endovascular extraction from the pulmonary artery reported.[1] (The title of this article mentions endovascular management of bullet embolization to the heart.)

D. J. Dries, MSE, MD

Reference

1. Chen JJ, Mirvis SE, Shanmuganathan K. MDCT diagnosis and endovascular management of bullet embolization to the heart. *Emerg Radiol.* 2007;14:127-130.

Epidemiology and risk factors of sepsis after multiple trauma: An analysis of 29,829 patients from the Trauma Registry of the German Society for Trauma Surgery

Wafaisade A, Trauma Registry of the German Society for Trauma Surgery (Univ of Witten/Herdecke, Cologne, Germany; et al)

Crit Care Med 39:621-628, 2011

Objectives.—The objectives of this study were 1) to assess potential changes in the incidence and outcome of sepsis after multiple trauma in Germany between 1993 and 2008 and 2) to evaluate independent risk factors for posttraumatic sepsis.

Design.—Retrospective analysis of a nationwide, population-based prospective database, the Trauma Registry of the German Society for Trauma Surgery.

Setting.—A total of 166 voluntarily participating trauma centers (levels I-III).

Patients.—Patients registered in the Trauma Registry of the German Society for Trauma Surgery between 1993 and 2008 with complete data sets who presented with a relevant trauma load (Injury Severity Score of ≥9) and were admitted to an intensive care unit (n = 29,829).

Interventions.—None.

Measurements and Main Results.—Over the 16-yr study period, 10.2% (3,042 of 29,829) of multiply injured patients developed sepsis during their hospital course. Annual data were summarized into four subperiods: 1993–1996, 1997–2000, 2001–2004, and 2005–2008. The incidences of sepsis for the four subperiods were 14.8%, 12.5%, 9.4%, and 9.7% ($p < .0001$), respectively. In-hospital mortality for all trauma patients decreased for the respective subperiods (16.9%, 16.0%, 13.7%, and 11.9%; $p < .0001$). For the subgroup of patients with sepsis, the mortality rates were 16.2%, 21.5%, 22.0%, and 18.2% ($p = .054$), respectively. The following independent risk factors for posttraumatic sepsis were calculated from a multivariate logistic regression analysis: male gender, age, preexisting medical condition, Glasgow Coma Scale Score of ≤8 at scene, Injury Severity Score, Abbreviated Injury Scale$_{THORAX}$ Score of ≥3, number of injuries, number of red blood cell units transfused, number of operative procedures, and laparotomy.

Conclusions.—The incidence of sepsis decreased significantly over the study period; however, in this decade the incidence remained unchanged. Although overall mortality from multiple trauma has declined significantly since 1993, there has been no significant decrease of mortality in the subgroup of septic trauma patients. Thus, sepsis has remained a challenging complication after trauma during the past 2 decades. Recognition of the identified risk factors may guide early diagnostic workup and help to reduce septic complications after multiple trauma (Figs 1-3).

▶ This is an impressive review of data entered in the German Trauma Registry. There are 2 important messages. First, although improvement is seen in

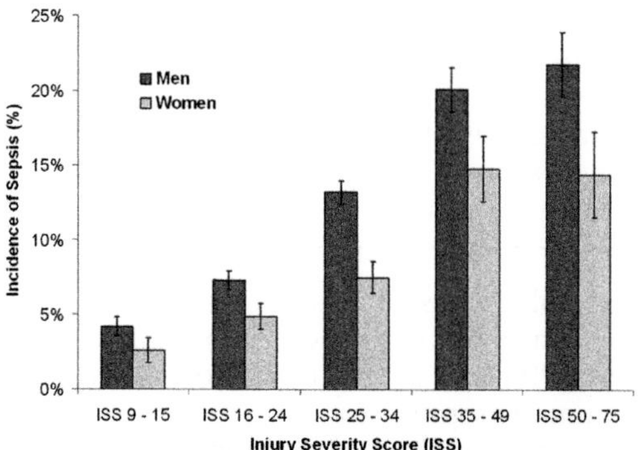

FIGURE 1.—Incidence of sepsis in multiple trauma patients, grouped for male and female gender and stratified for Injury Severity Score subgroups (n = 29,829; 1993–2008); $p < .0001$. Error bars represent 95% confidence intervals. (Reprinted from Wafaisade A, Trauma Registry of the German Society for Trauma Surgery. Epidemiology and risk factors of sepsis after multiple trauma: an analysis of 29,829 patients from the Trauma Registry of the German Society for Trauma Surgery. *Crit Care Med.* 2011;39:621-628, with permission from the Society of Critical Care Medicine and Lippincott Williams & Wilkins.)

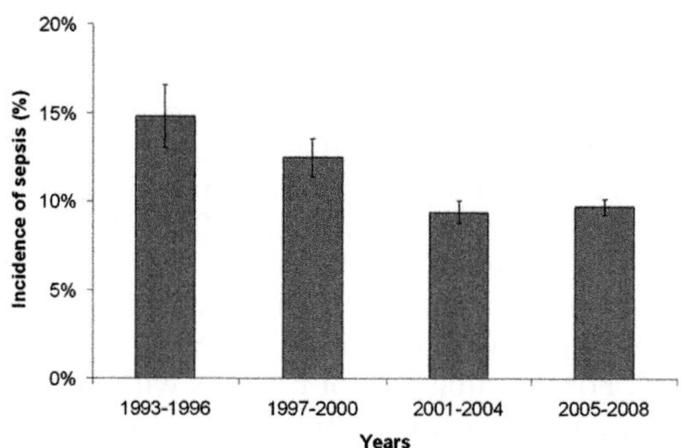

FIGURE 2.—Incidence of sepsis after multiple trauma from 1993 to 2008 (n = 29,829); $p < .0001$. Linear regression analysis showed a decrease of −0.46% per year for sepsis incidence. Error bars represent 95% confidence intervals. (Reprinted from Wafaisade A, Trauma Registry of the German Society for Trauma Surgery. Epidemiology and risk factors of sepsis after multiple trauma: an analysis of 29,829 patients from the Trauma Registry of the German Society for Trauma Surgery. *Crit Care Med.* 2011;39:621-628, with permission from the Society of Critical Care Medicine and Lippincott Williams & Wilkins.)

outcome with injury, the outcome of sepsis following injury is unchanged. Second, although multiple factors associated with sepsis following trauma are identified, our data are not sufficiently sophisticated to identify specific infectious complications and associate them with specific patterns of injury.[1,2]

There are a number of reasons for caution in review of these data. First, although the patients studied were placed in the registry between 1993 and 2008, the vast majority of patients were enrolled between 2005 and 2008. The quality of earlier data may be questionable. Second, the authors suggest identification of risk factors to guide early diagnostic workup and reduce septic complications after multiple trauma. The massive data included here do not

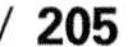

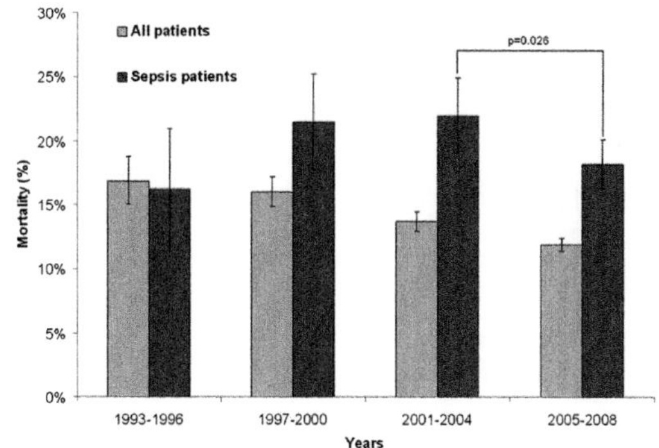

FIGURE 3.—Mortality in all trauma patients (*light gray columns;* n = 29,829; $p < .0001$) and in the subgroup of trauma patients who developed sepsis (*dark gray columns;* n = 3042; $p = .054$) from 1993 until 2008. In patients with sepsis, differences between two subsequent periods did not reach statistical significance except for the two latest subperiods, as depicted ($p = .026$). Linear regression analyses showed a slope of −0.433% per year for overall mortality and a slope of +0.155% per year for sepsis mortality. Error bars represent 95% confidence intervals. (Reprinted from Wafaisade A, Trauma Registry of the German Society for Trauma Surgery. Epidemiology and risk factors of sepsis after multiple trauma: an analysis of 29,829 patients from the Trauma Registry of the German Society for Trauma Surgery. *Crit Care Med.* 2011;39:621-628, with permission from the Society of Critical Care Medicine and Lippincott Williams & Wilkins.)

allow this. Far too many risk factors are identified, and specific etiologies for sepsis are not discussed.

D. J. Dries, MSE, MD

References

1. Saltzherr TP, Visser A, Ponsen KJ, Luitse JS, Goslings JC. Complications in multitrauma patients in a Dutch level 1 trauma center. *J Trauma.* 2010;69:1143-1146.
2. van Ruler O, Schultz MJ, Reitsma JB, Gouma DJ, Boermeester MA. Has mortality from sepsis improved and what to expect from new treatment modalities: review of current insights. *Surg Infect (Larchmt).* 2009;10:339-348.

Epidemiology of U.K. Military Burns

Foster MA, Moledina J, Jeffery SLA (Inst of Res and Development, Birmingham, UK)

J Burn Care Res 32:415-420, 2011

The authors review the etiology of U.K. military burns in light of increasing hybrid warfare. Analysis of the nature of these injured personnel will provide commanders with the evidence to plan for on-going and future operations. Case notes of all U.K. Armed Forces burn injured patients who were evacuated to the Royal Centre for Defence Medicine were reviewed. Demographics, burn severity, pattern, and mortality details were included. There were 134 U.K. military personnel with burns requiring return to the United Kingdom during 2001–2007. The median age was 27 (20–62) years.

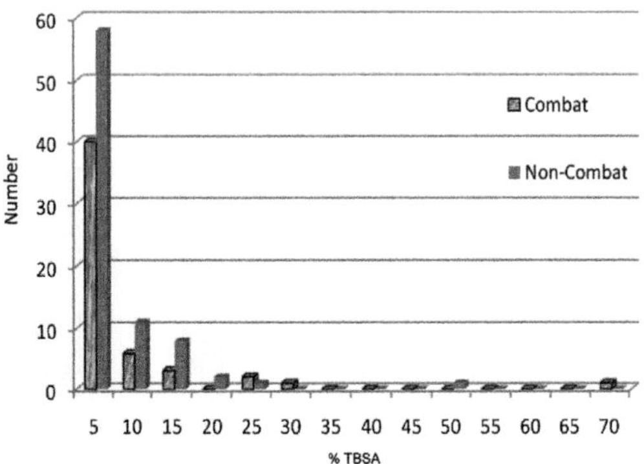

FIGURE 1.—%TBSA of combat and noncombat burns (2001–2007). (Reprinted from Foster MA, Moledina J, Jeffery SLA. Epidemiology of U.K. military burns. *J Burn Care Res.* 2011;32:415-420, with permission from the American Burn Association.)

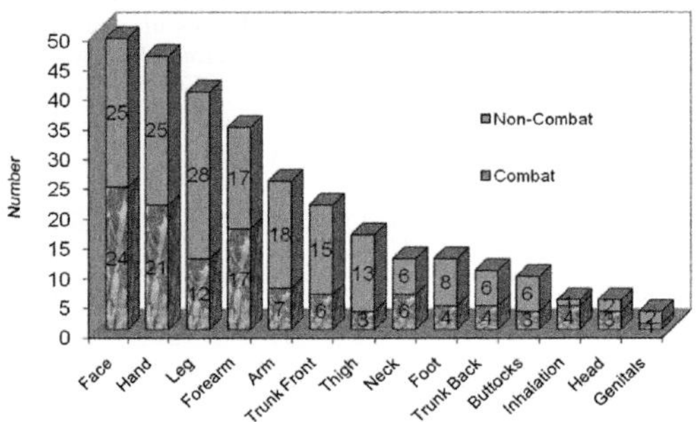

FIGURE 2.—The distribution of body area burned (2001–2007). (Reprinted from Foster MA, Moledina J, Jeffery SLA. Epidemiology of U.K. military burns. *J Burn Care Res.* 2011;32:415-420, with permission from the American Burn Association.)

Overall, 60% of burns seen were "accidental." Burning waste, misuse or disrespect of fuel, and scalds were the most prevalent noncombat burns. Areas commonly burned were the face, legs, and hands. During 2006–2007 in the two major conflicts, more than 59% (n = 36) of the burned patients evacuated to the United Kingdom were injured during combat. Burns sustained in combat represent 5.8% of all combat casualties and were commonly associated with other injuries. Improvised explosive device, minestrike, and rocket-propelled grenade were common causes. The mean TBSA affected for both groups was 5% (1–70). The majority of combat burn injuries have been small in size. Greater provision of flame retardant equipment and clothing may reduce the extent and number of combat burns in the future. The numbers of noncombat burns are being reduced by good military discipline (Figs 1 and 2, Table 2).

▶ The messages here are simple. The size and number of burns in current Middle Eastern conflicts is small.[1] However, important areas of the body are involved,

TABLE 2.—The Mechanism of Burn Separated Into Combat and Noncombat Injury During 2001–2007

Mechanism	N
Combat	
Improvised explosive device	26
Rocket propelled grenade	7
Mine strike	7
Indirect fire	6
Helicopter crash	3
Ammunition—breech explosion	2
Petrol bombs	3
Noncombat	
Scald	16
Burning rubbish	15
Electrical burns	12
Fuel misuse	9
BBQ	4
Under the influence of alcohol	4
Regimental badge branding	3
Threw lit cigarette into toilet	3
Others	14

particularly the face and hands. Thus, injury to even a small portion of the body surface area can lead to a soldier lost from combat duty. Improved combat protective gear protects the majority of the trunk and the proximal extremities.

As in other conflicts, the numbers of noncombat and combat burns are roughly comparable.[2] The majority of injuries are flash or flame burns. Scald and contact injuries are far less frequent. Of the combat injuries, improvised explosive devices cause the largest portion of insults.

D. J. Dries, MSE, MD

References

1. Kauvar DS, Wade CE, Baer DG. Burn hazards of the deployed environment in wartime: epidemiology of noncombat burns from ongoing United States military operations. *J Am Coll Surg*. 2009;209:453-460.
2. Wolf SE, Kauvar DS, Wade CE, et al. Comparison between civilian burns and combat burns from Operation Iraqi Freedom and Operation Enduring Freedom. *Ann Surg*. 2006;243:786-795.

Is pre-hospital thoracotomy necessary in the military environment?

Morrison JJ, Mellor A, Midwinter M, et al (Birmingham Res Park, UK; The James Cook Univ Hosp, Middlesbrough, UK)
Injury 42:469-473, 2011

Introduction.—Exsanguination from penetrating torso injury is a major source of mortality on the battlefield. Advanced Life Support guidelines suggest 'on-scene' thoracotomy for patients in cardiac arrest following penetrating chest trauma. This requires significant resourcing and training.

Experience from published series (31 pre-hospital thoracotomies with 3 survivors) suggests that when this manoeuvre is applied to a well selected group it is a significant and life-saving procedure. Can this be applied to military injuries?

Methods.—Over a 12 month period on Operation Herrick all patients who sustained significant thoracic trauma were retrospectively reviewed. Parameters were recorded to allow detailed analysis of injury pattern and operative management. Our main objective was to determine if an early (pre-hospital) thoracotomy would have influenced the outcome.

Results.—Over the period, 81 patients required operative intervention following thoracic trauma: 8 patients underwent emergency thoracotomy (performed as part of the resuscitation) and 14 underwent urgent thoracotomy (performed after physiology partly restored). There were 9 fatalities—7 undergoing emergency thoracotomy and 2 post-operatively from multi-organ failure. Of the 7 intra-operative deaths 4/7 patients had thoracic injury and 6/7 had additional abdominal injuries. The median predicted survival of fatalities was 2.0% using Trauma Injury Severity Scoring.

Discussion.—Emergency thoracotomy should be performed in cardiac arrest following penetrating trauma as soon as possible. Highest survival rates in both in-hospital and pre-hospital thoracotomy are found in isolated cardiac stab wounds (19.4%). Poorest survival is found in multiply, ballistic injured patients (0.7%). The latter best reflects the injury pattern

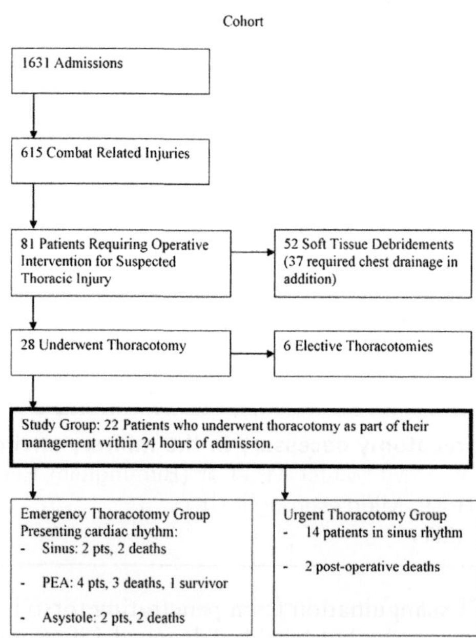

FIGURE 1.—Flow chart detailing patient cohort. (Reprinted from Morrison JJ, Mellor A, Midwinter M, et al. Is pre-hospital thoracotomy necessary in the military environment? *Injury.* 2011;42:469-473, Copyright 2011, with permission from Elsevier.)

of military patients who have cardiac arrest following penetrating torso injury.

Conclusion.—As our injury pattern suggests, any pre-hospital thoracotomy on military patients is likely to require complex intervention in very challenging environments. Our evidence does not support the notion that earlier thoracotomy could improve survival (Fig 1).

▶ The authors reveal military and civilian data to examine the role of aggressive early thoracotomy in the management of injuries where a penetrating mechanism predominates. Although civilian practice supports selective use of emergency thoracotomy, in the military setting, benefit seems unlikely.

Two factors may explain this outcome. First, the use of body armor limits torso injury to all but the most severe events. Thus, isolated or limited multiorgan injury where thoracotomy is most likely to be effective is unlikely in the military setting where multisystem trauma predominates. Second, initial care for the injured solider is frequently in an austere environment. Even if thoracotomy could be performed with some initial response, it is unlikely that resources to provide the second level of sophisticated and labor-intensive resuscitation would be immediately available.[1,2]

D. J. Dries, MSE, MD

References

1. *Advanced Trauma Life Support*, 7th ed., American College of Surgeons Committee on Trauma, 2004. American College of Surgeons, Chicago, IL.
2. Rhee PM, Acosta J, Bridgeman A, Wang D, Jordan M, Rich N. Survival after emergency department thoracotomy: review of published data from the past 25 years. *J Am Coll Surg*. 2000;190:288-298.

Topical negative pressure and military wounds—A review of the evidence

Fries CA, Jeffery SLA, Kay AR (Selly Oak Hosp, Birmingham, UK; Frenchay Hosp, Bristol, UK)

Injury 42:436-440, 2011

Background.—Topical negative pressure (TNP) has been used as a method of wound management for some years. Use of TNP is accepted best practice at Role 4. There are advocates of using TNP after initial wound surgery at Role 3 or 2E. The evidence to support forward use of TNP is not comprehensive, especially when considering this narrow cohort of patients and injury pattern. It is the aim of this review to evaluate the current evidence for the use of TNP in all wounds, and to find what evidence there is that may be applicable to military wounds.

Methods.—A literature search of Cinahl, Embase, Medline, ProQuest and the Cochrane Library was conducted; references were cross-referenced. All Randomised Controlled Trials (RCTs) were included in all languages over a comprehensive time period. An interim review was conducted by the Wound Management Working Group of the Academic

Box 1: Classification of Medical Support Structure

Role 1: Medical Support moving within fighting units.
Role 2: Dressing stations (can be enhanced with surgical capability).
Role 3: Field hospital with surgical support.
Role 4: Hospital away from combat zone with full range of medical and surgical support – in the UK this is University Hospital Birmingham.

Department of Military Surgery and Trauma. A further literature review was conducted to find all papers relating to the use of TNP on military wounds.

Results.—17 reports were reviewed relating to 14 studies including 662 patients. Of these 131 were reported to have had traumatic injuries. Significant results were reported with respect to time to wound healing, patient comfort and reduction in wound volumes. Bacterial load was not affected, in the 3 trials which commented on this, but in 1 there was a significant reduction in wound infections in the TNP group. Several of the trials were small, methodology was not consistent therefore no meta-analysis was possible. 2 papers were found describing case series of military patients being treated with TNP.

Conclusions.—There is very little published evidence in the form of RCTs to support the use of TNP in the acute traumatic military setting. This review supports the requirement for further investigation to evaluate whether this method of wound management has a place forward of Role 4 (Box 1).

▶ Topical negative pressure dressings have received significant attention in civilian practice for enhanced wound healing and accelerated granulation tissue formation.[1,2] There are relatively little data regarding the use of these dressings in traumatic wounds and even less information regarding the relevance in the military setting. This review questions whether bacterial load is reduced and whether a consistent pattern of improved healing can be demonstrated. It may be most appropriate, at this point, to send wounds that have been debrided at multiple early levels of care to centers providing definitive care of injury, where topical negative pressure management is most appropriate.

At the conclusion of this review, a group of British authors recommend regular application of topical negative pressure in role 4 hospitals (Box 1). The role for these dressings in dressing stations of field hospitals and other forward units remains unclear. Careful evaluation of any use of topical negative pressure beyond role 4 facilities is necessary.

D. J. Dries, MSE, MD

References

1. Morykwas MJ, Argenta LC, Shelton-Brown EI, McGuirt W. Vacuum-assisted closure: a new method for wound control and treatment: animal studies and basic foundation. *Ann Plast Surg*. 1997;38:553-562.
2. Ubbink DT, Westerbos SJ, Nelson EA, Vermeulen H. A systematic review of topical negative pressure therapy for acute and chronic wounds. *Br J Surg*. 2008;95:685-692.

War as a Laboratory For Trauma Research

Bohannon J

Science 331:1261-1263, 2011

Background.—War offers the richest laboratory for research into trauma medicine. In trauma cases the most crucial interventions are usually needed immediately. Advances seen in war include the motorized ambulances of World War I that moved solders back to the hospitals quickly, the World War II advances in the large-scale use of antibiotics, the Korean War's pioneering work in vascular surgery repair and grafting techniques, and the portable radiology equipment and ventilators first used in the Vietnam War. In the most current conflicts, improvised explosive devices (IEDs) are the primary risk, causing injuries combining burns, deep lacerations, and brain trauma from blast waves. Such injuries are too rare to be studied in peacetime, and the military keeps exhaustive data on preinjury health and postinjury outcome. Through the Joint Combat Casualty Research Team (JC2RT), medical research is being conducted in Iraq and Afghanistan and is yielding rapid interventions involving tourniquet use and the use of drugs and blood products. Many insights gained have made their way into civilian emergency medicine. However, controversy has arisen as journalists charge that researchers rush experimental treatments into use without proper ethical review or sufficient safety testing, possibly risking soldiers' lives. The process of overseeing research projects in war zones, the changes produced, and the charges brought against medical research were documented.

Process.—The eight-member JC2RT screens all projects submitted by researchers from the military plus any university-based scientific partners. This screening identifies problems, such as feasibility, with those writing the proposals unaware that there is no way to conduct the research they have envisioned. The use of experimental medical devices is also a fatal flaw because informed consent is required, and many wounded soldiers cannot grant consent. After prescreening, the project must be approved by an independent US Army institutional review board (IRB), which performs the same rigorous process as any other research institution, sourcing outside experts as needed. The JC2RT identifies issues that will cause problems with reviewers so researchers can fix them and streamlines the process of applying research results to patient treatment.

Results.—About 100 projects have been done in the field. All benefit from the US military's Joint Theater Trauma Registry (JTTR), a continuously updated record of trauma cases in Iraq and Afghanistan with about 40,000 case histories, including finely detailed medical observations, treatments, and outcomes. Most research incrementally improves existing treatments, but some have overturned paradigms of trauma care, such as blood transfusions and damage control surgery. For blood transfusions, the standard approach is to begin with concentrated red blood cells in saline solution, adding plasma containing platelets and clotting factors sparingly later. Waiting for clotting factors has led to extreme blood loss, so for severe injuries requiring massive transfusions the patient receives the equivalent of whole blood immediately with a full complement of clotting factors, with mortality reduced from 65% to 17%. In addition, some injuries are left open with the blood vessels tied off, then vigorously cleansed with saline solution until closure a few days or so later. This avoids massive infections and sepsis. Other problems being studied include preventing compartment syndrome (a pool of fluid between tissue layers that can cause amputation or death) by monitoring tissue oxygen levels and diagnosing brain trauma via ultrasound measurement of eye vessel blood pressure.

Charges and Conclusions.—The JC4RT was criticized by *The Baltimore Sun* in 2009 for exposing soldiers to the risks of unproved, probably useless

TABLE 1.—Trauma Research on the Battlefield

Research Topic	Summary	Example of Output or Project Status
Damage control resuscitation	Methods for resuscitating patients with massive blood loss	M. A. Borgman *et al.*, The ratio of blood products transfused affects mortality in patients receiving massive transfusions at a combat support hospital. *J Trauma* **63**, 805 (2007).
Compartment syndrome	Using oxygen concentration and other markers to detect dangerous fluid buildup in injured limbs	Ongoing
Prehospital lifesaving interventions	Assessing the performance of immediate interventions in trauma care	Ongoing
Vascular surgery	Comparing the effectiveness of vascular injury treatment for wounded soldiers	S. M. Gifford *et al.*, Effect of temporary shunting on extremity vascular injury: an outcome analysis from the Global War on Terror vascular injury initiative. *J Vasc Surg* **50**, 549 (2009).
Traumatic brain injury	Biomarkers and quantitative EEG for detecting brain injury and characterizing immunodeficiency	Ongoing
Critical Care Air Transport Team (CCATT)	Analysis of resuscitation and early clinical outcomes as a function of aeromedical platform	M. D. Goodman *et al.*, Traumatic brain injury and aeromedical evacuation: when is the brain fit to fly? *J Surg Res* **164**, 286 (2010).
Combat medicine training	Assessing the effectiveness of medical training in the context of Iraq and Afghanistan	J. A. Tyler *et al.*, Current US military operations and implications for military surgical training. *J Am Coll Surg* **211**, 658 (2010).
Tourniquets	Optimizing the use of tourniquets for improving survival and reducing amputations	J. F. Kragh Jr. *et al.*, Survival with emergency tourniquet use to stop bleeding in major limb trauma. *Annals of Surgery* **249**, 1 (2009).
Soft tissue injury	Assessing the effectiveness of the vacuum assisted device and other innovative treatments for soft tissue damage	R. Fang *et al.*, Feasibility of negative pressure wound therapy during intercontinental aeromedical evacuation of combat casualties. *J Trauma* **69**, S140 (2010).
Explosive mass casualty	Developing guidelines for intensive care for multiple casualties caused by explosions	B. W. Propper *et al.*, Surgical response to multiple casualty incidents following single explosive events. *Annals of Surgery* **250**, 311 (2009).

Editor's Note: Please refer to original journal article for full references.

treatments. Two bioethicists, their colleagues, and documents they consulted were used to examine the issues raised by this criticism and evaluate whether JC4RT's procedures for battlefield research were handled ethically. None of the examples of unethical research cited in *The Sun*'s report were valid. Reviewers found that the JC4RT's ethical approach reflected a continuous dedication to assess practices with real-time evaluations and weekly morbidity and mortality conferences. Their quality-improvement program was labeled second to none. The extra scrutiny was deemed justified in light of the history of using military personnel as guinea pigs for research and acknowledging that trauma patients often cannot give informed consent. Doctors from the military who reenter civilian practice are incorporating some of the protocols they learned in the war. For example, the military's massive blood transfusion protocol is being tested at 11 civilian trauma centers across the United States (Table 1).

▶ This summary reviews the recent progress and controversy surrounding battlefield research in contemporary Middle Eastern conflicts. The table demonstrates multiple projects that have influenced not only military but also civilian trauma practice. I note also that the majority of the projects cited have produced peer-reviewed publications. Thus, not only has the research project undergone review before execution, but the manuscripts produced passed the rigorous process of peer-review by both civilian and military experts.

One of the great advantages in military research dealing with injury is the extensive data on preinjury health of soldiers involved. This adds invaluable background information. In addition, because soldiers tend to be healthy young males, physiologic derangement caused by injury can be attributed to injury rather than to comorbid conditions.

Wartime medical research has a checkered history going back to the Second World War. However, projects reported here are examined critically by both civilian and military experts. The product of this work is improved care for all injured patients.

D. J. Dries, MSE, MD

Orthopedic Management of Children With Multiple Injuries

Abdelgawad AA, Kanlic EM (Texas Tech Univ Health Science Ctr at El Paso)

J Trauma 70:1568-1574, 2011

Background.—Children who suffer severe trauma usually sustain multiple, possibly life-threatening abdominal, head, and chest injuries, but also may have extremity injuries and fractures. Although orthopedic injuries are rarely life-threatening, when encountered in children with multiple injuries, they can lead to long-term morbidity and disability. The musculoskeletal management of multiply injured pediatric patients was reviewed.

Pediatric Issues.—Pediatric bone and skeletally mature bone differs. The thicker periosteum in pediatric patients usually remains intact on one side of the bone, so closed reduction easier and fewer fractures are displaced. Pediatric bone has a growth plate (physis) that, if injured, alters bone growth by closing completely, shortening affected bone and causing limb length discrepancies, or incompletely, causing angular deformity. Children's body surface area relative to their mass is greater than adults, making them more likely to develop hypothermia. Less fat and muscle mass offers less protection to the bone. The child's relatively large head circumference, especially when under age 8 years, means the neck is flexed when lying flat. Adjustments on pediatric backboards avoid cervical spine flexion. Children are also abuse victims, with abuse always a concern in multiple injuries. Orthopedic injuries found in abuse are humerus fracture in a child under age 3 years or femur fracture in a child under age 1 year.

Injuries and Treatment.—The most frequent orthopedic conditions seen in children with multiple injuries are open fractures, compartment syndrome, pelvic injuries, multiple bone fractures, fracture-associated vascular injuries, and spinal fractures. The management of these injuries is guided by Advanced Life Trauma Support principles.

Open fractures account for about 10% of fractures in children with multiple injuries. They may be type I (less than 1 cm long, minimal soft tissue crushing), type II (1 to 10 cm long with more soft tissue injury secondary to higher energy), or type III (caused by high-energy forces, more than 10 cm long, with extensive muscle damage). Type III fractures are further subclassified as IIIA, with limited periosteal and muscle stripping from bone; IIIB, with extensive periosteal stripping and plastic reconstructive procedures needed for bone coverage; or IIIC, with vascular injury requiring repair. Primary management of open fractures involves applying a sterile dressing to cover the wound and aligning and splinting the limb. Broken bone ends protruding from skin wounds are irrigated with sterile saline solution and gross contamination removed before they are reduced through the skin in the emergency department, avoiding deep tissue contamination. Debridement is carried out in the operating room. If urgent bone end reduction without cleansing is needed, thorough formal surgical debridement is done as soon as possible and includes meticulous cleansing of the bone ends and deep tissues. Open fractures are then managed with tetanus prophylaxis, antibiotics, and surgical management. Antibiotic use varies with degree of contamination. Types I and II require first-generation cephalosporin and an aminoglycoside is added for type III. Penicillin is used when the wound has gross contamination, is a farm injury, or is deep. Antibiotics are given for 48 to 72 hours, then repeated depending on what other procedures are done. Surgical treatment includes debridement, fracture fixation, and soft tissue management. Debridement is done as early as possible and repeated to control infection. Fracture fixation is often done with internal fixation. Soft tissue coverage may use negative pressure, keeping the field relatively and stimulating granulation tissue repair. Other methods include acute bone shortening and bone lengthening from a distal segment.

Compartment syndrome is elevated interstitial pressure in a closed osteofascial compartment that compromises microvascular structures. Careful examination is needed to detect it but it is suspected in all children having high-energy extremity trauma. Often the affected compartment exhibits tense noncompressible swelling. A child who requires higher doses of narcotics to remain comfortable likely has compartment syndrome. Another characteristic is severe pain with passive stretch of the distal joints; paresthesias, pulselessness, and paralysis are found later, but absence of these signs does not exclude compartment syndrome. It is more common in children with leg and forearm fractures and can occur with an open fracture. For nonresponsive children with multiple injuries, a pressure needle may be used to measure compartment pressure. Values over 30 mm Hg or a difference between patient diastolic pressure and compartment pressure less than 30 mm Hg indicates the syndrome. Continuous monitoring devices help for high-risk cases. If the condition is suspected, the cast and splints, plus padding, are removed or split immediately. The affected extremity remains below the level of the heart to maintain limb perfusion. Wide release of the affected compartments (fasciotomy) is needed within 8 hours for a good prognosis. Forearm compartment syndrome is released through a long volar incision, the dorsal compartment is reassessed, and a dorsal incision is added as needed. The four compartments in the lower leg require two incisions for release: one made midway between the anterolateral border of the tibial and anterior border of the fibula releases the anterior and lateral compartments and one done 1 inch posterior to the posteromedial border of the tibia releases the others. Fasciotomy wounds are left open for wet to dry dressing or negative pressure wound dressing. A few days later either delayed primary closure of split-thickness skin graft is done.

High-energy injuries can produce pelvic fractures, which are usually managed nonsurgically. Most pelvic fractures are stable and treated with early mobilization and weight bearing, followed by radiographs to check for displacement. Unstable pelvic fractures require surgical stabilization; an external fixator provides minimal discomfort and easy access to the abdomen. Visceral structures adjacent to the pelvis can suffer life-threatening injuries, so pelvic fracture management is done only once the child is stable. Temporary stabilization is done using a pelvic binder, sheet, or C-clamp.

Operative stabilization of children with multiple bone fractures shortens hospital stays and reduces complications related to immobilization. Bone fractures that would be treated conservatively if found alone are addressed surgically when associated with multiple injuries. Closed long bone injuries are managed within 48 to 72 hours if possible; delays permit secondary complications and make the repair more difficult. Operative fracture management can be piggy-backed to surgery on other body systems if needed. With children whose condition is unstable, most fractures are splinted and surgical management postponed until primary resuscitative efforts are complete. Splinted extremities are closely monitored for compartment syndrome. Traction provides temporary stabilization of femoral and pelvic fractures; injured extremities may have external fixation, which is converted to rigid nailing when the child's condition permits.

Children with supracondylar fracture of the humerus or fracture of the distal femur are more vulnerable to vascular injury. Limb vascularity distal to the fracture is closely monitored. Characteristics of associated vascular injury include pulselessness, pain, pallor, paresthesias, paralysis, and hypothermia. If closed reduction does not restore adequate blood flow, surgery is done to repair or reconstruct the arterial injury. Open reduction and fixation of the fracture is needed immediately.

Spinal trauma is assumed to be present in children with multiple injuries until ruled out by physical and radiographic evaluation. Spine and neurological status are carefully evaluated, palpating each spinous process and noting tenderness, gaps, or deviations. To avoid flexion of the cervical spine, the child's head is placed in a cutout in the transfer board or the body is elevated on a pad. Although controversial, many children are given high-dose steroids for 24 to 48 hours after a spinal cord injury. Clinicians should be aware that children, especially those under age 8 years, may have spinal cord injury without radiographic abnormality (SCIWORA). Characteristic normal findings of the pediatric spinal cord include pseudosubluxation of the vertebrae, where the anterior border of the vertebra above is anterior to the vertebra below. A continuous line along the anterior border of the posterior spinous processes indicates proper alignment. Magnetic resonance imaging (MRI) scans are advised to clear the child's cervical spine. Computed tomography (CT) scans are inadequate to visualize the cartilaginous spinal areas of young children, but if CT examination is chosen, it is performed using the lowest reasonable dose of radiation possible and focusing on obtaining the highest quality images. Repeat CT is limited to the area of interest when absolutely required.

Conclusions.—Trauma surgeons and general orthopedic surgeons should recognize typical orthopedic injuries in children with multiple injuries and deliver treatment in accordance with emergency protocols to permit maximal functional recovery.

▶ This is an excellent overview of treatment principles particular to the pediatric patient with orthopedic trauma. I will attempt to emphasize some of the highlights.

Debilitating injury can occur without obvious bony damage on standard imaging and examination if the lesion involves the growth plate. Closure of the physis may compromise longitudinal growth with premature closure, leading to shortening of the affected bone and limb length discrepancy. Another possible outcome of growth plate injury is angular deformity of affected bone.

Historically, open fractures have been sent for early operative debridement in all situations. More recent studies suggest that with lesser degrees of contamination and early administration of antibiotics, operative debridement up to 24 hours after injury may be safe. Patients with most severe contamination should still be debrided within 6 hours. A greater emphasis is placed on internal fixation with less emphasis on external fixation in these patients. Negative pressure dressings can be very effective in children by stimulation of soft tissue healing.

Pelvic fracture management is similar to that of adults. Sheets and pelvic binders are appropriate to reduce the pelvic volume and control bleeding with a tamponade effect. In general, pelvic fracture stabilization is not an emergency.

Advantages to early fracture stabilization have been reported in children, as previously noted in adults. The stable child with long bone injury should be treated within 48 to 72 hours. Complications and resource use are reduced with appropriate early surgical therapy.[1]

Finally, MRI may be a particularly valuable imaging modality in the pediatric cervical spine, ligamentous laxity contributes to the impression of subluxation, and CT is nondiagnostic. The importance of avoiding ionizing radiation in this age group is also emphasized.

D. J. Dries, MSE, MD

Reference

1. Lasanianos NG, Kanakaris NK, Dimitriou R, Pape HC, Giannoudis PV. Second hit phenomenon: existing evidence of clinical implications. *Injury*. 2011;42:617-629.

The timing of definitive fixation for major fractures in polytrauma—A matched-pair comparison between a US and European level I centres: Analysis of current fracture management practice in polytrauma

Schreiber VM, Tarkin IS, Hildebrand F, et al (Univ of Pittsburgh, PA; Hannover Med School, Germany; et al)

Injury 42:650-654, 2011

Purpose.—Early definitive stabilisation is usually the treatment of choice for major fractures in polytrauma patients. Modifications may be made when patients are in critical condition, or when associated injuries dictate the timing of surgery. The current study investigates whether the timing of fracture treatment is different in different trauma systems.

Materials and Methods.—Consecutive patients treated a Level I trauma centre were documented (Group US) and a matched-pair group was gathered from the German Trauma Registry (Group GTR). Inclusion criteria: New Injury Severity Score (NISS) >16, >2 major fractures and >1 organ/soft tissue injury. The timing and type of surgery for major fractures was recorded, as were major complications.

Results.—114 patients were included, $n = 57$ Group US (35.1% F, 64.9% M, mean age: 44.1 yrs ± 16.49, mean NISS: 27.4 ± 8.65, mean ICU stay: 10 ± 7.49) and $n = 57$ Group GTR (36.8% F, 63.1% M, mean age: 41.2 yrs ± 15.35, mean NISS: 29.4 ± 6.88, mean ICU stay: 15.6 ± 18.25). 44 (57.1%) out of 77 fractures in Group US received primary definitive fracture fixation compared to 61 (65.5%) out of 93 fractures in Group GTR (n.s.). The average duration until definitive treatment was comparable in all major extremity fractures (pelvis: 5 days ± 2.8 Group US, 7.1 days ± 9.6 Group GTR (n.s.), femur: 7.9 days ± 8.3 Group US, 5.5 days ± 7.9 (n.s.), tibia: 6.2 days ± 5.6 Group US, 6.2 days ± 9.1 Group GTR (n.s.),

TABLE 3.—Distribution of Initial Treatments for Major Fractures Regardless of the Localisation

Primary Treatment	USA $n = 77$	GER $n = 93$	p-Value
Definitive stabilisation	44 (57.1%)	61 (65.6%)	n.s.
Traction	7 (9.1%)	1 (1.1%)	n.s.
Temporizing Ext. fixation	19 (24.8%)	21 (22.6%)	n.s.
Ext. fix as def. treatment	7 (9.1%)	10 (10.8%)	n.s.

TABLE 4.—Mean Duration Until Definitive Treatment of Major Fractures, Specified According to Body Regions

Duration Until Definitive Treatment	USA $n = 77$	GER $n = 93$	p-Value
All fractures	5.5 days ± 4.2	6.6 days ± 8.7	n.s.
Humerus fractures	5 days ± 3.7	6.6 days ± 6.1	n.s.
Radius fractures	6 days ± 4.7	6.1 days ± 8.7	n.s.
Femur fractures	7.9 days ± 8.3	5.5 days ± 7.9	n.s.
Tibia fractures	6.2 days ± 5.6	6.2 days ± 9.1	n.s.
Pelvis fractures	5 days ± 2.8	7.1 days ± 9.6	n.s.

humerus: 5 days ± 3.7 Group US, 6.6 days ± 6.1 Group GTR (n.s.), radius: 6 days ± 4.7 Group US, 6.1 days ± 8.7 Group GTR (n.s.).

Conclusion.—The current matched-pair analysis demonstrates that the timing of initial definitive fixation of major fractures is comparable between the US and Europe. Certain fractures are stabilised internally in a staged fashion regardless the trauma system, thus discounting previous apparent contradictions (Table 3 and 4).

▶ This brief report provides data regarding the current state-of-the art in timing and type of acute fracture management. A relatively small data set is used from the United States provided by a single center. A sampling from the large German Trauma Registry is provided for a European sample. These data are relevant because they come from 2 different systems with a variety of practitioners managing orthopedic injuries.

A review of the tables provided with this comment finds that both the United States and Germany move directly to definitive fracture stabilization approximately 60% of the time. Traction is infrequently used, and both groups of practitioners make use of temporizing external fixation (Table 3). I was surprised to see that several days pass until fractures are stabilized in both systems (Table 4). This seems to argue against specific care system limitations despite different provider organizations. Thus, in both the United States and Western Europe, emphasis is given to stabilization of fractures as allowed by the need for advanced cardiopulmonary support.[1-3]

D. J. Dries, MSE, MD

References

1. Border JR. Death from severe trauma: open fractures to multiple organ dysfunction syndrome. *J Trauma*. 1995;39:12-22.
2. Pape HC, Rixen D, Morley J, et al. Impact of the method of initial stabilization for femoral shaft fractures in patients with multiple injuries at risk for complications (borderline patients). *Ann Surg*. 2007;246:491-499.
3. Scalea TM, Boswell SA, Scott JD, Mitchell KA, Kramer ME, Pollak AN. External fixation as a bridge to intramedullary nailing for patients with multiple injuries and with femur fractures: damage control orthopedics. *J Trauma*. 2000;48:613-621.

A Small Dose of Arginine Vasopressin in Combination with Norepinephrine is a Good Early Treatment for Uncontrolled Hemorrhagic Shock After Hemostasis

Li T, Fang Y, Zhu Y, et al (Third Military Med Univ, Chongqing, P.R. China)

J Surg Res 169:76-84, 2011

Background.—Limited fluid resuscitation has been proven to have a good effect on uncontrolled hemorrhagic shock. Arginine vasopressin (AVP) and norepinephrine (NE) were used to treat vasodilatory or septic shock, and were used to reduce the fluid requirement for uncontrolled hemorrhagic shock. Based on their pressor and hemodynamic stabilization effects, it is speculated that AVP and NE may be a good treatment for uncontrolled hemorrhagic shock at early stage after hemostasis.

Methods.—Experiments were conducted in two parts. Each part had control, lactated Ringer's solution (LR), whole blood, NE, arginine vasopressin (AVP), NE+AVP, and AVP+, NE+ whole blood. Rats ($n = 8-10$/group), respectively, received LR, whole blood, NE (1 μg/kg) and AVP (0.1 U/kg) infusion alone, or in combination after 60 min hypotensive resuscitation (50 mmHg). The volume in each group was two times the volume of shed blood.

Results.—Whole blood improved all observed parameters, particularly the tissue blood flow and mitochondrial function of liver and kidney, and the 12-h survival (50%). NE only increased the hemodynamics. 0.1 U/kg of AVP had a similar effect with whole blood on hemodynamics, tissue blood flow, mitochondrial function, and the 12-h survival. AVP+NE significantly improved all observed variables ($P < 0.05$ or 0.01), the 12-h survival was 70%. Whole blood further potentiated the beneficial effect of AVP+NE, and 12-h animal survival rate in this group was 80%.

Conclusion.—AVP+NE is a good treatment for uncontrolled hemorrhagic shock at the early stage after hemostasis if blood is unavailable. Whole blood transfusion can potentiate this beneficial effect of AVP+NE (Fig 2).

▶ This is a small animal study with all inherent limitations of rodent trials. Obviously, it is difficult to replicate the clinical scenario with this type of study. I am impressed, however, that the authors do utilize an injury model with splenic

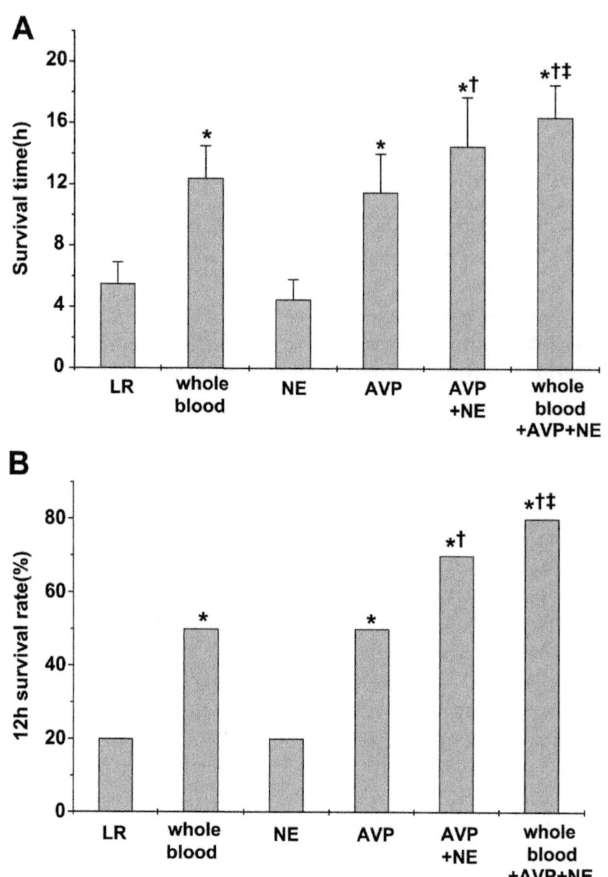

FIGURE 2.—Effects of different treatments on survival time (A) and 12-h survival (B) of uncontrolled hemorrhagic shock in rats after hemostasis. $^{*}P < 0.05$ *versus* LR group; $^{\dagger}P < 0.05$ *versus* NE group, $^{\ddagger}P < 0.05$ *versus* AVP. (Reprinted from Li T, Fang Y, Zhu Y, et al. A small dose of arginine vasopressin in combination with norepinephrine is a good early treatment for uncontrolled hemorrhagic shock after hemostasis. *J Surg Res*. 2011;169:76-84, with permission form Elsevier.)

disruption rather than the traditional controlled bleed via a catheter. Because the authors truly use a model of injury, I was attracted to this article. A second advantage is evidence of meticulous technique used.

A number of conclusions can be drawn. First, lactated Ringer's solution (LR) is an inefficient and possibly ineffective resuscitation solution in the setting of significant hemorrhage. This study reaffirms limitations of LR raised in previous laboratory tests.[1] Second, arginine vasopressin should be used in the setting of hemorrhagic shock, not just sepsis. This study confirms the value of arginine vasopressin in hemorrhagic shock.[2,3] Third, norepinephrine is also a reasonable therapeutic choice in the setting of significant hemorrhage.[4] Finally, although the authors do not emphasize this, it is clear from their data that whole blood is a powerful resuscitation solution and contributes significantly to the impressive outcome seen with arginine vasopressin and norepinephrine.[5]

What are we to take away? First, significant blood loss requires blood replacement. If blood is unavailable or present in small amounts, arginine vasopressin and norepinephrine may be reasonable components of an early resuscitation cocktail (Fig 2).

D. J. Dries, MSE, MD

References

1. Koustova E, Stanton K, Gushchin V, Alam HB, Stegalkina S, Rhee PM. Effects of lactated Ringer's solutions on human leukocytes. *J Trauma*. 2002;52:872-878.
2. Robin JK, Oliver JA, Landry DW. Vasopressin deficiency in the syndrome of irreversible shock. *J Trauma*. 2003;54:S149-S154.
3. Holmes CL, Patel BM, Russell JA, Walley KR. Physiology of vasopressin relevant to management of septic shock. *Chest*. 2001;120:989-1002.
4. De Backer D, Biston P, Devriendt J, et al. Comparison of dopamine and norepinephrine in the treatment of shock. *N Engl J Med*. 2010;362:779-789.
5. Dries DJ. The contemporary role of blood products and components used in trauma resuscitation. *Scan J Trauma Resusc Emerg Med*. 2010;18:63.

Second hit phenomenon: Existing evidence of clinical implications

Lasanianos NG, Kanakaris NK, Dimitriou R, et al (Leeds Biomedical Res Unit, UK; Leeds Teaching Hosps NHS Trust, UK; et al)

Injury 42:617-629, 2011

The last two decades extensive research evidence has been accumulated regarding the pathophysiology of trauma and the sequelae of interventions that follow. Aim of this analysis has been to collect and categorise the existing data on the so-called "second hit" phenomenon that includes the biochemical and physiologic alterations occurring in patients having surgery after major trauma.

Articles were extracted from the PubMed database and the retrieved reports were included in the study only if pre-specified eligibility criteria were fulfilled. Moreover, a constructed questionnaire was utilised for quality assessment of the outcomes.

Twenty-six articles were eligible for the final analysis, referring to a total of 8262 patients that underwent surgery after major trauma. Sixteen retrospective clinical studies including 7322 patients and 10 prospective ones, including 940 patients were evaluated.

Several variables able to reproduce a post-operative second hit were identified; mostly related to pulmonary dysfunction, coagulopathy, fat or pulmonary embolism, and the inflammatory immune system. Indicative conclusions were extracted, as well as the need for further prospective randomised trials. Suggestions on the content and the rationale of future studies are provided (Table 8).

▶ This article is an extensive compendium of data describing the evidence that therapeutic interventions after injury may perpetuate and magnify the physiologic impact of the original insult. As one might expect, there is great heterogeneity in

TABLE 8.—Weaknesses of the Review Due to Studies Characteristics

a/a	Weakness Description	Examples–Comments
1	Differences to the criteria and definitions of the utilised subgroup analysis	The use of a time threshold for early fixation was not uniform (most commonly was 24 h,[6,8–10,12,15,22,26,30,32,35,48,53,54,56,71,73,76] in some 48 h,[4,59] or in others not defined). The ISS threshold of polytrauma was not uniform in all studies (in most is $\geq$16, in others >18 or higher[6,12,73]). In several studies[4,6,30,35,63,71] examining cardio-pulmonary dysfunction, a subgroup of those with chest injuries was not analysed separately.
2	Differences to the definitions of the examined variables	Pneumonia, ARDS or MOF were defined uniformly with small differences from one study to another adding potential bias to the results. If for example the ratio of PaO_2/FiO_2 is used as an ARDS criterion in patients not mechanically ventilated, a very high incidence of ARDS is recorded.
3	Mixed group analysis of the polytrauma population	The impact of polytrauma on the degree of hypoxemia, cellular injury and associated inflammatory response is not comparable with those of isolated injuries. In a number of studies the non-polytrauma/isolated fracture groups were not differentiated from the more severely injured.[26,48,71] In several studies[22,32,35,53,59,63,68,71] the type of intramedullary fixation (reamed or unreamed) of femoral fractures was not described.
4	Biased selection of patients to be included in different groups	Homogeneity in patients between different groups of treatment may be unobtainable. More severely injured patients usually receive what is believed to be the safest possible surgical treatment. In studies examining damage control orthopaedics groups vs. Early total care groups the DCO patients usually have significantly more severe trauma.
5	Lack of prospective studies	Thirteen out of the 23 studies examined and especially those of the 1980s and 1990s were retrospective. Prospective studies with polytrauma patients may be difficult to be organised. Consent and randomization of patients that may be in a high risk for their life, cannot be so easily performed resulting in a problematic enrolment procedures.

Editor's Note: Please refer to original journal article for full references.

the studies performed and the outcomes obtained (Table 8). It is important to note that the surgical insults studied are generally based on orthopedic fracture stabilization.

There are a number of conclusions to consider. First, in adequately resuscitated patients, early operative intervention is reasonable and may be advisable. Second, the impact of head injury is inadequately studied as a trigger for adverse outcomes. Third, it appears that the timing of operation has a greater role than the type of procedure, based on this extensive review. Finally, I note that the studies do not use consistent criteria to quantify the impact of secondary insults.

D. J. Dries, MSE, MD

Association of 6% hetastarch resuscitation with adverse outcomes in critically ill trauma patients

Lissauer ME, Chi A, Kramer ME, et al (Univ of Maryland Med Ctr, Baltimore)

Am J Surg 202:53-58, 2011

Background.—Six percent hetastarch is used as a volume expander but has been associated with poor outcomes. The aim of this study was to evaluate trauma patients resuscitated with hetastarch.

Methods.—A retrospective review was performed of adult trauma patients. Demographics, injury severity, laboratory values, outcomes, and hetastarch use were recorded.

Results.—A total of 2,225 patients were identified, of whom 497 (22%) received hetastarch. There were no differences in age, gender, injury mechanism, lactate, hematocrit, or creatinine. The mean injury severity score was different: 29.7 ± 12.6 with hetastarch versus 27.5 ± 12.6 without hetastarch. Acute kidney injury developed in 65 hetastarch patients (13%) and in 131 (8%) without hetastarch (relative risk, 1.73; 95% confidence interval [CI], 1.30–2.28). Hetastarch mortality was 21%, compared with 11% without hetastarch (relative risk, 1.84; 95% CI, 1.48–2.29). Multivariate logistic regression demonstrated hetastarch use (odds ratio, 1.96; 95% CI, 1.49–2.58) as independently significant for death. Hetastarch use was independently significant for renal dysfunction as well (odds ratio, 1.70; 95% CI, 1.22–2.36).

Conclusions.—Because of the detrimental association with renal function and mortality, hetastarch should be avoided in the resuscitation of trauma patients.

▶ The ideal resuscitation fluid for injured patients has been extensively discussed and remains a subject of debate. Isotonic crystalloids are typically used initially. Expansive administration of these fluids, however, is associated with a significant risk of complications including compartment syndromes. With significant bleeding, massive blood product administration is appropriate. The optimal fluid for the patient without significant blood product requirements who has reached the limits of crystalloid administration is debated.[1-3]

This retrospective work from the large data set of the University of Maryland argues that 6% hetastarch is associated with adverse outcomes, including renal insufficiency and other end organ injury, particularly in patients who are not taken to the operating room. It is important to note that the Injury Severity Score is greater in patients receiving starch than those receiving other strategies. In addition, as a retrospective study, fluids given are not based on a consistent protocol. Further review of the data presented by these investigators, however, suggests that hetastarch, like albumin, may also be deleterious in the setting of head injury.[3] Thus, where aggressive blood product administration is not indicated, the role and optimal type of supplemental colloid remains unclear.

D. J. Dries, MSE, MD

References

1. Cotton BA, Guy JS, Morris JA Jr, Abumrad NN. The cellular, metabolic, and systemic consequences of aggressive fluid resuscitation strategies. *Shock*. 2006; 26:115-121.
2. Rhee P, Koustova E, Alam HB. Searching for the optimal resuscitation method: Recommendations for the initial fluid resuscitation of combat casualties. *J Trauma*. 2003;54:S52-S62.
3. Finfer S, Bellomo R, Boyce N, et al. A comparison of albumin and saline for fluid resuscitation in the intensive care unit. *N Engl J Med*. 2004;350:2247-2256.

HIV and Hepatitis in an Urban Penetrating Trauma Population: Unrecognized and Untreated

Seamon MJ, Ginwalla R, Kulp H, et al (Cooper Univ Hosp, Camden, NJ; Johns Hopkins Hosp, Baltimore, MD; Temple Univ School of Medicine, Philadelphia, PA; et al)
J Trauma 71:306-311, 2011

Background.—Despite limited prospective data, it is commonly believed that human immunodeficiency virus (HIV) and hepatitis infections are widespread in the penetrating trauma population, placing healthcare workers at risk for occupational exposure. Our primary study objective was to measure the prevalence of HIV (anti-HIV), hepatitis B (HB surface antigen [HBsAg]), and hepatitis C virus (anti-HCV) in our penetrating trauma population.

Methods.—We prospectively analyzed penetrating trauma patients admitted to Temple University Hospital between August 2008 and February 2010. Patients ($n = 341$) were tested with an oral swab for anti-HIV and serum evaluated for HBsAg and anti-HCV. Positives were confirmed with western blot, neutralization immunoassay, and reverse transcription polymerase chain reaction, respectively. Demographics, risk factors, and clinical characteristics were analyzed.

Results.—Of 341 patients, 4 patients (1.2%) tested positive for anti-HIV and 2 had a positive HBsAg (0.6%). Hepatitis C was the most prevalent measured infection as anti-HCV was detected in 26 (7.6%) patients. Overall, 32 (9.4%) patients were tested positive for anti-HIV, HBsAg, or anti-HCV. Twenty-eight (75%) of these patients who tested positive were undiagnosed before study enrollment. When potential risk factors were analyzed, age (odds ratio, 1.07, $p = 0.031$) and intravenous drug use (odds ratio 14.4, $p < 0.001$) independently increased the likelihood of anti-HIV, HBsAg, or anti-HCV-positive markers.

Conclusions.—Greater than 9% of our penetrating trauma study population tested positive for anti-HIV, HBsAg, or anti-HCV although patients were infrequently aware of their seropositive status. As penetrating trauma victims frequently require expedient, invasive procedures, universal precautions are essential. The prevalence of undiagnosed HIV and hepatitis in penetrating trauma victims provides an important opportunity

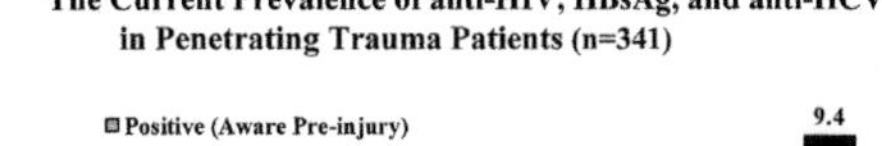

The Current Prevalence of anti-HIV, HBsAg, and anti-HCV
in Penetrating Trauma Patients (n=341)

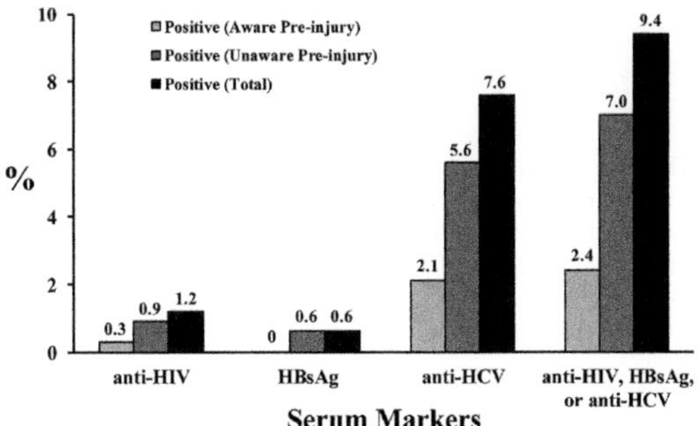

FIGURE 1.—The prevalence of anti-HIV, HBsAg, and anti-HCV were evaluated in 341 patients with penetrating injuries. Most (75%) seropositive patients were undiagnosed before study participation. (Reprinted from Seamon MJ, Ginwalla R, Kulp H, et al. HIV and hepatitis in an urban penetrating trauma population: unrecognized and untreated. *J Trauma*. 2011;71:306-311, with permission from Lippincott Williams & Wilkins.)

for education, screening, and earlier treatment of this high-risk population (Fig 1).

▶ These data are the result of a survey taken at an urban trauma center with a significant volume of penetrating trauma cases. Nearly 10% of patients were positive for hepatitis B, surface antigen, anti–hepatitis C virus and anti-human immunodeficiency virus.[1-3] These data may represent underestimates, as the investigators did not include patients with self-inflicted penetrating injury or injury by means other than a knife or gun. In addition, patients who are transfused >10 units of blood products were excluded as well as those who died before study enrollment. While elimination of the last group makes some sense, individuals receiving many units of blood products typically require extensive and aggressive resuscitation and may pose greater risk of injury to caregivers. The authors did report an impressive 88.3% participation among patients approached for enrollment.

The study population represented youth and male gender. However, patients who tested positive tended to be older and were more commonly white with a history of intravenous drug use. Notably, no patient 21 years and younger was pathogen positive, whereas 25% of patients age 40 years or older were seropositive for 1 of the pathogens of concern. Nearly 70% of patients who admitted to intravenous (IV) drug abuse tested positive for a measured serum marker, while only 6.5% of patients who denied IV drug abuse had a positive test result.

It is important to recognize that this sample of trauma patients comes from an urban center, and results may not be applicable to trauma patients from other regions. Clearly, patients who give a history of intravenous drug abuse need to be very closely followed up with during the course of resuscitation and hospitalization because of a dramatic increase in the presence of pathogens of interest. A clear majority of these patients are unaware of infection status in this report (Fig 1).

D. J. Dries, MSE, MD

References

1. Kelen GD, Fritz S, Qaqish B, et al. Unrecognized human immunodeficiency virus infection in emergency department patients. *N Engl J Med.* 1988;318:1645-1650.
2. Kelen GD, Green GB, Purcell RH, et al. Hepatitis B and hepatitis C in emergency department patients. *N Engl J Med.* 1992;326:1399-1404.
3. Kaplan AJ, Zone-Smith LK, Hannegan C, Norcross ED. The prevalence of hepatitis C in a regional level I trauma center population. *J Trauma.* 1992;33: 126-129.

Mechanism of Injury Affects Acute Coagulopathy of Trauma in Combat Casualties

Simmons JW, White CE, Ritchie JD, et al (United States Army Inst of Surgical Res, San Antonio, TX)
J Trauma 71:S74-S77, 2011

Background.—Recent evidence suggests trauma involving total body tissue damage increases the acute coagulopathy of trauma (ACOT) by various mechanisms, especially in massive transfusion (MT). Our hypothesis was that MT patients injured by explosion will have a higher international normalization ratio (INR) at admission than MT patients injured by gunshot wound (GSW).

Methods.—A retrospective review was performed on US military injured in Operation Iraqi Freedom/Operation Enduring Freedom from March 2003 to September 2008, who received MT (≥10 red blood cells in 24 hours) and had an INR on admission. Two cohorts were created based on mechanism. Admission vital signs, labs, transfusion, and mortality data were compared.

Results.—Seven hundred fifty-one MT patients were identified. Four hundred fifty patients had admission INR and were injured by either GSW or explosion. Patients demonstrated similar injury severity scale and Glasgow Coma Scale. Patients injured by explosion presented with higher INR, greater base deficit, and more tachycardic than patients injured by GSW. Transfusion of blood products was similar between both groups.

Conclusions.—The primary finding of this study is that patients injured by explosion presented with a higher INR than those injured by GSW, even with similar injury severity scale. In addition, patients injured by explosion presented more tachycardic and with a greater base deficit. These findings support the theory that ACOT is affected by the amount of tissue injured. Further research is needed into the pathophysiology of ACOT because this may impact care of patients with total body tissue damage/hypoxia and

TABLE 1.—Analysis by Cohort

	GSW (N = 78)	Explosion (N = 372)	*p*
Demographics			
Age (yr)	25 ± 6	26 ± 6	0.641
ISS	23 ± 10	24 ± 12	0.291
Vitals			
Pulse	101 ± 36	114 ± 34	0.006
SBP (mm Hg)	100 ± 37	105 ± 36	0.291
Temperature (°F)	97.5 ± 1.9	97.5 ± 6.5	0.999
GCS	11 ± 5	12 ± 5	0.686
Labs			
Hgb (g/dL)	11.7 ± 2.5	11.3 ± 2.8	0.285
BD (mEq/L)	−5.8 ± 6.2	−8.2 ± 7.2	0.006
INR	1.5 ± 0.5	1.8 ± 1.0	<0.001
INR >1.5	37%	50%	0.048
Mortality	24%	21%	0.508

improve the treatment of their coagulopathy while minimizing the attendant complications (Table 1).

▶ Historically, prehospital treatment of shock consists of crystalloid-based fluid resuscitation. This had been believed to dilute clotting factors causing coagulopathy. Brohi and coworkers challenge this classical teaching and have shown that shock and pattern of tissue injury may have greater impact on coagulopathy after injury.[1] Hypothermia has also been implicated. However, hypothermia has limited effect on function or clinical bleeding above 33°C.[2] Similarly, clinically important academia, as a contributor to coagulopathy after injury, seems to be limited for a pH > 7.2.[3]

This work is based on contemporary data from the current Middle Eastern conflicts and answers a simple question regarding the impact of volume of injured tissue on presenting coagulopathy. There were no differences in mortality or blood product administration. However, patients with higher volume of tissue injury (the explosion group) had a greater base deficit and international normalization ratio. While the clinical difference in these numbers may seem to be small, the authors have utilized a unique dataset to strengthen data supporting a physiologic rationale for the development of shock after injury. Thus, even in the setting of comparable resuscitation outcomes, there is a metabolic gradient associated with volume of tissue injured (Table 1).

D. J. Dries, MSE, MD

References

1. Brohi K, Singh J, Heron M, Coats T. Acute traumatic coagulopathy. *J Trauma.* 2003;54:1127-1130.
2. Meng ZH, Wolberg AS, Monroe DM 3rd, Hoffman M. The effect of temperature and pH on the activity of factor VIIa: implications for the efficacy of high-dose factor VIIa in hypothermic and acidotic patients. *J Trauma.* 2003;55:886-891.
3. Wolberg AS, Meng ZH, Monroe DM 3rd, Hoffman M. A systematic evaluation of the effect of temperature on coagulation enzyme activity and platelet function. *J Trauma.* 2004;56:1221-1228.

Mission to Eliminate Postinjury Abdominal Compartment Syndrome

Balogh ZJ, Martin A, van Wessem KP, et al (John Hunter Hosp and Univ of Newcastle, Australia)

Arch Surg 146:938-943, 2011

Objectives.—To determine the current incidence of postinjury abdominal compartment syndrome (ACS), the effect of intra-abdominal hypertension (IAH) on trauma outcomes, and the independent predictors of postinjury IAH.

Design.—Prospective cohort study.

Setting.—University-affiliated level 1 trauma center.

Patients.—Eighty-one consecutive shock/trauma patients admitted to the intensive care unit (mean [SD] values: age, 41 [2] years; 70% male; injury severity score, 29 [1]; base deficit, 6 [0.5] mmol/L; lactate level, 29.73 [4.5] mg/dL; transfusions of packed red blood cells, 5 [0.5] U in first 24 hours; mortality rate, 2.5%; and multiple organ failure [MOF], 6%) had second hourly intraabdominal pressure (IAP) monitoring.

Main Outcome Measures.—Intensive care unit length of stay, ACS, IAH, MOF, mortality.

Results.—The mean (SD) IAP was 14 (1) mm Hg. No patients developed ACS. Sixty-one patients (75%) had sustained IAH. Both patients with IAH and those without had similar demographics and injury severity. Patients with IAH had worse metabolic acidosis ($P = .02$), received more crystalloids ($P = .03$), and underwent laparotomy more frequently ($P = .005$). One patient with IAH and one without died. MOF occurred in 1 patient without IAH (5%) vs 4 with IAH (7%). The mean (SD) intensive care unit length of stay was 11 (3) days in patients without IAH vs 8 (1) days in those with IAH. Intraabdominal hypertension was poorly predictive of MOF (odds ratio, 1.17; 95% confidence interval, 0.96-1.43; $P = .13$). Of the 30 variables in multiple logistic regression analysis, only base deficit, laparotomy, and emergency department crystalloids were identified as weak predictors of IAP greater than 12 mm Hg. No predictors were found for the clinically more relevant IAP greater than 15 mm Hg and IAP greater than 18 mm Hg.

Conclusions.—Most of the severe shock/trauma patients developed sustained IAH. Based on univariate and multivariate analyses, there was no difference in outcomes between the trauma patients with IAH and those without. Multiple logistic regression analysis failed to show IAH as a predictor of MOF. The attenuation of the deadly ACS to a less deleterious IAH could be considered a success of the last decade in trauma and critical care.

▶ Early publications on abdominal compartment syndrome report high mortality and multiple organ failure. Recent advances in trauma and critical care, including hemostatic resuscitation and use of open abdomen strategies, have reduced the incidence and mortality rate associated with abdominal compartment syndrome. This report comes from one of the centers that has led this work.[1] Abdominal hypertension and abdominal compartment syndrome are described as previously reported by the World Society of Abdominal Compartment Syndrome.[2,3] While details of the resuscitation strategy used by these authors are not provided, they indicate that crystalloid limits of resuscitation are 2 L of crystalloids in the emergency department and a total of <4 L of crystalloids before admission to the intensive care unit. Patients requiring additional resuscitation receive various colloids with a focus on blood component therapy. I note in reviewing inclusion criteria that patients requiring massive transfusion (10 units of packed red blood cells in 24 hours) were not prominent. Thus, patients requiring the most aggressive resuscitation strategies were not frequently represented in these results.

Remarkably, intra-abdominal hypertension (IAH) did not change outcome in this prospective patient cohort. While a significant number of patients developed IAH, with careful limits to resuscitation, these patients did not progress to abdominal compartment syndrome, develop organ failure or reach high-grade IAH (Fig in original article). IAH levels are defined as grade 1, intra-abdominal pressure (IAP) 12–5 mm Hg; grade 2, IAP 16–20 mm Hg; grade 3, IAP 21–25 mm Hg; grade 4, >25 mm Hg).[1-4]

Resuscitation for injury was based on a practice of giving 3 times crystalloid resuscitation volume to presumed blood volume loss. This strategy, dating to the 1960s and 1970s, led to visceral edema and abdominal compartment syndrome. In this millennium, the switch of resuscitation strategies away from massive crystalloid administration is one of the major causes for decrease in IAH and abdominal compartment syndrome.

D. J. Dries, MSE, MD

References

1. Malbrain ML, Cheatham ML, Kirkpatrick A, et al. Results from the international conference of experts on intra-abdominal hypertension and abdominal compartment syndrome I: definitions. *Intensive Care Med.* 2006;32:1722-1732.
2. Cheatham ML, Malbrain ML, Kirkpatrick A, et al. Results from the international conference of experts on intra-abdominal hypertension and abdominal compartment syndrome II: recommendations. *Intensive Care Med.* 2007;33:951-962.
3. Sauaia A, Moore EE, Johnson JL, Ciesla DJ, Biffl WL, Banerjee A. Validation of postinjury multiple organ failure scores. *Shock.* 2009;31:438-447.
4. Balogh Z, McKinley BA, Cox CS Jr, et al. Abdominal compartment syndrome: the cause or effect of postinjury multiple organ failure. *Shock.* 2003;20:483-492.

Femoral Shaft Fracture Fixation and Chest Injury After Polytrauma

Bone LB, Giannoudis P (Erie County Med Ctr, Buffalo, NY; Leeds General Infirmary, Clarendon Wing, UK)

J Bone Joint Surg Am 93:311-317, 2011

Background.—Multiply injured patients who have fractures were traditionally placed in a splint or skeletal traction until they could be stabilized sufficiently to have fracture fixation surgery. Numerous complications developed in these cases, including adult respiratory distress syndrome, infection, pneumonia, malunion, nonunion, and death, especially in patients with a high Injury Severity Score (ISS). Based on these outcomes and further study, various approaches have been developed related to the patient's status.

Approaches.—Bilateral femoral fracture in a hemodynamically stable patient is safely handled using intramedullary nailing as long as the patient's oxygenation and hydration are closely monitored during the initial nail placement to verify the patient's stable condition is maintained. Patients who have bilateral femoral fracture and pulmonary contusion but are well oxygenated are better managed using either bilateral external fixation or intramedullary nailing of one femur and external fixation or plate fixation of the other, which is the preferred approach. Patients whose oxygenation is questionable should be managed with external fixation whether the femoral fracture is unilateral or bilateral.

Patients with femoral fracture who have an ISS of 18 or higher have no undue risk of complications and should undergo immediate intramedullary nailing. If the patient remains unstable after resuscitation or is in extremis (at the point of death), temporary stabilization of the long-bone fracture is achieved with external fixation. Femoral fracture, ISS of

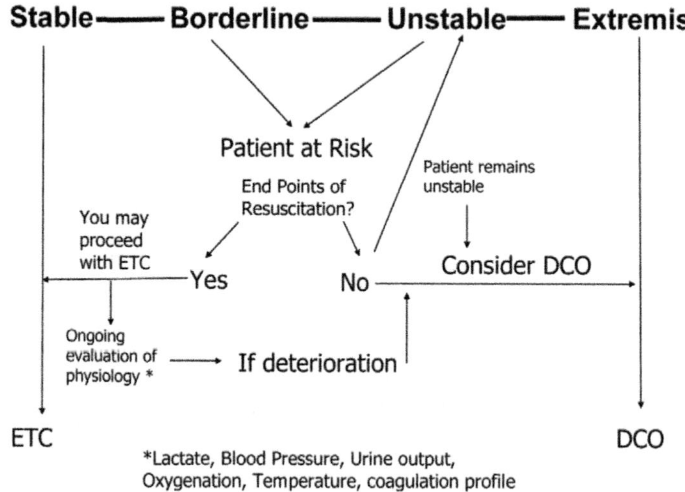

FIGURE 1.—The condition of a trauma patient on admission can range from hemodynamically stable to in extremis—i.e., in the process of dying. The stable patient is best managed with early definitive stabilization of the fractures (early total care [ETC]). The patient in extremis requires rapid temporary stabilization with external fixation. A "patient at risk" is a patient with a higher Injury Severity Score (ISS), an initial systolic blood pressure of <100 mm Hg, a lactate level of >2.5 mmol/L, and associated chest and abdominal injuries. These patients need aggressive resuscitation, and if they can be stabilized with fluid and blood replacement and ventilatory assistance definitive stabilization can be done. If they do not stabilize, they require damage control orthopaedics (DCO). The unstable patient, defined as one who remains hypotensive but who also may have hypothermia, coagulation abnormalities, and decreased oxygenation, needs constant reassessment, aggressive resuscitation, warming, and improvement of the coagulation profile. If this can be achieved in a timely fashion, the patient may also have definitive surgery. If not, then damage control stabilization is required. The grade of recommendation for the treatment strategy presented in this figure is B. (Reprinted from Bone LB, Giannoudis P. Femoral shaft fracture fixation and chest injury after polytrauma. *J Bone Joint Surg Am.* 2011;93:311-317, with permission from The Journal Of Bone and Joint Surgery, Inc.)

18 or greater, and substantial lung injury in a patient who is hemodynamically stable, not hypothermic, and well oxygenated and has a lactate level of about 2.2 mmol/L can also safely be managed with acute intramedullary femoral nail placement.

Advantages and Disadvantages.—Definitive stabilization allows the patient to be mobilized more quickly, which improves lung function. This approach is best for patients who are sufficiently stable and offers the additional advantages of spending less time in the intensive care unit, on ventilation support, and in the hospital, as well as seldom requiring a second operation. However, not all unstable patients do well with definitive stabilization and some multiply injured patients should not be managed with acute intramedullary fixation of femoral fractures. Temporary stabilization is better for these patients because it substantially reduces the degree of insult accompanying a second surgery. Unstable patients must be closely monitored to ensure they can undergo definitive treatment. Patients who are hemodynamically unstable, have coagulation abnormalities, are

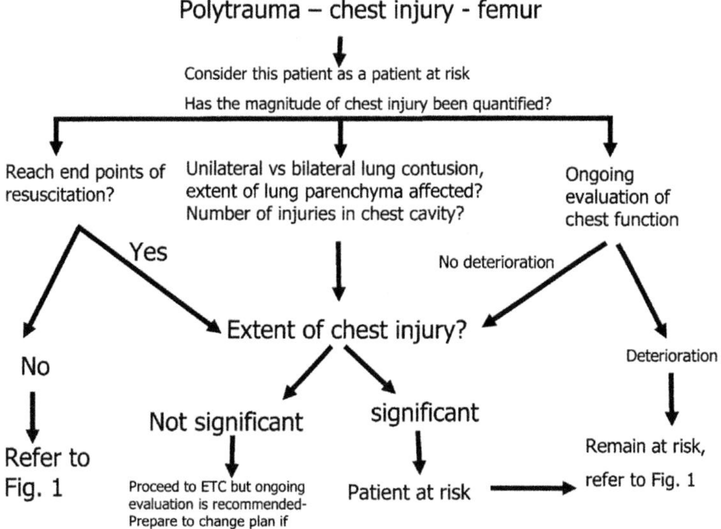

FIGURE 2.—Any patient with a chest injury with an AIS (Abbreviated Injury Scale[46]) score of ≥2 and a femoral fracture should be considered a patient at risk. A computed tomography (CT) scan of the chest should be performed to quantify the extent of chest involvement. If the patient can reach a satisfactory end point of resuscitation with stable blood pressure, adequate oxygenation, and a reduced lactate level, he or she may proceed to definitive early total care (ETC) but will require ongoing evaluation. If the patient cannot reach an adequate end point of resuscitation, he or she is considered an unstable patient and requires the damage control approach. If the extent of the chest injury is shown to be substantial by magnetic resonance imaging evaluation—i.e., >25% of the lung is injured—the patient is at substantial risk and should have damage control orthopaedics. Throughout the resuscitation period, and any surgical intervention, the chest injury needs ongoing evaluation. If no deterioration occurs, then definitive stabilization can proceed. If lung function deteriorates, then the patient becomes "at risk" and requires damage control orthopaedics. The grade of recommendation for the treatment strategy presented in this figure is B. (Reprinted from Bone LB, Giannoudis P. Femoral shaft fracture fixation and chest injury after polytrauma. *J Bone Joint Surg Am.* 2011;93:311-317, with permission from The Journal Of Bone and Joint Surgery, Inc.)

TABLE 1.—Definition of "Patient at Risk"

Multiply injured patient with ISS of >20 and thoracic trauma
Multiply injured patient with hemorrhagic shock (initial systolic blood pressure of <90 mm Hg)
Bilateral pulmonary contusion
Initial mean pulmonary artery pressure of >24 mm Hg

hypothermic, or demonstrate poor oxygenation or ventilation should have temporary fracture fixation, with definitive repair delayed until their general condition is stabilized (Figs 1, 2 and Table 1).

▶ This common sense review includes a number of treatment algorithms. The observations of the authors can be summarized simply. The patient with femur fractures and chest injury must be assessed for hemodynamic as well as pulmonary stability prior to fracture stabilization.[1,2] The simple presence of chest injury and femur fractures does not preclude definitive plating or intramedullary nailing. Given our current knowledge, the additive contribution of fat emboli to pulmonary dysfunction after injury is not sufficient to automatically refuse operative stabilization.

D. J. Dries, MSE, MD

References

1. Lefaivre KA, Starr AJ, Stahel PF, Elliott AC, Smith WR. Prediction of pulmonary morbidity and mortality in patients with femur fracture. *J Trauma.* 2010;69: 1527-1536.
2. O'Toole RV, O'Brien M, Scalea TM, Habashi N, Pollak AN, Turen CH. Resuscitation before stabilization of femoral fractures limits acute respiratory distress syndrome in patients with multiple traumatic injuries despite low use of damage control orthopedics. *J Trauma.* 2009;67:1013-1021.

Impact of Improved Combat Casualty Care on Combat Wounded Undergoing Exploratory Laparotomy and Massive Transfusion

Simmons JW, White CE, Eastridge BJ, et al (United States Army Inst of Surgical Res, Fort Sam Houston, TX; et al)
J Trauma 71:S82-S86, 2011

Background.—Studies have shown decreased mortality after improvements in combat casualty care, including increased fresh frozen plasma (FFP):red blood cell (RBC) ratios. The objective was to evaluate the evolution and impact of improved combat casualty care at different time periods of combat operations.

Methods.—A retrospective review was performed at one combat support hospital in Iraq of patients requiring both massive transfusion (≥10 units RBC in 24 hours) and exploratory laparotomy. Patients were divided into two cohorts based on year wounded: C1 between December 2003 and June 2004, and C2 between September 2007 and May 2008.

Admission data, amount of blood products and fluid transfused, and 48 hour mortality were compared. Statistical significance was set at $p < 0.05$.

Results.—There was decreased mortality in C2 (47% vs. 20%). Patients arrived warmer with higher hemoglobin. They were transfused more RBC and FFP in the emergency department (5 units ± 3 units vs. 2 units ± 2 units; 3 units ± 2 units vs. 0 units ± 1 units, respectively) and received less crystalloid in operating room (3.3 L ± 2.2 L vs. 8.5 L ± 4.9 L). The FFP:RBC ratio was also closer to 1:1 in C2 (0.775 ± 0.32 vs. 0.511 ± 0.21).

Conclusions.—The combination of improved prehospital care, trauma systems approach, performance improvement projects, and improved transfusion or resuscitation practices have led to a 50% decrease in mortality for this critically injured population. We are now transfusing blood products in a ratio more consistent with 1 FFP to 1 RBC. Simultaneously, crystalloid use has decreased by 61%, all of which is consistent with hemostatic resuscitation principles (Tables 2 and 5).

▶ Contemporary military activities are unique in that they have spawned formation of formal trauma systems to support combatants. With trauma system formation, a programmatic approach to transport, resuscitation, and hospital organization has been made possible. In addition, registries within this trauma system have been developed to facilitate unparalleled review of results and provide opportunities for improvement in care.[1,2] These authors compare 2 cohorts of patients receiving resuscitation and emergency laparotomy. An obvious decrease in mortality is identified. With data gathered by the registry mechanism, factors contributing to this improvement in outcome can be delineated.

Prehospital care has been modified to reduce crystalloid administration by paramedics in the field. Now small boluses of crystalloids are given only to the extent that a radial pulse is restored. Comparison of the base deficit between

TABLE 2.—The Patient Population was Split Into Two Groups Based on Time Wounded

	December 2003–June 2004 (N = 30)	September 2007–May 2008 (N = 66)	*p*
Demographics			
Age (yrs)	30 ± 11	30 ± 18	0.483
Military ISS	27 ± 17	30 ± 15	0.500
Vital signs			
SBP (mm Hg)	88 ± 35	99 ± 36	0.147
Pulse (bpm)	122 ± 25	124 ± 33	0.621
Respirations (per min)	29 ± 14	28 ± 20	0.310
GCS	10 ± 5	12 ± 5	0.328
Temperature (°F)	94.3 ± 2.9	97.2 ± 9.3	<0.001
Laboratory results			
Hgb (g/dL)	9.3 ± 2.7	10.9 ± 2.4	0.003
Plt (10^3 cells/mm^3)	187 ± 107	225 ± 123	0.178
INR	1.9 ± 0.8	1.8 ± 1.1	0.207
Base deficit (mEq/L)	−13.2 ± 8.3	−9.1 ± 6.1	0.010
pH	7.1 ± 0.2	7.2 ± 0.1	0.025

SBP, systolic blood pressure; GCS, Glasgow Coma Scale; INR, International Normalization Ratio.
Data were presented as mean ± SD.

TABLE 5.—Cumulative FFP:RBC Ratios

	December 2003–June 2004	September 2007–May 2008	p
ED ratio	0.238 ± 0.768	0.541 ± 0.17	0.088
OR ratio	0.421 ± 0.312	0.769 ± 0.207	<0.001
Total ratio	0.511 ± 0.32	0.775 ± 0.211	<0.001

Data were presented as mean ± SD.

the 2 cohorts suggests that improvement in prehospital resuscitation is associated with less severe presentation of acidosis in hospital (Table 2).

Second, control of blood loss with the use of tourniquet technology has seen significant resurgence. In the field, every soldier now carries a combat tourniquet system so that blood loss due to major extremity injury can be reduced even before arrival of medical personnel. Third, hypothermia, part of the physiologic basis for poor resuscitation outcome, is now managed with hypothermia prevention/management kits that are mandatory on rotor-wing and ground evacuation patients. A variety of devices are now available and readily employed for rewarming of patients before arrival at hospital. Whenever possible, warmed intravenous (IV) fluids are also provided. Combat medics are trained to use portable heating systems to warm IV fluids in the field. This work also follows the trend toward increasing use of blood products with comparable ratio administration of fresh frozen plasma to packed red blood cells[3,4] (Table 5).

Finally, a formal stepwise system of incremental care is now available to the combat casualty. Thus, patient needs and medical resources are better matched.

D. J. Dries, MSE, MD

References

1. Eiseman B. Combat casualty management in Vietnam. *J Trauma.* 1967;7:53-63.
2. Eastridge BJ, Jenkins D, Flaherty S, Schiller H, Holcomb JB. Trauma system development in a theater of war: Experiences from Operation Iraqi Freedom and Operation Enduring Freedom. *J Trauma.* 2006;61:1366-1373.
3. Borgman MA, Spinella PC, Perkins JG, et al. The ratio of blood products transfused affects mortality in patients receiving massive transfusions at a combat support hospital. *J Trauma.* 2007;63:805-813.
4. Tien HC, Jung V, Rizoli SB, Acharya SV, MacDonald JC. An evaluation of tactical combat casualty care interventions in a combat environment. *J Am Coll Surg.* 2008;207:174-178.

Comparison of Nonoperative Management With Renorrhaphy and Nephrectomy in Penetrating Renal Injuries

Bjurlin MA, Jeng EI, Goble SM, et al (Cook County Hosp, Chicago, IL; Univ of Illinois at Chicago; American College of Surgeons, Chicago, IL; et al)
J Trauma 71:554-558, 2011

Background.—We reviewed our experience with penetrating renal injuries to compare nonoperative management of penetrating renal injuries with renorrhaphy and nephrectomy in light of concerns for unnecessary explorations and increased nephrectomy rates.

Methods.—In this retrospective study, we reviewed the records of 98 penetrating renal injuries from 2003 to 2008. Renal injuries were classified according to the American Association for the Surgery of Trauma and analyzed based on nephrectomy, renorrhaphy, and nonoperative management. Patient characteristics and outcomes measured were compared between management types. Continuous variables were summarized by means and compared using t test. Categorical variables were compared using χ^2 test.

Results.—Nonoperative management was performed in 40% of renal injuries, followed by renorrhaphy (38%) and nephrectomy (22%). Of renal gunshot wounds (n = 79), 26%, 42%, and 32% required nephrectomy, renorrhaphy, and were managed nonoperatively, respectively. No renal stab wound (n = 16) resulted in a nephrectomy and 81% were managed conservatively. Renal injuries managed nonoperatively had a lower incidence of transfusion (34 vs. 95%, $p < 0.001$), shorter mean intensive care unit (ICU) (3.0 vs. 9.0 days, $p = 0.028$) and mean hospital length of stay (7.9 vs. 18.1 days, $p = 0.006$), and lower mortality rate (0 vs. 20%, $p = 0.005$) compared with nephrectomy but similar to renorrhaphy (transfusion: 34 vs. 36%, $p = 0.864$; mean ICU: 3.0 vs. 2.8 days, $p = 0.931$; mean hospital length of stay: 7.9 vs. 11.2 days, $p = 0.197$; mortality: 0 vs. 6%, $p = 0.141$). The complication rate of nonoperative management was favorable compared with operative management.

Conclusions.—Selective nonoperative management of penetrating renal injuries resulted in a lower mortality rate, lower incidence of blood transfusion, and shorter mean ICU and hospital stay compared with patients

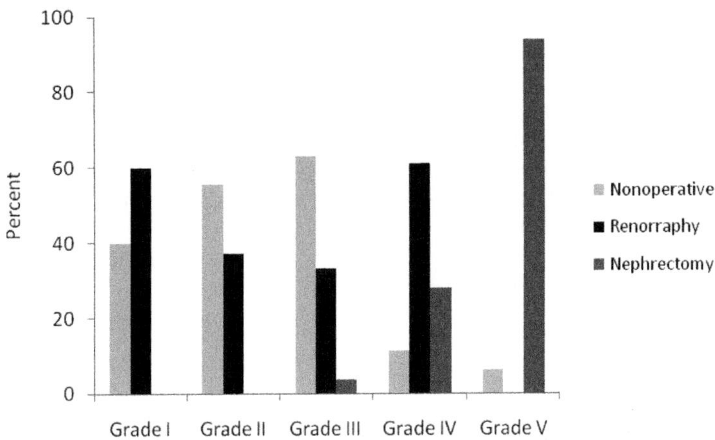

FIGURE 1.—Incidence of nonoperative management, renorrhaphy, and nephrectomy of penetrating renal injury grades I to V. (Reprinted from Bjurlin MA, Jeng EI, Goble SM, et al. Comparison of nonoperative management with renorrhaphy and nephrectomy in penetrating renal injuries. *J Trauma*. 2011;71: 554-558, with permission from Lippincott Williams & Wilkins.)

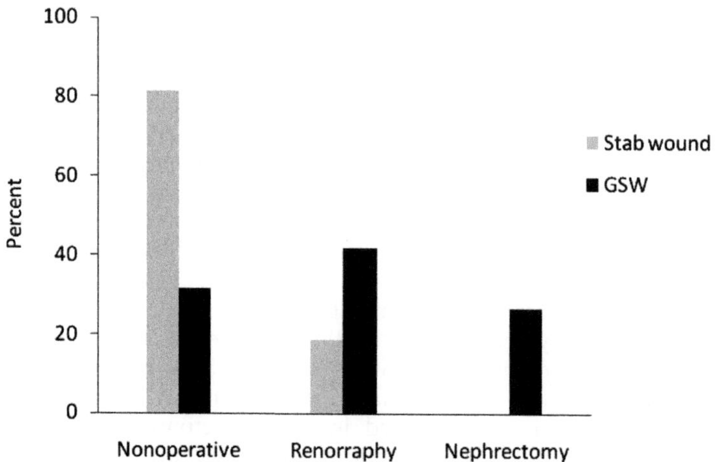

FIGURE 2.—Incidence of renal stab wound and GSW managed nonoperatively, with renorrhaphy, and nephrectomy. (Reprinted from Bjurlin MA, Jeng EI, Goble SM, et al. Comparison of nonoperative management with renorrhaphy and nephrectomy in penetrating renal injuries. *J Trauma*. 2011;71:554-558, with permission from Lippincott Williams & Wilkins.)

managed by nephrectomy but similar to renorrhaphy. Complication rates were low and similar to operative management (Figs 1 and 2).

▶ This study suggests that nonoperative management is appropriate in selected penetrating renal injuries. I emphasize that stab wounds clearly can be managed in this way. The likelihood of a renal repair is much higher when gunshot injury is involved (Fig 2).[1]

It is also important to note that the severity of injury directly relates to the type of treatment required (Fig 1). High-grade renal injury is much more likely to be associated with operative repair or nephrectomy. Low-grade injury, on the other hand, can frequently be managed nonoperatively regardless of etiology.[2,3]

The authors allude to two important limitations of this work. First, late complications, including fistula formation, scarring, chronic pyelonephritis, and hypertension, are not adequately characterized. Second, and more important, minimally invasive techniques, including embolization, percutaneous drainage, and ureteral stenting, are not characterized from the standpoint of outcome in this population.

D. J. Dries, MSE, MD

References

1. Voelzke BB, McAninch JW. Renal gunshot wounds: clinical management and outcome. *J Trauma*. 2009;66:593-601.
2. Santucci RA, Fisher MB. The literature increasingly supports expectant (conservative) management of renal trauma—a systematic review. *J Trauma*. 2005;59: 493-503.
3. Wright JL, Nathens AB, Rivara FP, Wessells H. Renal and extrarenal predictors of nephrectomy from the national trauma data bank. *J Urol*. 2006;175:970-975.

Management of Gunshot Pelvic Fractures With Bowel Injury: Is Fracture Debridement Necessary?

Rehman S, Slemenda C, Kestner C, et al (Temple Univ Hosp, Philadelphia, PA)

J Trauma 71:577-581, 2011

Background.—Low-velocity pelvic gunshot injuries occur commonly in urban trauma centers, occasionally involving concomitant intestinal viscus injury leading to potential fracture site contamination. Surgical debridement of the fractures may be necessary to prevent osteomyelitis, although not routinely performed in many centers. The purpose of this study was to determine whether fracture debridement should be done to prevent osteomyelitis in these injuries.

Methods.—A 5-year retrospective review of all patients older than 12 years with low-velocity gunshot pelvic fractures was performed at an urban Level I trauma center. Medical records and radiographs/computed tomographic scans were reviewed, and data regarding fracture location, concomitant intestinal viscus injury, orthopedic surgical intervention, antibiotic treatment, and bone and/or joint infection were recorded.

Results.—Of a total of 103 patients identified, 19 had expired within 48 hours and were excluded, resulting in a total of 84 study subjects for review. Fifty of 84 patients (59%) had a perforated viscus with 31 large bowel injuries and 30 small bowel injuries. Eighteen patients (21%) had intra-articular fractures, 15 of which involved the hip joint. Orthopedic surgical fracture debridement was done only in intra-articular fractures with retained bullet fragments (seven cases). Deep infection occurred in one patient with a missile injury to the hip joint with concomitant intestinal spillage. Immediate joint debridement was performed in this case, but successful missile fragment removal was not achieved until the second

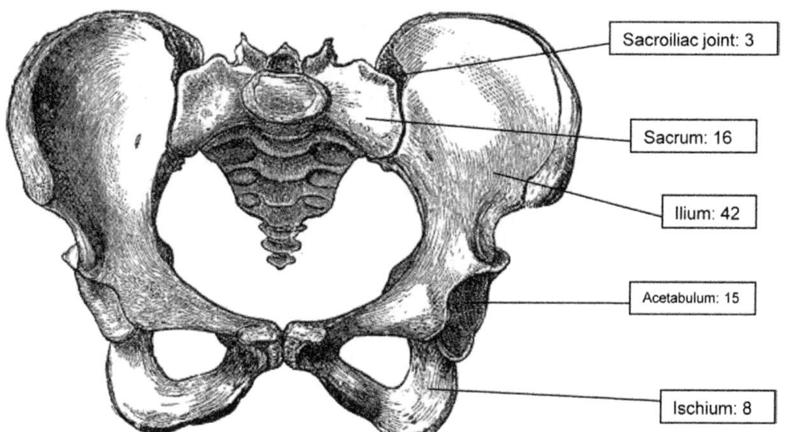

FIGURE 4.—Anatomic locations of gunshot pelvic fractures in this series. (Reprinted from Rehman S, Slemenda C, Kestner C, et al. Management of gunshot pelvic fractures with bowel injury: is fracture debridement necessary? *J Trauma*. 2011;71:577-581, Lippincott Williams & Wilkins.)

debridement after 48 hours. No infections occurred in any extra-articular fractures, regardless of the presence of intestinal spillage.

Conclusions.—Extra-articular gunshot pelvic fractures do not require formal orthopedic fracture debridement even in cases with concomitant intestinal viscus injury. However, debridement with bullet removal should be done in cases with intra-articular involvement, particularly if there are retained bullet fragments in the joint, to prevent deep infection (Fig 4).

▶ These authors address a simple and important question. It appears that only retained fragments in joint spaces warrant debridement, regardless of the spillage of intestinal content. However, I note, first, that relatively few injuries occurred in the joint space (Fig 4). The majority of fractures studied did not involve a joint. Therefore, the important part of this dataset is quite small. Second, the authors note that they explored involved joints even if a foreign body was not present. Therefore, some joint infections might have been prevented by this prophylactic joint exploration. Third, as the authors admit, the conclusions drawn here may not apply to all types of ammunition. At the very least, we can say that if a missile does not affect the joint space, acute exploration may not be needed.

D. J. Dries, MSE, MD

Early Surgical Stabilization of Flail Chest With Locked Plate Fixation

Althausen PL, Shannon S, Watts C, et al (Reno Orthopaedic Clinic, NV; Univ of Nevada Med School, Reno; et al)

J Orthop Trauma 25:641-648, 2011

Objectives.—To compare the results of surgical stabilization with locked plating to nonoperative care of flail chest injuries.

Design.—Retrospective case–control study.

Setting.—Level II trauma center.

Patients/Participants.—From January 2005 to January 2010, 22 patients with flail chest treated with locked plate fixation were compared with a matched cohort of 28 nonoperatively managed patients at our institution.

Intervention.—Open reduction internal fixation of rib fractures with 2.7-mm locking reconstruction plates.

Main Outcome Measurements.—Demographic data, such as age, sex, injury severity score, number of fractures, and lung contusion severity, were recorded. Intensive care unit data concerning length of stay (LOS), tracheostomy, and ventilator days were noted. Operative data, such as time to OR, operative time, and estimated blood loss, were recorded. Hospital data, including total hospital LOS, need for reintubation, and home oxygen requirements, were documented.

Results.—Average follow-up period of operatively managed patients was 17.84 ± 4.51 months, with a range of 13–22 months. No case of hardware failure, hardware prominence, wound infection, or nonunion was reported.

Operatively treated patients had shorter intensive care unit stays (7.59 vs. 9.68 days, $P = 0.018$), decreased ventilator requirements (4.14 vs. 9.68 days, $P = 0.007$), shorter hospital LOS (11.9 vs. 19.0 days, $P = 0.006$), fewer tracheostomies (4.55% vs. 39.29%, $P = 0.042$), less pneumonia (4.55% vs. 25%, $P = 0.047$), less need for reintubation (4.55% vs. 17.86%, $P = 0.34$), and decreased home oxygen requirements (4.55% vs. 17.86%, $P = 0.034$).

Conclusions.—This study demonstrates the potential benefits of surgical stabilization of flail chest with locked plate fixation. When compared with case-matched controls, operatively managed patients demonstrated improved clinical outcomes. Locked plate fixation seems to be safe as no complications associated with hardware failure, plate prominence, wound infection, or nonunion were noted.

▶ This study from a level II trauma center has an impressive number of patients with flail chest and, I presume, contusions.[1] A relatively recent series of patients with surgical plate fixation were compared with a historical cohort of patients who were treated without operative procedure. A number of clinical parameters, summarized in the abstract, suggest strongly positive outcomes with fracture stabilization.

Further review of the methods suggests that the authors have become inclusive in recent years when selecting patients for plate fixation.[2,3] They have developed excellent operative technique, and their short-term outcomes are good. I was surprised at the poor outcomes in their historical controls and the number of flail chest patients seen at a single level II trauma center. We are not told the period of time during which the nonoperatively treated patients were admitted. I am concerned that the pattern of care and decision for procedures such as tracheostomy and diagnosis for common problems such as pneumonia were not consistent among groups.[4,5]

This article can be recommended for data provided on operative technique. However, my concerns about controls as used by these authors raise concern about some of the claims made by these surgeons.

D. J. Dries, MSE, MD

References

1. Cohn SM. Pulmonary contusion: review of the clinical entity. *J Trauma*. 1997;42: 973-999.
2. Marasco SF, Sutalo ID, Bui AV. Mode of failure of rib fixation with absorbable plates: a clinical and numerical modeling study. *J Trauma*. 2010;68:1225-1233.
3. Strumwasser A, Chu E, Yeung L, Miraflor E, Sadjadi J, Victorino GP. A novel CT volume index score correlates with outcomes in polytrauma patients with pulmonary contusion. *J Surg Res*. 2011;170:280-285.
4. Michelet P, Couret D, Brégeon F, et al. Early onset pneumonia in severe chest trauma: a risk factor analysis. *J Trauma*. 2010;68:395-400.
5. Truitt MS, Mooty RC, Amos J, et al. Out with the old, in with the new: a novel approach to treating pain associated with rib fractures. *World J Surg*. 2010;34: 2359-2362.

Penetrating neck trauma: a case for conservative approach

Zaidi SMH, Ahmad R (SMHS Hosp Karan Nagar, Srinagar, J & K, India)
Am J Otolaryngol 32:591-596, 2011

Background.—Selective conservative management of penetrating neck trauma is a commonly adopted procedure to manage patients of such trauma. However, at places where trauma services are inadequate on different counts and a low-intensity military conflict is on, relevance of this approach without compromising the safety and well-being of the patient remains to be evaluated.

Objectives.—The study aimed to address the relevance of selective conservative management of penetrating neck trauma in a low-intensity military conflict of Kashmir.

Patients and Methods.—This was a prospective case study of patients presenting to the ENT Head & Neck Surgery department with penetrating neck trauma for a 2-year period from June 2003 to May 2005. After a careful physical examination in the emergency room, immediate surgical intervention or a careful observation is planned. Relevant investigations in the latter group if indicated by clinical examination determined whether to operate or to continue such approach. The data were collected and analyzed.

Results.—Forty-six patients fulfilled the criteria to be included in the study. Eight patients (17.4%) underwent immediate surgical intervention, whereas the remaining patients (78.26%) were carefully observed for a minimum of 24 hours. Two patients of the active observation group required delayed exploration because of the close proximity of projectile to vessels. None of the patients in either group died. There was significant difference between the 2 groups in terms of hospital stay, use of diagnostic tests, and complications.

Conclusions.—Selective conservative management is a cost-effective approach for penetrating neck trauma even in areas where there is relative paucity of advanced trauma services. These results further reinforce the validity of careful physical examination as a reliable tool to guide further management without necessarily resorting to expensive and at times difficult to do diagnostic tests (Tables 2, 3, and 5).

▶ Three anatomic zones of the neck provide an important guideline for management of penetrating injuries. Zone I is that area between the clavicles and cricoid cartilage, including the thoracic outlet vasculature and the vertebral and proximal carotid arteries. Lung, trachea, esophagus, spinal cord, thoracic duct, and major cervical trunks may also be found in Zone I. Zone II lies between cricoid cartilage and the angle of the mandible. Jugular veins, vertebral and common carotid arteries, and the external and internal branches of the carotid artery are also located in this zone. Trachea, esophagus, spinal cord, and larynx traverse this area. The most cephalad area, Zone III, lies between the angle of the mandible and the base of the skull. The pharynx is located in this zone with jugular veins, vertebral arteries, and the distal internal carotid arteries. Zones I and III are bounded by bony structures and, if penetrating injury is suspected, evaluated

TABLE 2.—Clinical Features at the Time of Admission

Symptom/Sign	No. of Patients
Hemoptysis	14
Hoarseness of voice	13
Odynophagia/dysphagia	26
Hematemesis	1
Subcutaneous emphysema	9
Active bleeding not responding to conservative measures	3
Shock	3
Expanding hematoma	1
Respiratory distress	3
Mild discomfort	20

TABLE 3.—Comparison of Different Investigations

Investigation Positive Report	Immediate Exploration	Active Observation
Soft tissue neck	7 (n = 10)	20 (n = 36)
CT scan	6 (n = 7)	5 (n = 11)
Barium swallow	Nil	1 (n = 3)
Fiber-optic airway endoscopy	3 (n = 10)	5 (n = 25)

TABLE 5.—Complications in 2 Groups

Complication	Immediate Exploration (n = 10)	Active Observation (n = 36)
Significant airway reduction (<50%)	1	None
Permanent voice problems (at 6 mo)	3	None
Neural deficit	2	1
Wound infection	2	3
Pharyngocutaneous fistula	None	1

with a variety of imaging techniques. Zone II can be evaluated more rapidly in the operating room should an injury present. Traditional teaching includes opening the neck for Zone II injuries that appear to penetrate the platysma.[1]

These authors present a series of 46 patients. Approximately 60% of injures were in Zone II, and the majority of these injuries came from projectiles. Patients with obvious airway or vascular compromise of a critical nature were taken to the operating room. The majority of these patients (36 of 46) were admitted for active observation without extensive imaging. Patients presenting with signs of injury including reversible shock, static hematomas, dysphonia, dysphasia, and subcutaneous emphysema or brief episodes of hematemesis or hemoptysis were observed with serial physical examination and limited diagnostic studies.

Remarkably, there was no difference in complication pattern between the 2 groups. Clinical assessment successfully segregated patients requiring urgent operative intervention from those tolerating expectant management. Two patients in the observation group were later taken to the operating room because of foreign bodies located in immediate proximity to vascular structures, and projectiles were removed. There was no acute mortality in either group.

The authors demonstrate success in carefully selected patients followed with minimal imaging and careful physical examination in the setting of injury penetrating the platysma. With greater public sensitivity to avoidance to radiation, particularly in children, an approach incorporating careful clinical observation has merit.[2-4]

D. J. Dries, MSE, MD

References

1. Britt LD, Weireter LJ, Cole FJ. Management of acute neck injuries. In: Feliciano FV, Mattox KL, Moore EE, eds. *Trauma*. 6th ed. McGraw Hill; 2008: 467-477.
2. Brenner DJ, Hall EJ. Computed tomography—an increasing source of radiation exposure. *N Engl J Med*. 2007;357:2277-2284.
3. Brenner DJ, Hricak H. Radiation exposure from medical imaging: time to regulate? *JAMA*. 2010;304:208-209.
4. Smith-Bindman R, Lipson J, Marcus R, et al. Radiation dose associated with common computed tomography examinations and the associated lifetime attributable risk of cancer. *Arch Intern Med*. 2009;169:2078-2086.

Emergency department predictors of tracheostomy in patients with isolated traumatic brain injury requiring emergency cranial decompression

Shamim MS, Qadeer M, Murtaza G, et al (Aga Khan Univ Hosp, Karachi, Pakistan)

J Neurosurg 115:1007-1012, 2011

Object.—Patients with severe traumatic brain injury (TBI) frequently require a tracheostomy for prolonged mechanical ventilation and/or pulmonary toilet. It is now proven that the earlier the procedure is done, the more beneficial it is to the patient. The present study was carried out to determine if the requirement of a tracheostomy can be predicted on arrival of a patient to the emergency department. The prediction can potentially aid in combining the procedure with cranial decompression. In this study, the authors' aim was to determine the emergency department predictors of tracheostomy in patients with isolated TBI requiring emergency cranial decompression.

Methods.—The authors performed a retrospective chart review of all patients who underwent surgery for isolated TBI and required more than 4 days of mechanical ventilation. Multivariate logistic regression analysis was used for predictive indicators.

Results.—In patients with isolated severe TBI, a patient age of 31–50 years, the presence of preexisting medical comorbid conditions, a delay in emergency department arrival exceeding 1.5 hours, an abnormal pupil response on arrival, and a preoperative neurological worsening during hospital stay were independent predictors of the requirement for tracheostomy. These findings were validated in a small cohort of patients and were found to be significant.

Conclusions.—Requirement of a tracheostomy can be predicted in patients with severe TBI on arrival to the emergency department. These results were validated in a small cohort of patients, and it was found that the positive predictive value of requirement of tracheostomy was directly proportional to the number of predictors present. Larger prospective studies with appropriate control groups are further recommended to validate the authors' findings (Figs 1 and 2).

▶ The authors have identified a small number of predictors, readily picked up in the clinical setting, which can predict the need for tracheostomy during hospitalization. Both retrospective and prospective datasets are provided. It appears that most tracheostomies are performed within the early days of hospitalization, assuming that the patient is still on mechanical ventilation at hospital day 4. While a variety of outcome data are provided, strict criteria for determination of the need for tracheostomy are not given. The key factor appears to be judgment of the attending neurosurgeon or the attending intensivist.

I was also concerned that patients included for this evaluation all required craniotomy with or without replacement of the bone flap. A large number of patients with significant head injury do not require an early neurosurgical procedure.[1-3] Thus, this dataset may not apply to a large number of head-injured patients.

Finally, the next important step for these or other investigators interested in this question is to evaluate the impact of this tracheostomy algorithm on infectious, mechanical, and other complications. The authors provide a predictor for

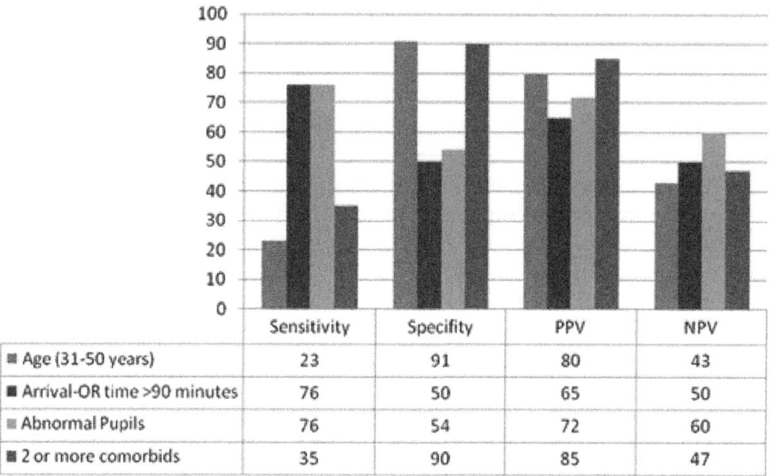

	Sensitivity	Specifity	PPV	NPV
Age (31-50 years)	23	91	80	43
Arrival-OR time >90 minutes	76	50	65	50
Abnormal Pupils	76	54	72	60
2 or more comorbids	35	90	85	47

FIGURE 1.—Validation of results. Sensitivity, specificity, positive predictive value (PPV), and negative predictive value (NPV) for each significant variable. OR = operating room. (Reprinted from Shamim MS, Qadeer M, Murtaza G, et al. Emergency department predictors of tracheostomy in patients with isolated traumatic brain injury requiring emergency cranial decompression. *J Neurosurg*. 2011;115:1007-1012.)

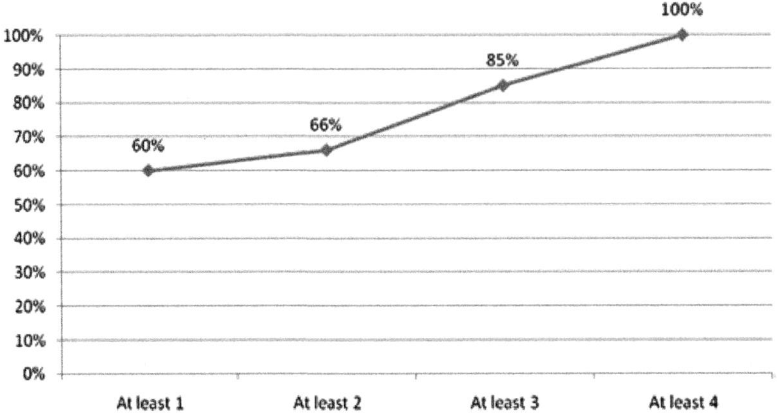

FIGURE 2.—Validation of results. Cumulative positive predictive value of significant variables. The number of factors is shown on the x axis. (Reprinted from Shamim MS, Qadeer M, Murtaza G, et al. Emergency department predictors of tracheostomy in patients with isolated traumatic brain injury requiring emergency cranial decompression. *J Neurosurg*. 2011;115:1007-1012.)

the need to place a surgical airway. We need to show that these criteria, with airway placement, are also associated with improvement in reported outcomes.

D. J. Dries, MSE, MD

References

1. Martins ET, Linhares MN, Sousa DS, et al. Mortality in severe traumatic brain injury: a multivariated analysis of 748 Brazilian patients from Florianópolis City. *J Trauma*. 2009:85-90.
2. Petroni G, Quaglino M, Lujan S, et al. Early prognosis of severe traumatic brain injury in an urban argentinian trauma center. *J Trauma*. 2010;68:564-570.
3. Chelly H, Chaari A, Daoud E, et al. Diffuse axonal injury in patients with head injuries: an epidemiologic and prognosis study of 124 cases. *J Trauma*. 2011;71: 838-846.

Costs of Postoperative Sepsis: The Business Case for Quality Improvement to Reduce Postoperative Sepsis in Veterans Affairs Hospitals

Vaughan-Sarrazin MS, Bayman L, Cullen JJ (Univ of Iowa College of Medicine)
Arch Surg 146:944-951, 2011

Objective.—To estimate the incremental costs associated with sepsis as a complication of general surgery, controlling for patient risk factors that may affect costs (eg, surgical complexity and comorbidity) and hospital-level variation in costs.

Design.—Database analysis.

Setting.—One hundred eighteen Veterans Health Affairs hospitals.

Patients.—A total of 13 878 patients undergoing general surgery during fiscal year 2006 (October 1, 2005, through September 30, 2006).

Main Outcome Measures.—Incremental costs associated with sepsis as a complication of general surgery (controlling for patient risk factors and hospital-level variation of costs), as well as the increase in costs associated with complications that co-occur with sepsis. Costs were estimated using the Veterans Health Affairs Decision Support System, and patient risk factors and postoperative complications were identified in the Veterans Affairs Surgical Quality Improvement Program database.

Results.—Overall, 564 of 13 878 patients undergoing general surgery developed postoperative sepsis, for a rate of 4.1%. The average unadjusted cost for patients with no sepsis was $24 923, whereas the average cost for patients with sepsis was 3.6 times higher at $88 747. In risk-adjusted analyses, the relative costs were 2.28 times greater for patients with sepsis relative to patients without sepsis (95% confidence interval, 2.19-2.38), with the difference in risk-adjusted costs estimated at $26 972 (ie, $21 045 vs $48 017). Sepsis often co-occurred with other types of complications, most frequently with failure to wean the patient from mechanical ventilation after 48 hours (36%), postoperative pneumonia (31%), and reintubation for respiratory or cardiac failure (29%). Costs were highest when sepsis occurred with pneumonia or failure to wean the patient from mechanical ventilation after 48 hours.

Conclusion.—Given the high cost of treating sepsis, a business case can be made for quality improvement initiatives that reduce the likelihood of postoperative sepsis.

▶ The incremental costs associated with treating sepsis can be substantial, with estimates ranging from $10 500 to $40 000 per case. As postoperative complications account for 30% of severe sepsis cases, the authors of this study cite the importance of reducing the incidence of postsurgical sepsis by creating a business case for quality improvement initiatives. The study estimates the incremental costs of sepsis as a complication of general surgery in 118 Veterans Health Affairs hospitals.

This retrospective study included 13 678 general surgery patients in which 564 (4.1%) developed sepsis. The sepsis rate in the study was found to increase with age and patient characteristics, including the presence of diabetes mellitus, wound infection, blood transfusion, pneumonia, and ventilator dependence. The average unadjusted cost for the 564 patients who experienced sepsis was 3.6 times higher ($88 747 vs $24 923). Assuming a 10% reduction in postoperative sepsis rates, extrapolating this cost savings across the approximately 4 million general surgery procedures in US hospital annually could save more than $421 million.

Several initiatives were cited to reduce the rate of sepsis in postoperative patients including the Surgical Infection Prevention system and the Surviving Sepsis Campaign. Poor compliance, however, was identified as a source for improvement, as < 30% of inpatients with severe sepsis receive the recommended care. Additionally, studies have found a relationship between postoperative complication rates and hospital staffing. Hospitals with higher nursing staffing ratios and more highly educated nurses providing care for high-risk surgery patients have lower morbidity and resource utilization compared with other hospitals. Meaningful reductions in postoperative complications will require a team approach by practitioners and hospital administrators to improve outcomes and reduce expenses.

R. Perez, MD
S. L. Zanotti-Cavazzoni, MD

Test Characteristics of Focused Assessment of Sonography for Trauma for Clinically Significant Abdominal Free Fluid in Pediatric Blunt Abdominal Trauma

Fox JC, Boysen M, Gharahbaghian L, et al (Univ of California at Irvine, Orange; Stanford Univ, Palo Alto, CA; et al)
Acad Emerg Med 18:477-482, 2011

Objectives.—Focused assessment of sonography in trauma (FAST) has been shown useful to detect clinically significant hemoperitoneum in adults, but not in children. The objectives were to determine test characteristics for clinically important intraperitoneal free fluid (FF) in pediatric blunt abdominal trauma (BAT) using computed tomography (CT) or surgery as criterion reference and, second, to determine the test characteristics of FAST to detect any amount of intraperitoneal FF as detected by CT.

Methods.—This was a prospective observational study of consecutive children (0–17 years) who required trauma team activation for BAT and received either CT or laparotomy between 2004 and 2007. Experienced physicians performed and interpreted FAST. Clinically important FF was defined as moderate or greater amount of intraperitoneal FF per the radiologist CT report or surgery.

Results.—The study enrolled 431 patients, excluded 74, and analyzed data on 357. For the first objective, 23 patients had significant hemoperitoneum (22 on CT and one at surgery). Twelve of the 23 had true-positive FAST (sensitivity = 52%; 95% confidence interval [CI] = 31% to 73%). FAST was true negative in 321 of 334 (specificity = 96%; 95% CI = 93% to 98%). Twelve of 25 patients with positive FAST had significant FF on CT (positive predictive value [PPV] = 48%; 95% CI = 28% to 69%). Of 332 patients with negative FAST, 321 had no significant fluid on CT (negative predictive value [NPV] = 97%; 95% CI = 94% to 98%). Positive likelihood ratio (LR) for FF was 13.4 (95% CI = 6.9 to 26.0) while the negative LR was 0.50 (95% CI = 0.32 to 0.76). Accuracy was 93% (333 of 357, 95% CI = 90% to 96%). For the second objective, test characteristics were as follows: sensitivity = 20% (95% CI = 13% to 30%), specificity = 98% (95% CI = 95% to 99%), PPV = 76% (95% CI = 54% to 90%), NPV = 78% (95% CI = 73% to 82%), positive LR = 9.0 (95% CI = 3.7

to 21.8), negative LR = 0.81 (95% CI = 0.7 to 0.9), and accuracy = 78% (277 of 357, 95% CI = 73% to 82%).

Conclusion.—In this population of children with BAT, FAST has a low sensitivity for clinically important FF but has high specificity. A positive FAST suggests hemoperitoneum and abdominal injury, while a negative FAST aids little in decision-making.

▶ Focused assessment with sonography in trauma (FAST) is a true staple in the assessment of trauma patients with both blunt and penetrating injuries. Although its strengths and weaknesses have been described well for adults, there is a paucity of literature in the pediatric population. This study sought to describe the test characteristics of FAST in detecting clinically important free fluid in pediatric blunt abdominal trauma (BAT) patients. Consecutive pediatric patients sustaining BAT were enrolled if parents would consent. Three hundred fifty-seven patients were included in the data analysis. Of 23 patients with significant hemoperitoneum, FAST was positive in 12, yielding a sensitivity of 52% (95% confidence interval 31%–73%). FAST was negative in 321 of 334 patients with no significant hemoperitoneum with specificity of 96% (95% confidence interval 93%–98%). A motivated group of sonographers led the study, and the results are likely representative of a best-case scenario. The low sensitivity may cause alarm at first sight. However, much like most diagnostic tests in medicine, they should be used in context of the patient with some consideration of pretest probability. It would have been interesting to see the sensitivity in unstable patients, because this is where the FAST has shown most benefit in adult patients. Among pediatric BAT patients, the authors summarize it best: "A positive FAST suggests hemoperitoneum and abdominal injury, while a negative FAST aids little in decision-making."

M. D. Zwank, MD

Selective Use of Computed Tomography Compared With Routine Whole Body Imaging in Patients With Blunt Trauma

Gupta M, Schriger DL, Hiatt JR, et al (Univ of California, Los Angeles; David Geffen School of Medicine at UCLA)

Ann Emerg Med 58:407-416, 2011

Study Objective.—Routine pan–computed tomography (CT, including of the head, neck, chest, abdomen/pelvis) has been advocated for evaluation of patients with blunt trauma based on the belief that early detection of clinically occult injuries will improve outcomes. We sought to determine whether selective imaging could decrease scan use without missing clinically important injuries.

Methods.—This was a prospective observational study of 701 patients with blunt trauma at an academic trauma center. Before scanning, the most senior emergency physician and trauma surgeon independently indicated which components of pan-CT were necessary. We calculated the proportion of scans deemed unnecessary that: (a) were abnormal and resulted in a pre-defined critical action or (b) were abnormal.

Results.—Pan-CT was performed in 600 of the patients; the remaining 101 underwent limited scanning. One or both physicians indicated a willingness to omit 35% of the individual scans. An abnormality was present in 18% of scans, including 22% of desired scans and 10% of undesired scans. Among the 95 patients who had one of the 102 undesired scans with abnormal results, 3 underwent a predefined critical action. There is disagreement among the authors about the clinical significance of the abnormalities found on the 99 undesired scans that did not lead to a critical action.

Conclusion.—Selective scanning could reduce the number of scans, missing some injuries but few critical ones. The clinical importance of injuries missed on undesired scans was subject to individual interpretation, which varied substantially among authors. This difference of opinion serves as a microcosm of the larger debate on appropriate use of expensive medical technologies.

▶ This is the first article to my knowledge in which the authors could not agree on an interpretation of the results and thus wrote 2 opposing conclusions. This highlights an ongoing debate regarding the use of CT scan in blunt trauma patients. On one side of the debate is great concern of radiation exposure to these often young patients and doubt as to the significance of injuries that are often found with CT. On the other side of the debate is the counterpoint that blunt trauma patients often have serious injuries that can only be discerned by CT scan. This study examined a cohort of 600 trauma patients. Physicians decided before CT scanning whether a given CT was "necessary" based on history and physical examination. After CT scan, injuries were noted and tabulated by whether the CT was previously deemed necessary. Nine hundred ninety-two (35%) of 2804 CT scans were deemed unnecessary by at least 1 physician. Of these 992 808 were obtained, and 102 (10%) were abnormal. Three of these scans indicated an injury that led to a predefined critical action (2 chest tubes and 1 reversal of coagulopathy for intracranial hemorrhage). Not surprisingly, emergency physicians were much less likely to desire any given CT. On the other hand, many of the CT scans that they didn't want ended up abnormal with wide-ranging injuries as severe as grade 3 splenic and liver lacerations. There was debate among the authors as to the significance of the many missed injuries. Although this study doesn't answer the debate, it certainly informs it. More limited CT scan use in blunt trauma patients is certain to "miss" injuries, although many physicians might be comfortable with that fact knowing that more aggressive CT scan use comes with its own morbidity.

M. D. Zwank, MD

Endovascular Treatment of Penetrating Traumatic Injuries of the Extracranial Carotid Artery

Herrera DA, Vargas SA, Dublin AB (Universidad de Antioquia, Medellin, Colombia; UC Davis Med Ctr, Sacramento, CA)

J Vasc Interv Radiol 22:28-33, 2011

Purpose.—To describe the clinical and angiographic results of endovascular therapy for traumatic injuries of the extracranial carotid artery.

Materials and Methods.—The clinical and angiographic features of 36 traumatic injuries of the carotid artery during a 12-year period were reviewed. There were 35 male patients (97.2%) and 1 female patient (2.8%) with an average age of 28.8 years (range 13–60 years). Of the 36 lesions of the carotid artery, 29 (80.6%) were the result of gunshot injury, and 7 (19.4%) were secondary to stab wounds. In 24 (66.7%) instances, the injury resulted in a pseudoaneurysm; in 7 (19.4%), in an arteriovenous fistula (AVF); in 4 (11.1%), in a dissection; and in 1 (2.8%), in inactive bleeding. All patients were treated with an endovascular approach using different techniques (balloon occlusion, embolization, or stent deployment).

Results.—Endovascular therapy resulted in documented lesion occlusion in 34 (94.4%) patients. Two patients declined any follow-up postprocedural imaging; however, they have remained asymptomatic. Clinical improvement was documented in 35 (97.2%) patients, and there was one procedure-related complication with fatal consequences.

Conclusions.—In this series, endovascular techniques were an effective method of treatment. It was possible to use different endovascular

TABLE 1.—Clinical Presentation and Angiographic Findings of Penetrating Lesions of the Extracranial Carotid Artery

	$N = 36$	%
Mechanism of trauma		
Gunshot	29	80.6%
Stab wound	7	19.4%
Presentation		
Bleeding	14	38.9%
Pulsatile mass	7	19.4%
Neck bruit	7	19.4%
Hematoma	4	11.1%
Stroke	3	8.3%
Dementia syndrome	1	2.8%
Injured vessel		
ECA	15	41.7%
ICA	14	38.9%
CCA	7	19.4%
Type of lesion		
Pseudoaneurysm	24	66.7%
Carotid-jugular AVF	7	19.4%
Dissection	4	11.1%
Active bleeding	1	2.8%

reconstructive techniques or parent artery occlusion depending on the degree of vessel damage, with resolution of clinical symptoms and avoidance of surgery in most cases (Table 1).

▶ In this small series, the authors note greater than 90% good outcomes with lesions involving the external, internal, and common carotid arteries. Stents can also be used to manage bleeding from branches of these 3 vessels. Only one of the patients treated was bleeding. Obviously, stents are appropriate for pseudoaneurysms and other lesions resulting from concussive injury to the extracranial carotid vasculature.

While the authors do not address this point, it is also interesting to note that evolving endovascular technology may facilitate access to injuries that at present have no good open surgical therapy. These include injuries traversing the skull base or immediately adjacent to the skull base. However, consistent with the literature in stent placement for vascular injury in the aorta, this patient group is young, and maturity of the patient with stents in place has not yet been investigated.

Patients in this series were treated with both covered and bare stent grafts. One patient with an uncovered graft failed to continue antiplatelet medications and suffered graft thrombosis. Graft thrombosis was not associated with neurologic injury. Reliability of the trauma population with respect to chronic anticoagulation has always been questionable.

D. J. Dries, MSE, MD

Abdominal trauma in primary blast injury

Owers C, Morgan JL, Garner JP (Rotherham NHS Foundation Trust, UK)
Br J Surg 98:168-179, 2011

Background.—Blast injury is uncommon, and remains poorly understood by most clinicians outside regions of active warfare. Primary blast injury (PBI) results from the interaction of the blast wave with the body, and typically affects gas-containing organs such as the ear, lungs and gastrointestinal tract. This review investigates the mechanisms and injuries sustained to the abdomen following blast exposure.

Methods.—MEDLINE was searched using the keywords 'primary blast injury', 'abdominal blast' and 'abdominal blast injury' to identify English language reports of abdominal PBI. Clinical reports providing sufficient data were used to calculate the incidence of abdominal PBI in hospitalized survivors of air blast, and in open- and enclosed-space detonations.

Results.—Sixty-one articles were identified that primarily reported clinical or experimental abdominal PBI. Nine clinical reports provided sufficient data to calculate an incidence of abdominal PBI; 31 (3·0 per cent) of 1040 hospitalized survivors of air blast suffered abdominal PBI, the incidence ranging from 1·3 to 33 per cent. The incidence for open- and enclosed-space detonations was 5·6 and 6·7 per cent respectively. The terminal ileum and caecum were the most commonly affected organs.

Surgical management of abdominal PBI is similar to that of abdominal trauma of other causes.

Conclusion.—Abdominal PBI is uncommon but has the potential for significant mortality and morbidity, which may present many days after blast exposure. It is commoner after blast in enclosed spaces and under water (Fig 2, Tables 1-3).

▶ This is an excellent literature review of the epidemiologic, diagnostic, and clinical issues that persist in challenging the clinician to optimally manage the patient with abdominal trauma in primary blast injury. Perhaps the most important confounding epidemiologic factor is the lack of large clinical series from patients with isolated injury. Disaster scenes or the battlefield can be a difficult classroom.[1] Many patients sustaining primary blast injury also have secondary or tertiary mechanisms of injury. Thus, the effects of primary blast injury, that is, because of the initial pressure wave, are harder to isolate.

Blast wave may encounter the body because of transmission through air (more common) or through water, which is less common.[2] In either case, initial symptoms include nausea and vomiting, bloody diarrhea, and testicular pain. Symptoms may persist, and perforation of the gastrointestinal tract may occur days after intestinal injury. There are no data on effective imaging techniques. In particular, CT scan, which is most helpful in solid organ injury, has been less effective in hollow viscus injury as seen in abdominal primary blast injury. In the setting of air blast injury or water emersion blast injury, solid organ injury typically involves the liver and spleen. Air blast patients have far greater frequency of solid organ injury reported than patients suffering water emersion blast. Both patient groups have high-volume hollow viscus injuries. The terminal ileum and cecum are most frequently affected.

Many of these patients may not develop transmural hollow viscus injury for days after blast trauma. Based on the limited literature available, intestinal perforation, if it will occur, generally occurs 3 to 5 days after injury. The duration

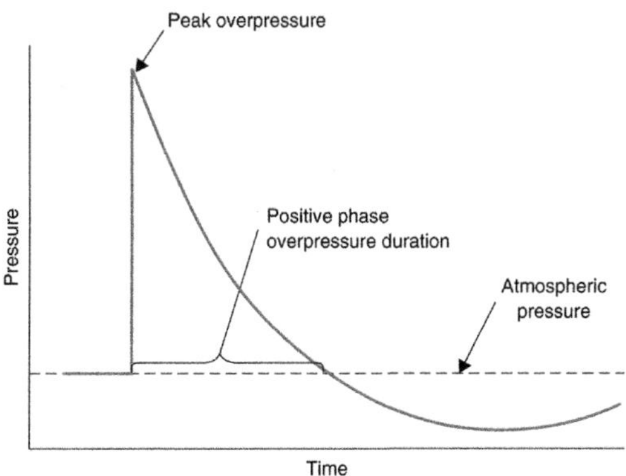

FIGURE 2.—Idealized pressure waveform at a single point from a free field air blast. (Reprinted from Owers C, Morgan JL, Garner JP. Abdominal trauma in primary blast injury. *Br J Surg*. 2011;98:168-179, Copyright © 2011, British Journal of Surgery Society Ltd. Reproduced with permission. Permission is granted by John Wiley & Sons Ltd on behalf of the BJSS Ltd.)

TABLE 1.—Zuckerman's Classification of Blast Injury[67]

Type of Blast Injury	Mechanism of Injury
Primary	Interaction of the blast wave with the body
Secondary	Energized fragments from the bomb itself or environmental debris accelerated by the blast wind
Tertiary	Physical displacement of the body by the blast wind, including tumbling and impact with stationary objects; crush from building collapse caused by blast wind
Quaternary	All other miscellaneous effects, including psychological effects of an explosion, burns and inhalational injury

Editor's Note: Please refer to original journal article for full references.

TABLE 2.—Relative Effects of 4-ms Exposure to Varying Blast Overpressures After Free Field Detonation[78]

Overpressure (kPa)	Effect
7	Damage to ordinary buildings and windows break
14	Slight risk of tympanic membrane perforation
100	50 per cent chance of tympanic membrane perforation
275	Reinforced buildings suffer significant damage
480	50 per cent chance of marked pulmonary injury
900	50 per cent chance of death

Editor's Note: Please refer to original journal article for full references.

TABLE 3.—Anatomical Distribution of Abdominal Injuries Found in Survivors or at Autopsy for Air and Immersion Blast Exposure[10,11,12,14–16,19,23,26,27,33]

	Air Blast		Immersion Blast	
	Operative Findings	Autopsy Findings	Operative Findings	Autopsy Findings
Hollow organs				
Stomach	10	1	0	1
Duodenum	4	0	1	1
Jejunum	10	0	3	1
Ileum	54	2	36	7
Bladder	3	0	0	0
Colon	13	4	54	4
Gastrointestinal haematoma (NOS)	5	5	41	9
Solid organs				
Liver	39	2	2	2
Spleen	47	7	2	2
Kidney	15	4	0	0
Testes	1	1	0	0
Mesentery	14	8	0	0

NOS, not otherwise specified.
Editor's Note: Please refer to original journal article for full references.

of observation prior to discharge or transfer of the patient to a lower level of care remains unclear.

D. J. Dries, MSE, MD

References

1. Trunkey DD, Johannigman JA, Holcomb JB. Lessons relearned. *Arch Surg*. 2008; 143:112-114.
2. DePalma RG, Burris DG, Champion HR, Hodgson MJ. Blast injuries. *N Engl J Med*. 2005;352:1335-1342.

Management of Penetrating Abdominal Trauma in the Conflict Environment: The Role of Computed Tomography Scanning

Morrison JJ, Clasper JC, Gibb I, et al (Royal Centre for Defence Medicine, Edgbaston, Birmingham, UK; Centre for Defence Imaging, Gosport, UK)
World J Surg 35:27-33, 2011

Background.—Computed tomography (CT) scanning is a vital imaging technique in selecting patients for nonoperative management of civilian penetrating abdominal trauma. This has reduced the rate of nontherapeutic laparotomies and associated complications. Battlefield abdominal injuries conventionally mandate laparotomy, and with the advent of field deployable CT scanners it is unclear whether some ballistic injuries can be managed conservatively.

Methods.—A retrospective 12 month cohort of patients admitted to a forward surgical facility in Afghanistan who sustained penetrating abdominal injury severe enough to warrant laparotomy or CT scan were studied. Patient details were retrieved from a prospectively maintained operative log and CT logs. Case notes were then reviewed and data pertaining to injury pattern, operative intervention, and survival were collected.

Results.—A total of 133 patients were studied: 73 underwent immediate laparotomy (Lap group) and 60 underwent CT scanning (CT group). Of those undergoing CT scanning 17 underwent laparotomy and 43 were selected for nonoperative management. There were 15 deaths in the Lap group and none in the CT group. The median New Injury Severity and Revised Trauma Score was 29 and 7.55 in the Lap group and 9 and 7.8408 in the CT group, which is statistically significantly different ($p < 0.001$). Five patients in the CT-Lap group had nontherapeutic laparotomies and 1 patient failed nonoperative management.

Conclusions.—Computed tomography scanning can be used in stable patients who have sustained penetrating battlefield abdominal injury to exclude peritoneal breach and identify solid abdominal organ injury that can be safely managed nonoperatively.

► While CT scanning is frequently used in the civilian practice of trauma to rule out peritoneal perforation and assess the magnitude of abdominal trauma in stable patients, this has not been the practice in military trauma surgery. These data are gathered in the British Military Hospital in Helmand Province, Afghanistan. Contemporary patterns of injury are, therefore, represented by these data.

The authors demonstrate that in stable patients, CT evaluation can be performed prior to consideration of operative intervention with military patients just as in civilian practice.[1-3] There was no mortality in patients receiving CT imaging, suggesting that the authors were able to appropriately identify individuals who were stable enough that the CT examination could be obtained. When CT was obtained, approximately three-fourths of the patients were spared laparotomy. There is no evidence of late complications because of delay to laparotomy.

As more CT scanners are portable and made available in the forward combat environment, this technique may demonstrate its value as a preoperative screen for the stable patient under consideration for laparotomy. CT did not eliminate the nontherapeutic laparotomy in this series of patients with penetrating injury, but I believe that the incidence of nontherapeutic laparotomy can be significantly reduced using selected CT imaging.

D. J. Dries, MSE, MD

References

1. Ramirez RM, Cureton EL, Ereso AQ, et al. Single-contrast computed tomography for the triage of patients with penetrating torso trauma. *J Trauma*. 2009;67: 583-588.
2. Wurmb TE, Frühwald P, Hopfner W, et al. Whole-body multislice computed tomography as the first line diagnostic tool in patients with multiple injuries: the focus on time. *J Trauma*. 2009;66:658-665.
3. Tillou A, Gupta M, Baraff LJ, et al. Is the use of pan-computed tomography for blunt trauma justified? A prospective evaluation. *J Trauma*. 2009;67:779-787.

Blunt Thoracic Aortic Injuries: An Autopsy Study

Teixeira PGR, Inaba K, Barmparas G, et al (Univ of Southern California, Los Angeles, CA)

J Trauma 70:197-202, 2011

Objective.—The objective of this study was to identify the incidence and patterns of thoracic aortic injuries in a series of blunt traumatic deaths and describe their associated injuries.

Methods.—All autopsies performed by the Los Angeles County Department of Coroner for blunt traumatic deaths in 2005 were retrospectively reviewed. Patients who had a traumatic thoracic aortic (TTA) injury were compared with the victims who did not have this injury for differences in baseline characteristics and patterns of associated injuries.

Results.—During the study period, 304 (35%) of 881 fatal victims of blunt trauma received by the Los Angeles County Department of Coroner underwent a full autopsy and were included in the analysis. The patients were on average aged 43 years ±21 years, 71% were men, and 39% had a positive blood alcohol screen. Motor vehicle collision was the most common mechanism of injury (50%), followed by pedestrian struck by auto (37%). A TTA injury was identified in 102 (34%) of the victims. The most common site of TTA injury was the isthmus and descending thoracic aorta, occurring in 67 fatalities (66% of the patients with TTA injuries). Patients with TTA injuries were significantly more likely to have other associated injuries: cardiac injury (44% vs. 25%, $p = 0.001$), hemothorax (86% vs. 56%, $p < 0.001$), rib fractures (86% vs. 72%, $p = 0.006$), and intra-abdominal injury (74% vs. 49%, $p < 0.001$) compared with patients without TTA injury. Patients with a TTA injury were significantly more likely to die at the scene (80% vs. 63%, $p = 0.002$).

Conclusion.—Thoracic aortic injuries occurred in fully one third of blunt traumatic fatalities, with the majority of deaths occurring at the scene. The risk for associated thoracic and intra-abdominal injuries is significantly increased in patients with thoracic aortic injuries (Fig 2 and Table 2).

▶ Using autopsy data, the authors present a contemporary picture of development and presentation of blunt thoracic aortic injury. This study is powerful in that a complete survey of blunt trauma data is provided for a large county with no patients having complete autopsy information excluded.

The authors were careful to describe injuries identified. Most injuries occurred at the isthmus or proximal descending aorta. The aortic arch was injured in 11% of patients, and aortic injury at multiple sites was noted in 18% of autopsies.

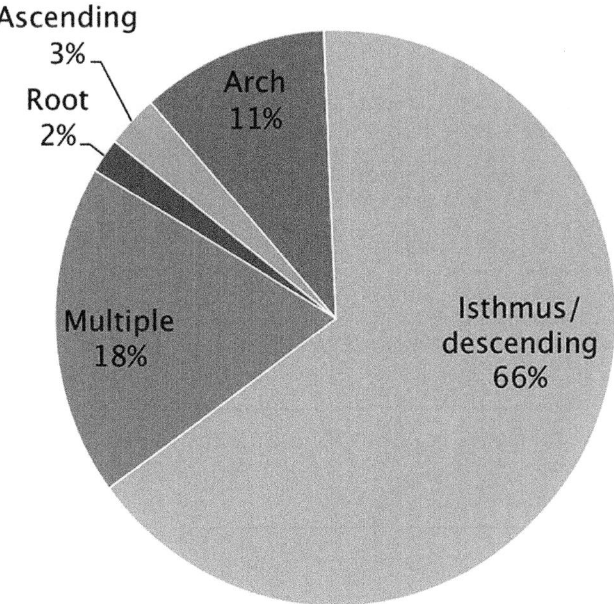

FIGURE 2.—Anatomic location of the thoracic aortic injuries. (Reprinted from Teixeira PGR, Inaba K, Barmparas G, et al. Blunt thoracic aortic injuries: an autopsy study. *J Trauma*. 2011;70:197-202, with permission from Lippincott Williams & Wilkins.)

TABLE 2.—Anatomic Location of the Traumatic Thoracic Aortic Injuries According to Mechanism

	MVC (53); % (n)	AVP (38); % (n)	MCC (7); % (n)	Fall (3); % (n)	Other (1); % (n)
Root	—	2.6 (1)	—	33.3 (1)	—
Ascending	1.9 (1)	2.6 (1)	14.3 (1)	—	—
Arch	11.3 (6)	13.2 (5)	—	—	—
Isthmus/descending	71.7 (38)	57.9 (22)	57.1 (4)	66.7 (2)	100 (1)
Multiple	15.1 (8)	23.7 (9)	28.6 (2)	—	—

AVP, auto vs. pedestrian; MCC, motorcycle collision.

Other torso injuries were more common than head injury in patients dying with blunt trauma.

Unfortunately, the authors provide a large amount of epidemiologic data but fail to indicate where aortic injury is the actual source of mortality in these patients.[1-3] Typical causes of early mortality include uncontrolled bleeding (as may occur with aortic injury) or catastrophic nervous system trauma. Clinicians evaluating patients for aortic injury should be aware that additional injuries focused on the torso are likely to be present. In addition to motor vehicle crash data, this large data set suggests a significant incidence of blunt thoracic aortic injury in pedestrians struck.

Finally, CT imaging remains the modality of choice in high-risk patients.[4]

D. J. Dries, MSE, MD

References

1. Siegel JH, Belwadi A, Smith JA, Shah C, Yang K. Analysis of the mechanism of lateral impact aortic isthmus disruption in real-life motor vehicle crashes using a computer-based finite element numeric model: with simulation of prevention strategies. *J Trauma*. 2010;68:1375-1395.
2. Demetriades D, Velmahos GC, Scalea TM, et al. Blunt traumatic thoracic aortic injuries: early or delayed repair—results of an American Association for the Surgery of Trauma prospective study. *J Trauma*. 2009;66:967-973.
3. Propper BW, Clouse WD. Thoracic aortic endografting for trauma: a current appraisal. *Arch Surg*. 2010;145:1006-1011.
4. Tillou A, Gupta Baraff LJ. Is the use of pan-computed tomography for blunt trauma justified? A prospective evaluation. *J Trauma*. 2009;67:779-787.

The Clinical Significance of Occult Thoracic Injury in Blunt Trauma Patients

Kaiser M, Whealon M, Barrios C, et al (Univ of California Irvine, Orange)
Am Surg 76:1063-1066, 2010

Increased use of thoracic CT (TCT) in diagnosis of blunt traumatic injury has identified many injuries previously undetected on screening chest x-ray (CXR), termed "occult injury." The optimal management of occult rib fractures, pneumothoraces (PTX), hemothoraces (HTX), and

TABLE 1.—Injuries Detected on Chest X-ray (CXR) and Thoracic CT (TCT)

	Rib Fractures	PTX	HTX	Pulmonary Contusions
CXR	112	24	18	94
TCT	184	106	75	184
Occult injuries (TCT−CXR)	72	82	57	90

PTX, pneumothorax; HTX, hemothorax.

TABLE 2.—Patient Characteristics at Admission

	No Thoracic Injury* (n = 1337)	Occult Thoracic Injury* (n = 205)	*P* (occult *vs* no thoracic injury)	Overt Thoracic Injury* (n = 227)	*P* (occult *vs* overt thoracic injury)
Age (years)	33.5 ± 23.3	33.3 ± 17.6	0.879	43.1 ± 20.1	<0.001
SBP (mm Hg)	135 ± 31.6	133 ± 22.0	0.215	135 ± 31	0.35
GCS	14.3 ± 2.1	14.2 ± 2.3	0.452	13.4 ± 3.5	0.007
RTS	7.67 ± 0.65	7.62 ± 0.85	0.352	7.3 ± 1.3	0.003

SBP, systolic blood pressure; GCS, Glasgow Coma Scale; RTS, Revised Trauma Score.
*Expressed as mean ± SD.

pulmonary contusions is uncertain. Our objective was to determine the current management and clinical outcome of these occult blunt thoracic injuries. A retrospective review identified patients with blunt thoracic trauma who underwent both CXR and TCT over a 2-year period at a Level I urban trauma center. Patients with acute rib fractures, PTX, HTX, or pulmonary contusion on TCT were included. Patient groups analyzed included: 1) no injury (normal CXR, normal TCT, n = 1337); 2) occult injury (normal CXR, abnormal TCT, n = 205); and 3) overt injury (abnormal CXR, abnormal TCT, n = 227). Patients with overt injury required significantly more mechanical ventilation and had greater mortality than either occult or no injury patients. Occult and no injury patients had similar ventilator needs and mortality, but occult injury patients remained hospitalized longer. No patient with isolated occult thoracic injury required intubation or tube thoracostomy. Occult injuries, diagnosed by TCT only, have minimal clinical consequences but attract increased hospital resources (Tables 1 and 2).

▶ While crude differences such as ventilator requirements and mortality are not different, this study demonstrates that occult injury is still an injury. Patients with occult trauma in this study did require increased hospital resource utilization. If patients are not fully imaged, occult injury will be missed.[1]

In an era in which we seek to reduce radiation exposure in our patients, we must accept missed injuries as long as life-threatening problems are absent.[2] In more than 1900 patients studied, 70% had no thoracic injury as defined by a normal chest x-ray and a normal thoracic CT. Did all these patients require imaging?

The authors also provide data on injuries detected on chest x-ray and thoracic CT. The difference in detection of rib fractures, pneumothorax, hemothorax, and pulmonary contusion is dramatic. For example, thoracic CT identified twice as many pulmonary contusions as plain chest x-ray did. The gradient is even more dramatic when hemothorax and pneumothorax are considered. Fifty percent more rib fractures are identified on thoracic CT than chest x-ray.

In addition to the limitations originating from retrospective data review, the authors admit to inconsistency in chest x-ray review with some data gathered by attending surgeons or senior surgical residents, while other images are formally reviewed by the attending radiologist at the time of thoracic CT imaging. Finally, recognizing that occult injury does not reflect the absence of injury, we must determine the optimal care pathways for patients with occult injury.[3]

D. J. Dries, MSE, MD

References

1. Tillou A, Gupta M, Baraff LJ, et al. Is the use of pan-computed tomography for blunt trauma justified? A prospective evaluation. *J Trauma*. 2009;67:779-787.
2. Markel TA, Kumar R, Koontz NA, Scherer LR, Applegate KE. The utility of computed tomography as a screening tool for the evaluation for pediatric blunt chest trauma. *J Trauma*. 2009;67:23-28.
3. Wurmb TE, Frühwald P, Hopfner W, et al. Whole-body multislice computed tomography as the first line diagnostic tool in patients with multiple injuries: the focus on time. *J Trauma*. 2009;66:658-665.

Biomarkers to Predict Wound Healing: The Future of Complex War Wound Management

Hahm G, Glaser JJ, Elster EA (Natl Naval Med Ctr, Bethesda, MD; Naval Med Res Ctr, Bethesda, MD; Uniformed Services Univ of Health Sciences, Silver Spring, MD)
Plast Reconstr Surg 127:21S-26S, 2011

Background.—Currently, no biological assay exists to objectively assess wounds to aid in timing of wound closure and guide therapy. In this article, the authors review military investigations in biomarkers as a method of objectively determining acute traumatic wound physiology and their applicability in predicting healing of complex soft-tissue wounds.

Methods.—The civilian literature related to biomarkers and wound physiology related to chronic and acute wounds was reviewed as a basis for current research into acute traumatic soft-tissue wounds.

Results.—Analysis of serum and wound effluent from traumatic extremity soft-tissue combat wounds revealed changes in specific proinflammatory matrix metalloproteinases associated with impaired wound healing. Forsberg et al. analyzed serum and wound effluent for chemokines and cytokines. An increase in serum procalcitonin levels correlated with wound dehiscence. Lastly, serum, wound effluent, and wound bed tissue biopsy specimens were analyzed by Hawksworth et al. Consistent with previous studies, elevation in proinflammatory cytokines was associated with wound dehiscence.

Conclusions.—Changes in levels of proteases, protease inhibitors, and inflammatory markers have been correlated with wound healing. These findings further support the idea that inflammatory dysregulation and a persistent inflammatory state leads to failure of wound healing in the acute setting. These findings highlight potential targets for the development of a biological assay to individualize management of complex soft-tissue wounds, based on patient physiology and response, that would be applicable to not only military trauma but also civilian trauma. Ultimately, this would result in earlier wound closure, reduction in the number of operating room trips, and reduced health care costs (Fig 1).

▶ This is a high-level conceptual discussion based on clinical and research data about the balance between proinflammatory cytokines, matrix metalloproteinases, and inhibitors of matrix metalloproteinases in relation to wound healing.[1,2]

There are limited data to suggest that imbalance of matrix metalloproteinases and their inhibitors or a preponderance of proinflammatory cytokines is more

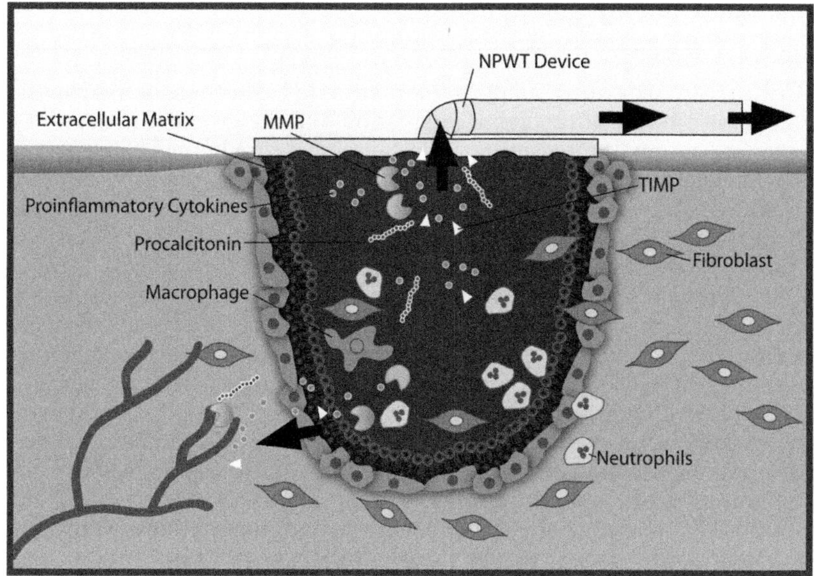

FIGURE 1.—This drawing depicts the complex interaction that exists in a soft-tissue wound bed between inflammatory cells (e.g., fibroblasts, neutrophils, macrophages) and their products. An orderly progression through the phases of wound healing (inflammation, proliferation, maturation) must take place for normal wound healing. Although these phases overlap, the biomarkers involved in wound healing offer the ability to assess a patient's physiologic status, from which management decisions can be derived. *MMP*, matrix metalloproteinase; *TIMP*, tissue inhibitor of metalloproteinase; *NPWT*, negative-pressure wound therapy. (Reprinted from Hahm G, Glaser JJ, Elster EA. Biomarkers to predict wound healing: the future of complex war wound management. *Plast Reconstr Surg*. 2011;127:21S-26S, with permission from the American Society of Plastic Surgeons.)

likely to be associated with failure of wound healing, perhaps most dramatically illustrated by fascial dehiscence.

These data are obviously without controls for pattern of injury or surgical technique. At best, the clinician may suspect that a preponderance of proinflammatory markers or matrix metalloproteinases suggests an increased likelihood of wound healing failure. Whether the use of mediator panels in evaluating wound status is any better than eyeball assessment by a skilled clinician is unclear.

D. J. Dries, MSE, MD

References

1. Broughton G 2nd, Janis JE, Attinger CE. The basic science of wound healing. *Plast Reconstr Surg*. 2006;117:12S-34S.
2. Utz ER, Elster EA, Tadaki DK, et al. Metalloproteinase expression is associated with traumatic wound failure. *J Surg Res*. 2010;159:633-639.

Challenging Issues in Surgical Critical Care, Trauma, and Acute Care Surgery: A Report From the Critical Care Committee of the American Association for the Surgery of Trauma

Napolitano LM, Fulda GJ, Davis KA, et al (Univ of Michigan, Ann Arbor)
J Trauma 69:1619-1633, 2010

Critical care workforce analyses estimate a 35% shortage of intensivists by 2020 as a result of the aging population and the growing demand for greater utilization of intensivists. Surgical critical care in the U.S. is particularly challenged by a significant shortfall of surgical intensivists, with only 2586 surgeons currently certified in surgical critical care by the American Board of Surgery, and even fewer surgeons (1204) recertified in surgical critical care as of 2009. Surgical critical care fellows (160 in 2009) represent only 7.6% of all critical care trainees (2109 in 2009), with the largest number of critical care fellowship positions in internal medicine (1472, 69.8%). Traditional trauma fellowships have now transitioned into Surgical Critical Care or Acute Care Surgery (trauma, surgical critical care, emergency surgery) fellowships. Since adult critical care services are a large, expensive part of U.S. healthcare and workforce shortages continue to impact our healthcare system, recommendations for regionalization of critical care services in the U.S. is considered. The Critical Care Committee of the AAST has compiled national data regarding these important issues that face us in surgical critical care, trauma and acute care surgery, and discuss potential solutions for these issues.

▶ This important article crosses critical care disciplines. Among the specialties providing critical care, there is a shortage of practitioners, and burnout of existing practitioners is widely documented.[1,2] Contrary to the popular rumor that certification and recertification in surgical critical care are unduly difficult, pass rates well in excess of 90% are noted in recent years for both the certification and recertification examinations. Thus, difficulty of examination material cannot logically be implicated.

Many other issues are present, however. In the face of growing demand for critical care resources, training programs in all disciplines are inadequate to provide practitioners in the present fragmented training approach. Regionalization and a consistent critical care curriculum, spanning the disciplines providing critical care, are essential.[3] Communication between the specialties providing critical care and between intensivists and the public is also flawed.

A common concern voiced by surgeons examining critical care training is the loss of operative practice. Trauma fellowships, which may complement critical care training, are not specifically recognized by the American Board of Surgery and do not allow participants to sit for a separate examination. A more recent development is Acute Care Surgery fellowship programs. Examinations in Acute Care Surgery are not yet available. Only 7 sites, as of the writing of this article, have been approved by the American Association for the Surgery of Trauma as Acute Care Surgery fellowship training sites. To paraphrase a concluding statement by the authors, the current status of critical care in the United States must change to effectively meet the needs of multiple disciplines and an increasingly demanding patient population. The public deserves no less.

D. J. Dries, MSE, MD

References

1. Angus DC, Kelley MA, Schmitz RJ, et al. Caring for the critically ill patient. Current and projected workforce requirements for care of the critically ill and patients with pulmonary disease: can we meet the requirements of an aging population? *JAMA*. 2000;284:2762-2770.
2. Krell K. Critical care workforce. *Crit Care Med*. 2008;36:1350-1353.
3. Dorman T, Angood PB, Angus DC, et al. Guidelines for critical care medicine training and continuing medical education. *Crit Care Med*. 2004;32:263-272.

Operative Treatment of Chest Wall Injuries: Indications, Technique, and Outcomes

Lafferty PM, Anavian J, Will RE, et al (Cooper Bone & Joint Inst, Camden, NJ; Brown Univ Med School, Providence, RI; Multicare Orthopaedic Surgery, Tacoma, WA; et al)

J Bone Joint Surg Am 93:97-110, 2011

Most injuries to the chest wall with residual deformity do not result in long-term respiratory dysfunction unless they are associated with pulmonary contusion.

Indications for operative fixation include flail chest, reduction of pain and disability, a chest wall deformity or defect, symptomatic nonunion, thoracotomy for other indications, and open fractures.

Operative indications for chest wall injuries are rare (Table 1).

▶ The vast majority of rib fractures can be managed without operative intervention. Operative stabilization, however, should be considered in patients with

TABLE 1.—Potential Indications and Considerations for Operative Fixation of Rib Fractures*

Operative Indications	Other Considerations
Flail chest	Failure to wean from ventilator
	Paradoxical movement visualized during weaning
	No substantial pulmonary contusion
	No substantial brain injury
Reduction of pain and disability	Painful, movable consecutive rib fractures
	Failure of narcotics or epidural pain catheter
	Fracture movement exacerbating pain, inhibiting respiratory effort
	Minimal associated injuries
Chest wall deformity/defect	Chest wall crush injury with collapse of the structure of the chest wall and marked loss of thoracic volume
	Severely displaced, multiple rib fractures or tissue defect that may result in permanent deformity or pulmonary hernia
	Severely displaced fractures substantially impeding lung expansion or fractured ribs impaling the lung
	Patient expected to survive other injuries
Symptomatic rib fracture nonunion	Radiographic evidence of fracture nonunion
	Patient reports persistent, symptomatic fracture movement
Thoracotomy for other indications in the setting of rib fractures	
Open rib fracture	

*The content in this table was obtained, and modified, from: Nirula R, Diaz JJ Jr, Trunkey DD, Mayberry JC. Rib fracture repair: indications, technical issues, and future directions. *World J Surg*. 2009;33:14-22. With kind permission from Springer Science+Business Media.

a number of conditions, including obvious chest wall deformity, severely displaced multiple rib fractures, fracture nonunion, persistent symptomatic fracture movement, or in the setting of multiple rib fractures, where prolonged mechanical ventilation can be predicted.[1,2]

As operative criteria are identified, it appears that early intervention will minimize the amount of fracture callus, which needs to be dissected. Early intervention also offers the opportunity for simultaneous evacuation of blood in the thorax, which can later contribute to fibrothorax.

There is no good randomized data to support a consistent pattern of recommendations for rib fracture stabilization at this time. Multiple disciplines including orthopedics, plastic and reconstructive surgery, thoracic surgery, and trauma surgeons have interest in the management of these patients. Therefore, turf wars may impede progress in this important area.[3]

D. J. Dries, MSE, MD

References

1. Campbell N, Conaglen P, Martin K, Antippa P. Surgical stabilization of rib fractures using Inion OTPS wraps—techniques and quality of life follow-up. *J Trauma*. 2009;67:596-601.
2. Bottlang M, Helzel I, Long WB, Madey S. Anatomically contoured plates for fixation of rib fractures. *J Trauma*. 2010;68:611-615.
3. Mayberry JC, Ham LB, Schipper PH, Ellis TJ, Mullins RJ. Surveyed opinion of American trauma, orthopedic, and thoracic surgeons on rib and sternal fracture repair. *J Trauma*. 2009;66:875-879.

Returning to Work After Severe Multiple Injuries: Multidimensional Functioning and the Trajectory From Injury to Work at 5 Years

Soberg HL, Roise O, Bautz-Holter E, et al (Oslo Univ Hosp, Norway; et al)
J Trauma 71:425-434, 2011

Background.—The process of returning to work (RTW) after multiple injuries is lengthy. Prospective studies with follow-up times of up to 5 years are necessary but lacking. The aim of this study was to describe the trajectory of RTW and to examine the factors that predicted RTW over 5 years for patients with multiple injuries using a prospective cohort design.

Methods.—One-hundred one patients aged 18 years to 67 years who had been admitted to a trauma referral center with a New Injury Severity Score >15 starting January 2002 through June 2003 were included. The follow-up rate at 5 years was 79%. Outcomes were assessed 6 weeks after discharge and at 1 year, 2 years, and 5 years postinjury. The instruments used to assess patient status were the Short Form 36, the World Health Organization Disability Assessment Schedule II cognitive subscale, a Cognitive Function Scale, and the Brief Approach/Avoidance Coping Questionnaire. Repeated measures analyses of categorical correlated data were applied.

Results.—Patient's mean age was 34.5 years (SD, 13.5); 83% were men and 25% had a university or college education; 66% were blue-collar workers. Mean New Injury Severity Score was 35.1 (SD, 12.7). RTW rates were 28% at 1 year, 43% at 2 years, and 49% at 5 years postinjury. There were differences among patients in RTW status, and personal factors and physical and psychosocial functioning. Predictors of RTW were as follows: measurement occasion, education (high/low), coping, and physical and cognitive functioning. The proportion of unexplained variation between subjects in the models was 31% to 55%.

Conclusion.—Of the patients included in this study, 49% achieved RTW, and 23% received full disability benefits. Higher education; better physical, social, and cognitive functioning; and coping strategies all predicted RTW (Fig 2).

▶ This is an extension of excellent Scandinavian work showing that factors related to injury alone do not explain the functional rehabilitation. Personal factors, including age, gender, education, type of work, coping strategies, and physical and psychosocial functioning, have an important impact. This study is most remarkable for the 5-year follow-up it includes and is a continuation of work previously done by these investigators.[1-3] I do caution the reader, however, to note the exclusions and the relatively small number of patients who are followed up.

Patients with previous injury, burn injury, substance addiction, and psychological disease, aphasia, or lack of language facility were excluded. In addition, the unemployed were excluded. Many trauma patients come from these demographic

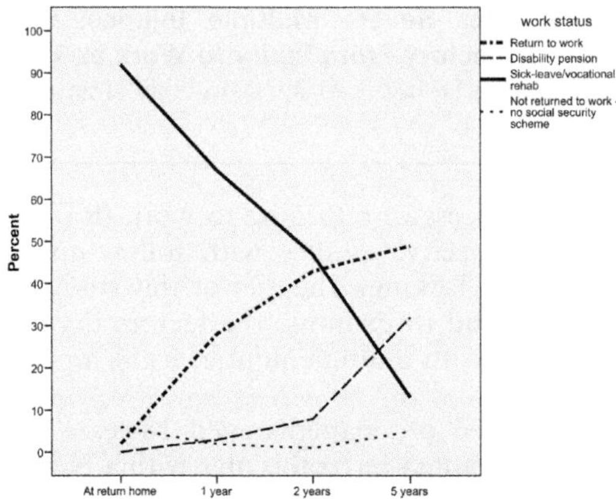

FIGURE 2.—Distribution of persons returned to work (complete return), on sick leave/vocational rehabilitation, disability pension, or not returned to work receiving no social security support (%). (Reprinted from Soberg HL, Roise O, Bautz-Holter E, et al. Returning to work after severe multiple injuries: multidimensional functioning and the trajectory from injury to work at 5 years. *J Trauma.* 2011;71:425-434, with permission from Lippincott Williams & Wilkins.)

groups. It is also important to note that this study comes from a university hospital, so we can assume sophistication in the rehabilitation process.

In the course of follow-up, those lost early in the course of the study were male. This is consistent with trauma practice around the world. When multivariate analysis was performed identifying predictors of favorable outcome, gender fell out but age remained as a predictor of poorer function. When the final analysis was done, nearly half of the patients had achieved complete return to pre-injury work status, but 30% had full- or part-time disability. Time in hospital or rehabilitation settings was not a significant predictor of return to work. The figure shows the trajectory of the various patient groups (Fig 2).

Specific rehabilitation strategies utilized in these patients were not examined. However, it appears that rehabilitation aimed at return to work after multiple injuries should include a focus on coping and response to psychosocial factors as well as physical function.

D. J. Dries, MSE, MD

References

1. Soberg HL, Finset A, Bautz-Holter E, Sandvik L, Roise O. Return to work after severe multiple injuries: a multidimensional approach on status 1 and 2 years post-injury. *J Trauma.* 2007;62:471-481.
2. Vles WJ, Steyerberg EW, Essink-Bot ML, van Beeck EF, Meeuwis JD, Leenen LP. Prevalence and determinants of disabilities and return to work after major trauma. *J Trauma.* 2005;58:126-135.
3. MacKenzie EJ, Morris JA Jr, Jurkovich GJ, et al. Return to work following injury: the role of economic, social, and job-related factors. *Am J Public Health.* 1998;88:1630-1637.

10 Neurologic: Traumatic and Non-traumatic

Detection of Blast-Related Traumatic Brain Injury in U.S. Military Personnel

Mac Donald CL, Johnson AM, Cooper D, et al (Washington Univ School of Medicine, St Louis, MO; et al)

N Engl J Med 364:2091-2100, 2011

Background.—Blast-related traumatic brain injuries have been common in the Iraq and Afghanistan wars, but fundamental questions about the nature of these injuries remain unanswered.

Methods.—We tested the hypothesis that blast-related traumatic brain injury causes traumatic axonal injury, using diffusion tensor imaging (DTI), an advanced form of magnetic resonance imaging that is sensitive to axonal injury. The subjects were 63 U.S. military personnel who had a clinical diagnosis of mild, uncomplicated traumatic brain injury. They were evacuated from the field to the Landstuhl Regional Medical Center in Landstuhl, Germany, where they underwent DTI scanning within 90 days after the injury. All the subjects had primary blast exposure plus another, blast-related mechanism of injury (e.g., being struck by a blunt object or injured in a fall or motor vehicle crash). Controls consisted of 21 military personnel who had blast exposure and other injuries but no clinical diagnosis of traumatic brain injury.

Results.—Abnormalities revealed on DTI were consistent with traumatic axonal injury in many of the subjects with traumatic brain injury. None had detectible intracranial injury on computed tomography. As compared with DTI scans in controls, the scans in the subjects with traumatic brain injury showed marked abnormalities in the middle cerebellar peduncles ($P < 0.001$), in cingulum bundles ($P = 0.002$), and in the right orbitofrontal white matter ($P = 0.007$). In 18 of the 63 subjects with traumatic brain injury, a significantly greater number of abnormalities were found on DTI than would be expected by chance ($P < 0.001$). Follow-up DTI scans in 47 subjects with traumatic brain injury 6 to 12 months after enrollment showed persistent abnormalities that were consistent with evolving injuries.

Conclusions.—DTI findings in U.S. military personnel support the hypothesis that blast-related mild traumatic brain injury can involve axonal injury. However, the contribution of primary blast exposure as compared with that of other types of injury could not be determined directly, since none of the subjects with traumatic brain injury had isolated primary blast injury. Furthermore, many of these subjects did not have abnormalities on DTI. Thus, traumatic brain injury remains a clinical diagnosis. (Funded by the Congressionally Directed Medical Research Program and the

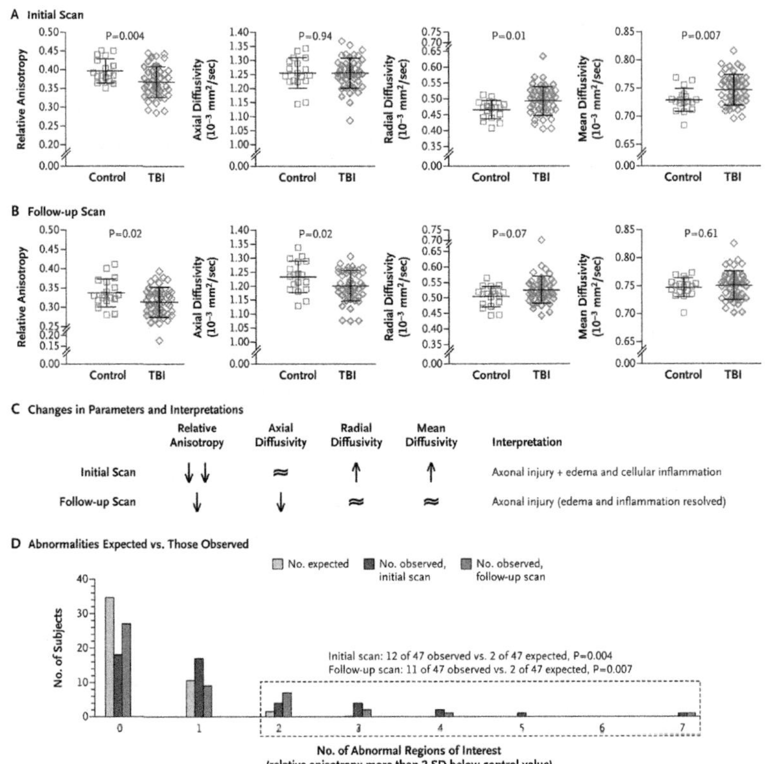

FIGURE 4.—Evolution of Abnormalities over Time as Assessed with Diffusion Tensor Imaging. All data in Panels A through D are from the 18 controls and 47 subjects with traumatic brain injury (TBI) who underwent both initial and follow-up diffusion tensor imaging (DTI). The formulas for calculating relative anisotropy, axial diffusivity, radial diffusivity, and mean diffusivity are available in Figure S1 and S8 in the Supplementary Appendix. In Panels A and B, the longer horizontal lines indicate the means and the I bars indicate standard deviations. Panel A shows the results of the initial scans (obtained within 90 days after injury) in the cingulum bundles, with reduced relative anisotropy, increased radial diffusivity, and increased mean diffusivity in the subjects with TBI as compared with the controls. Panel B shows the follow-up scans (obtained 6 to 12 months after study enrollment) in the cingulum bundles, with reduced relative anisotropy and reduced axial diffusivity. Panel C shows the changes in DTI parameters between initial and follow-up scanning in subjects with TBI as compared with controls and the interpretation of these changes (see also Fig. S4 in the Supplementary Appendix). The double arrows indicate more extensive reduction in relative anisotropy; the ≈ symbol indicates that there was no significant difference between subjects with TBI and controls. Panel D shows differences in observed versus expected DTI abnormalities on initial and follow-up scans in the 47 subjects with TBI. The dotted box indicates the group of subjects with two or more abnormal regions of interest. (Reprinted from Mac Donald CL, Johnson AM, Cooper D, et al. Detection of blast-related traumatic brain injury in U.S. military personnel. *N Engl J Med.* 2011;364:2091-2100, Copyright 2011, with permission from Massachusetts Medical Society. All rights reserved.)

National Institutes of Health; ClinicalTrials.gov number, NCT00785304.) (Fig 4).

▶ This is important but very preliminary work that begins to describe a major clinical legacy of the current conflicts in the Middle East.[1,2] A number of immediate observations must be made. Although there were no limitations based on severity of injury for enrollment, the need for patient consent limited this study to mild injuries. The criteria for enrollment included "clinical impression" of traumatic brain injury. Only 2 time points were studied. Unfortunately, it appears that changes noted on MRI were persistent over the course of this trial. CT scans were unremarkable; thus, the role of MRI in the evaluation of these patients is clear. Finally, the sample size is small, and longer-term outcomes are unavailable. Representative data plots are shown (Fig 4).

A number of additional simple, but important, questions can be asked. First, because these patients suffered multiple injuries, is blast-related traumatic brain injury truly caused by a multihit phenomenon? What are the effects of care? Transport physiology and the impact of pain control are poorly understood.[3,4] Third, we have at most 2 time points in a small sample set. What is the natural history of these men having minor brain trauma by clinical standards?

D. J. Dries, MSE, MD

References

1. DuBose JJ, Barmparas G, Inaba K, et al. Isolated severe traumatic brain injuries sustained during combat operations: demographics, mortality outcomes, and lessons to be learned from contrasts to civilian counterparts. *J Trauma*. 2011;70:11-16.
2. Ropper A. Brain injuries from blasts. *N Engl J Med*. 2011;364:2156-2157.
3. McGhee LL, Slater TM, Garza TH, Fowler M, DeSocio PA, Maani CV. The relationship of early pain scores and posttraumatic stress disorder in burned soldiers. *J Burn Care Res*. 2011;32:46-51.
4. Goodman MD, Makley AT, Lentsch AB, et al. Traumatic brain injury and aeromedical evacuation: when is the brain fit to fly? *J Surg Res*. 2010;164:286-293.

Correlation between Glasgow coma score components and survival in patients with traumatic brain injury

Kung W-M, Tsai S-H, Chiu W-T, et al (Taipei Med Univ-Wan Fang Hosp, Taiwan)

Injury 42:940-944, 2011

Background.—The Glasgow coma scale (GCS) score is used in the initial evaluation of patients with traumatic brain injury (TBI); however, the determination of an accurate score is not possible in all clinical situations. Our aim is to determine if the individual components of the GCS score, or combinations of them, are useful in predicting mortality in patients with TBI.

Methods.—The components of the GCS score and the receiver-operating characteristic (ROC) curves were analyzed from 27,625 cases of TBI in Taiwan.

TABLE 5.—Receiver-Operating Characteristic Analysis of Mortality Prediction

	Area Under ROC curve	95% Confidence Interval
E	0.863	0.847–0.878
M	0.900	0.875–0.903
V	0.890	0.877–0.903
E + *M*	0.877	0.865–0.890
V + *E*	0.904	0.892–0.916
V + *M*	0.903	0.891–0.916
GCS	0.885	0.873–0.897

ROC, receiver-operating characteristic; *E*, eye opening score; *M*, motor reaction score; *V*, verbal response score; GCS, Glasgow coma scale.

Results.—The relationship between the survival rate and certain eye (*E*), motor (*M*) and verbal (*V*) score combinations for GCS scores of 6, 11, 12 and 13 were statistically significant. The areas under ROC curve of *E* + *V*, *M* + *V* and *M* alone were 0.904, 0.903 and 0.900, respectively, representing the 3 most precise combinations for predicting mortality. The area under the ROC curve for the complete GCS score (*E* + *M* + *V*) was 0.885. Patients with lower *E*, *M* and *V* score respectively, and lower complete GCS scores had higher hazard of death than those with the highest scores.

Conclusion.—The results of this study indicate that the 3 fundamental elements comprising the Glasgow coma scale, *E*, *M*, and *V* individually, and in certain combinations are predictive of the survival of TBI patients. This observation is clinically useful when evaluating TBI patients in whom a complete GCS score cannot be obtained (Table 5).

► Since its origin in 1974, the Glasgow Coma Scale (GCS) score has continued to be the international standard of description for neurologic function.[1] A number of confounders must be considered, including alcohol and other drug use (underrepresented in this population) and mechanism of injury. Although this is a large patient set, this is a single-nation and single-population data set. The data have power in their homogeneity. Applicability in less developed societies and cultures where alcohol and weapons of penetrating trauma are more prevalent is unclear.

This article is to be recommended for statistical rigor but reinforces the value of description of patient activity—ideally without administration of sedating and neuromuscular blocking agents—to establish severity of traumatic brain injury. Although a score is helpful, it is fraught with opportunity for misinterpretation. Careful description of patient activity remains very helpful. I was surprised that receiver operating chacteristic curve analysis did not provide stronger support for collection of good motor data. Of the 3 components of the GCS, this has historically been the most helpful in predicting outcome of severe neurologic injury[2] (Table 5).

D. J. Dries, MSE, MD

References

1. Teasdale G, Jennett B. Assessment of coma and impaired consciousness. A practical scale. *Lancet.* 1974;2:81-84.
2. Healey C, Osler TM, Rogers FB, et al. Improving the Glasgow Coma Scale score: motor score alone is a better predictor. *J Trauma.* 2003;54:671-680.

Decompressive Craniectomy in Diffuse Traumatic Brain Injury

Cooper DJ, for the DECRA Trial Investigators and the Australian and New Zealand Intensive Care Society Clinical Trials Group (Alfred Hosp, Melbourne, Victoria, Australia)

N Engl J Med 364:1493-1502, 2011

Background.—It is unclear whether decompressive craniectomy improves the functional outcome in patients with severe traumatic brain injury and refractory raised intracranial pressure.

Methods.—From December 2002 through April 2010, we randomly assigned 155 adults with severe diffuse traumatic brain injury and intracranial hypertension that was refractory to first-tier therapies to undergo either bifrontotemporoparietal decompressive craniectomy or standard care. The original primary outcome was an unfavorable outcome (a composite of death, vegetative state, or severe disability), as evaluated on the Extended Glasgow Outcome Scale 6 months after the injury. The final primary outcome was the score on the Extended Glasgow Outcome Scale at 6 months.

Results.—Patients in the craniectomy group, as compared with those in the standard-care group, had less time with intracranial pressures above the treatment threshold ($P<0.001$), fewer interventions for increased intracranial pressure ($P<0.02$ for all comparisons), and fewer days in the intensive care unit (ICU) ($P<0.001$). However, patients undergoing craniectomy had worse scores on the Extended Glasgow Outcome Scale than those receiving standard care (odds ratio for a worse score in the craniectomy group, 1.84; 95% confidence interval [CI], 1.05 to 3.24; $P = 0.03$) and a greater risk of an unfavorable outcome (odds ratio, 2.21; 95% CI, 1.14 to 4.26; $P = 0.02$). Rates of death at 6 months were similar in the craniectomy group (19%) and the standard-care group (18%).

Conclusions.—In adults with severe diffuse traumatic brain injury and refractory intracranial hypertension, early bifrontotemporoparietal decompressive craniectomy decreased intracranial pressure and the length of stay in the ICU but was associated with more unfavorable outcomes. (Funded by the National Health and Medical Research Council of Australia and others; DECRA Australian Clinical Trials Registry number, ACTRN012605000009617.)

▶ Traumatic brain injury (TBI) is costly to US health care. According to the Centers for Disease Control, an estimated 1.5 million Americans suffer TBI each year, of which approximately 300 000 are hospitalized, and more than 50 000 will die.[1] A study assessing the role of decompressive craniectomy (DC) after TBI showed a trend toward beneficial outcome in these patients.[2] Based on this, Cooper et al studied the role of a rather unusual "bifronto-temporo-parietal" DC in eligible TBI patients versus standard maximal medical therapy in the intensive care unit. Limitations of this trial included the small number of patients randomly selected from the available number of subjects screened, which could reflect selection bias and the statistically significant preponderance of patients with non-pupillary reactivity within the surgical group, which may have explained the results of this trial. In this sense, this study does not put DC for intracranial pressure management after TBI to death but generates additional questions, such as what's the right subset of patients that would benefit from this intervention? Perhaps TBI patients without pupillary abnormalities?[3]

F. Rincon, MD

References

1. Brain Trauma Foundation, American Association of Neurological Surgeons, Congress of Neurological Surgeons. Guidelines for the management of severe traumatic brain injury. *J Neurotrauma*. 2007;24:S1-S106.
2. Sahuquillo J, Arikan F. Decompressive craniectomy for the treatment of refractory high intracranial pressure in traumatic brain injury. *Cochrane Database Syst Rev*. 2006;(1):CD003983.
3. Mack WJ, Hickman ZL, Ducruet AF, et al. Pupillary reactivity upon hospital admission predicts long-term outcome in poor grade aneurysmal subarachnoid hemorrhage patients. *Neurocrit Care*. 2008;8:374-379.

Cilostazol Versus Aspirin for Secondary Prevention of Vascular Events After Stroke of Arterial Origin

Kamal AK, Naqvi I, Husain MR, et al (Aga Khan Univ Hosp, Karachi, Pakistan)
Stroke 42:e382-e384, 2011

The objective of this review was to determine the relative effectiveness and safety of cilostazol compared directly with aspirin in the prevention of stroke and other serious vascular events in patients at high vascular risk for subsequent stroke, those with previous transient ischemic attack, or ischemic stroke of arterial origin.

This review of the available trials in the Asian population shows cilostazol to be superior to aspirin in the secondary prevention of vascular events (stroke, myocardial infarction, or vascular death), strokes of all type (ischemic or hemorrhagic), and hemorrhagic stroke subtype alone after stroke of arterial origin. Cilostazol is associated with fewer major bleeding events than aspirin.

▶ Cilostazol is both an antiplatelet and vasodilating agent for the prevention of recurrent ischemia studied in 2 clinical trials in Japan and China. This meta-analysis explores the efficacy and safety profile of this medication, which has been around for other indications such as peripheral vascular disease. On the basis of these results, cilostazol promises to be an alternative for the prevention of recurrent stroke. Additional clinical trials including subjects of other races and ethnicities are needed before recommendations can be made to support its use in stroke populations.

F. Rincon, MD

Cerebral Oxygen Transport Failure?: Decreasing Hemoglobin and Hematocrit Levels After Ischemic Stroke Predict Poor Outcome and Mortality: STroke: RelevAnt Impact of hemoGlobin, Hematocrit and Transfusion (STRAIGHT)—an Observational Study

Kellert L, Martin E, Sykora M, et al (Univ of Heidelberg, Germany; Comenius Univ, Bratislava, Slovakia)

Stroke 42:2832-2837, 2011

Background and Purpose.—Although conceivably relevant for penumbra oxygenation, the optimal levels of hemoglobin (Hb) and hematocrit (Hct) in patients with acute ischemic stroke are unknown.

Methods.—We identified patients from our prospective local stroke database who received intravenous thrombolysis based on multimodal magnet resonance imaging during the years 1998 to 2009. A favorable outcome at 3 months was defined as a modified Rankin Scale score ≤2 and a poor outcome as a modified Rankin Scale score ≥3. The dynamics of Hemoglobin (Hb), Hematocrit (Hct), and other relevant laboratory parameters as well as cardiovascular risk factors were retrospectively assessed and analyzed between these 2 groups.

Results.—Of 217 patients, 114 had a favorable and 103 a poor outcome. In a multivariable regression model, anemia until day 5 after admission (odds ratio [OR]=2.61; 95% CI, 1.33 to 5.11; P=0.005), Hb nadir (OR=0.81; 95% CI, 0.67 to 0.99; P=0.038), and Hct nadir (OR=0.93; 95% CI, 0.87 to 0.99; P=0.038) remained independent predictors for poor outcome at 3 months. Mortality after 3 months was independently associated with Hb nadir (OR=0.80; 95% CI, 0.65 to 0.98; P=0.028) and Hb decrease (OR=1.34; 95% CI, 1.01 to 1.76; P=0.04) as well as Hct decrease (OR=1.12; 95% CI, 1.01 to 1.23; P=0.027).

Conclusions.—Poor outcome and mortality after ischemic stroke are strongly associated with low and further decreasing Hb and Hct levels. This decrease of Hb and Hct levels after admission might be more relevant and accessible to treatment than are baseline levels.

▶ Anemia in general (hemoglobin [Hb] <12 g/dL in women and <13 g/dL in men) is highly prevalent in older patients. Given the risk factor profile of ischemic stroke, it is intuitive to consider stroke patients at higher risk of worsening anemia upon admission to the hospital. The effect of this trend on functional outcome was assessed by Kellert et al in this elegant retrospective cohort study of a prospective compiled and maintain registry of ischemic stroke patients. The results of this analysis, particularly the association between worsening anemia and poor functional outcome at 3 months, confirm the detrimental effects of lower Hb in critically ill neurological patients, which has been attributed to oxygen delivery failure around the ischemic penumbra. This study supports the notion that lower levels of Hb may not be tolerated as well as in other medical critical-illness conditions. However, this study does not answer the most important questions: what is the threshold for blood transfusion and would this practice be associated with better outcomes after ischemic stroke? Similarly, the study may have been confounded by other potential effects such as the interaction between anemia and other comorbid conditions, nutritional status (albumin level), age, gender, and the admission to the National Institutes of Health Stroke Scale (severe strokes may be more likely to do worse). The authors provide a good summary of their study weaknesses, including their sample size, potential areas for therapeutic improvement such as limiting blood sampling to the necessary minimum, avoiding fluid overload, preventing and treating infections early, and controlling kidney function.

F. Rincon, MD

Combination oral antiplatelet therapy may increase the risk of hemorrhagic complications in patients with acute ischemic stroke caused by large artery disease

Itabashi R, Mori E, Furui E, et al (Kohnan Hosp, Sendai, Miyagi, Japan; Tohoku Univ Graduate School of Medicine, Sendai, Miyagi, Japan)
Thromb Res 128:541-546, 2011

Introduction.—The association between the frequency or severity of bleeding complications and combination antiplatelet therapy for acute stroke treatment is not understood in detail. This retrospective study investigated whether combination oral antiplatelet therapy for cases with acute ischemic stroke due to large artery disease increased the incidence of hemorrhagic complications.

Materials and Methods.—We reviewed 1335 consecutive patients who were admitted to our department within 7 days of the onset of an ischemic stroke or transient ischemic attack between April 2005 and November 2009. We enrolled 167 patients with >50% stenosis or occlusion in culprit major vessels and who were administered oral antiplatelet agents within 48 hours of admission. Hemorrhagic complications were classified according to the bleeding severity index. We studied the association between the incidence and severity of hemorrhagic complications during hospitalization and the clinical characteristics, including antiplatelet therapy.

Results.—Fifty-nine and 108 patients were treated with only 1 antiplatelet agent and combination antiplatelet agents, respectively. Fourteen patients developed bleeds (3 major and 11 minor), and all of the major bleeds occurred in those given combination agents. The proportion of patients receiving combination agents was significantly higher in those with significant bleeds. Multivariate logistic regression analysis revealed that being older and receiving combination agents were independent predictors for significant bleeds during hospitalization.

Conclusions.—Despite the retrospective nature of this study, our findings suggest that the incidence of hemorrhagic complications increases in patients with acute ischemic stroke treated with combination antiplatelet agents.

▶ In this interesting study, the authors confirmed once again the effects of dual or multiple antiplatelet regimens for patients with ischemic stroke. The aspirin and clopidogrel compared with clopidogrel alone after recent ischemic stroke or transient ischaemic attack in high-risk patients (MATCH) trial showed the higher risk of hemorrhagic transformation in patients taking the combination clopidogrel and aspirin, particularly among diabetic and older patients.[1] At the time of deciding which agent to use for secondary prophylaxis, the alternatives remain aspirin, clopidogrel, or combination aspirin/dipyridamole. I prefer single-agent or aspirin/dipyridamole and try to optimize other risk factors first before I conclude that the medication has been ineffective.

F. Rincon, MD

Reference

1. Diener HC, Bogousslavsky J, Brass LM, et al. Aspirin and clopidogrel compared with clopidogrel alone after recent ischaemic stroke or transient ischaemic attack in high-risk patients (MATCH): randomised, double-blind, placebo-controlled trial. *Lancet.* 2004;364:331-337.

Early continuous hypertonic saline infusion in patients with severe cerebrovascular disease

Hauer E-M, Stark D, Staykov D, et al (Univ of Erlangen, Germany; et al)
Crit Care Med 39:1766-1772, 2011

Objective.—To study the safety and the effects of early continuous hypertonic saline infusion in patients with cerebral edema and underlying cerebrovascular disease.

Design.—Retrospective analysis.

Setting.—University medical center.

Patients.—Neurologic intensive care unit population with mixed cerebrovascular diseases.

Interventions.—None.

Measurements and Main Results.—Between May 2008 and December 2009, 100 patients with severe intracerebral hemorrhage, cerebral ischemia, or aneurysmal subarachnoid hemorrhage and signs of intracranial hypertension received within ≤72 hrs after symptom onset a continuous infusion of hypertonic saline (3%, target sodium 145–155 mmol/L, target osmolality 310–320 mOsm/kg) over 13 (4–23) days. We analyzed the frequency of episodes with elevated intracranial pressure (new anisocoria or intracranial pressure >20 mm Hg for ≥20 mins), inhospital mortality, and the occurrence of adverse effects theoretically associated with hypertonic saline. The findings were compared with those of a historical control group (n = 115,

2007–2008) with equal underlying disease. In the treatment group, fewer episodes of critically elevated intracranial pressure (92 vs. 167, $p = .027$) in fewer patients (50 of 100 = 50.0% vs. 69 of 115 = 60.0% patients, $p = .091$) were observed, and inhospital mortality was significantly decreased (17.0% vs. 29.6%, $p = .037$). Adverse events, including cardiac arrhythmia, heart, liver or renal dysfunction, or pulmonary edema, occurred in both groups to a similar extent.

Conclusions.—Early and continuous infusion of hypertonic saline in patients with severe cerebrovascular disease and impending intracranial hypertension is safe and might reduce the frequency of intracranial pressure crises and mortality rate. A randomized controlled trial is warranted to confirm our findings and to evaluate the effects of hypertonic saline on functional outcomes (Fig 2).

▶ In this interesting analysis, the authors studied the effects of continuous infusion of hypertonic saline (HTS, 3%) for the management of intracranial hypertension in patients with different types of brain injury. The authors demonstrated that continuous HTS has a good safety profile, providing improvement in hemodynamic profiles, reduction in intermittent use of other hyperosmolar agents, and a mortality benefit particularly in the intracerebral

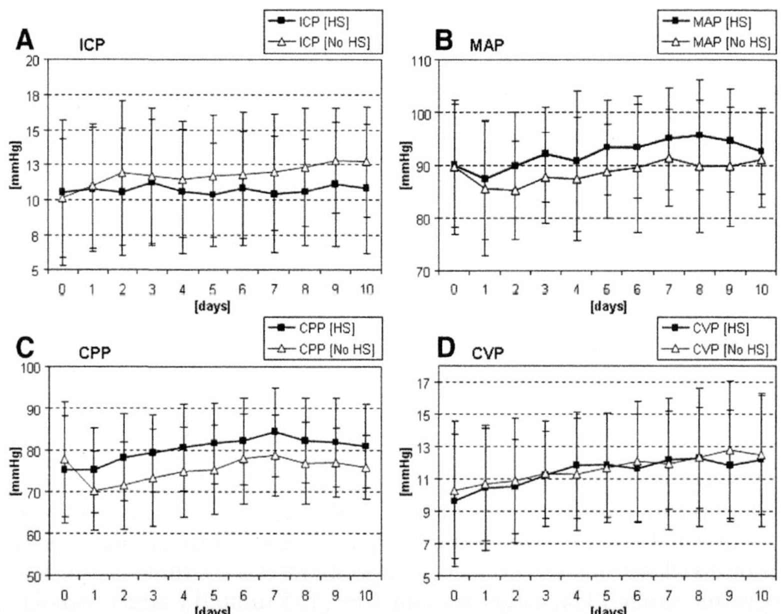

FIGURE 2.—Time course of intracranial pressure (*ICP*) (*A*), mean arterial pressure (*MAP*) (*B*), cerebral perfusion pressure (*CPP*) (*C*), and central venous pressure (*CVP*) (*D*) in the hypertonic saline (*HS*) group and no HS group. Data are expressed as mean ± SEM. (Reprinted from Hauer E-M, Stark D, Staykov D, et al. Early continuous hypertonic saline infusion in patients with severe cerebrovascular disease. *Crit Care Med.* 2011;39:1766-1772, with permission from the Society of Critical Care Medicine and Lippincott Williams & Wilkins.)

hemorrhage subgroup. Although the conclusions are in favor of HTS for intracranial pressure (ICP) control, several factors may have confounded the observed association. Of note is that the study used a younger historic control, which would have explained the differences in mortality and the observed complication rate. Nevertheless, this article is important and may support the use of continuous HTS in younger patients, but the interaction with age and additional comorbidities may need to be explored further. In my practice, I use continuous HTS for patients with cerebral edema, signs of intracranial hypertension, and good cardiovascular reserve, but I prefer intermittent boluses of HTS or hyperosmolar therapy for the management of ICP crisis and in those with history of heart failure or pulmonary complications. This study supports this approach.

F. Rincon, MD

Nicotine Replacement Therapy After Subarachnoid Hemorrhage Is Not Associated With Increased Vasospasm

Carandang RA, Barton B, Rordorf GA, et al (Univ of Massachusetts Med School/UMASS Memorial Med Ctr, Worcester; Harvard Med School/ Massachusetts General Hosp, Boston)

Stroke 42:3080-3086, 2011

Background and Purpose.—A significant number of patients with aneurysmal subarachnoid hemorrhage are active smokers and at risk for acute nicotine withdrawal. There is conflicting literature regarding the vascular effects of nicotine and theoretical concern that it may worsen vasospasm. The literature on the safety of nicotine replacement therapy and its effects on vasospasm is limited.

Methods.—A retrospective analysis was conducted of a prospectively collected database of aneurysmal subarachnoid hemorrhage patients admitted to the neurointensive care unit from 1994 to 2008. Paired control subjects matched for age, sex, Fisher score, aneurysm size and number, hypertension, and current medication were analyzed. The primary outcome was clinical and angiographic vasospasm and the secondary outcome was Glasgow Outcome Score on discharge. Conditional logistic models were used to investigate univariate and multivariate relationships between predictors and outcome.

Results.—Two hundred fifty-eight active smoking patients were included of which 87 were treated with transdermal nicotine replacement therapy. Patients were well matched for age, sex, gender, Fisher score, aneurysm size and number, hypertension, and current medications, but patients who received nicotine replacement therapy had less severe Hunt-Hess scores and Glasgow coma scores. There was no difference in angiographic vasospasm, but patients who received nicotine replacement therapy were less likely to have clinical vasospasm (19.5 versus 32.8%; $P=0.026$) and a Glasgow Outcome Score <4 on discharge (62.6% versus 81.6%; $P=0.005$) on multivariate analysis.

Conclusions.—Nicotine replacement therapy was not associated with increased angiographic vasospasm and was associated with less clinical vasospasm and better Glasgow Outcome Score scores on discharge.

▶ The use of nicotine replacement in critically ill subarachnoid hemorrhage (SAH) patients makes a lot of sense, because most of these patients are active smokers, and active delirium from nicotine withdrawal is associated with agitated delirium and worst outcomes. The results of this study confirm the safety and tolerability profile of nicotine replacement after SAH.[1] In practice, I screen all SAH patients for tobacco abuse and start early nicotine replacement. Importantly, patients with delirium from nicotine withdrawal may require higher doses of nicotine replacement (dual patch).[2]

F. Rincon, MD

References

1. Seder DB, Schmidt JM, Badjatia N, et al. Transdermal nicotine replacement therapy in cigarette smokers with acute subarachnoid hemorrhage. *Neurocrit Care.* 2011;14:77-83.
2. Mayer SA, Chong JY, Ridgway E, Min KC, Commichau C, Bernardini GL. Delirium from nicotine withdrawal in neuro-ICU patients. *Neurology.* 2001;57: 551-553.

Clinical practices, complications, and mortality in neurological patients with acute severe hypertension: Studying the Treatment of Acute hyperTension registry

Mayer SA, on behalf of the STAT Investigators (Columbia Univ College of Physicians and Surgeons, NY; et al)
Crit Care Med 39:2330-2336, 2011

Objective.—To determine the demographic and clinical features, hospital complications, and predictors of 90-day mortality in neurologic patients with acute severe hypertension.

Design.—Studying the Treatment of Acute hyperTension (STAT) was a multicenter (n = 25) observational registry of adult critical care patients with severe hypertension treated with intravenous therapy.

Setting.—Emergency department or intensive care unit.

Patients.—A qualifying blood pressure measurement >180 mm Hg systolic or >110 mm Hg diastolic (>140/90 mm Hg for subarachnoid hemorrhage) was required for inclusion in the STAT registry. Patients with a primary neurologic admission diagnosis were included in the present analysis.

Interventions.—All patients were treated with at least one parenteral (bolus or continuous infusion) antihypertensive agent.

Measurements and Main Results.—Of 1,566 patients included in the STAT registry, 432 (28%) had a primary neurologic diagnosis. The most common diagnoses were subarachnoid hemorrhage (38%), intracerebral hemorrhage (31%), and acute ischemic stroke (18%). The most common initial drug was labetalol (48%), followed by nicardipine (15%), hydralazine (15%), and sodium nitroprusside (13%). Mortality at 90 days was substantially higher in neurologic than in non-neurologic patients (24% vs. 6%, $p < .0001$). Median initial blood pressure was 183/95 mm Hg and did not differ between survivors and nonsurvivors. In a multivariable analysis, neurologic patients who died experienced lower minimal blood pressure values (median 103/45 vs. 118/55 mm Hg, $p < .0001$) and were less likely to experience recurrent hypertension requiring intravenous treatment (29% vs. 51%, $p = .0001$) than those who survived. Mortality was also associated with an increased frequency of neurologic deterioration (32% vs. 10%, $p < .0001$).

Conclusion.—Neurologic emergencies account for approximately 30% of hospitalized patients with severe acute hypertension, and the majority of those who die. Mortality in hypertensive neurologic patients is associated with lower minimum blood pressure values, less rebound hypertension, and a higher frequency of neurologic deterioration. Excessive blood pressure reduction may contribute to poor outcome after severe brain injury (Fig 1).

▶ In this interesting study, nearly 30% of 432 patients presenting to an emergency department (ED) with acute hypertension had a central nervous system

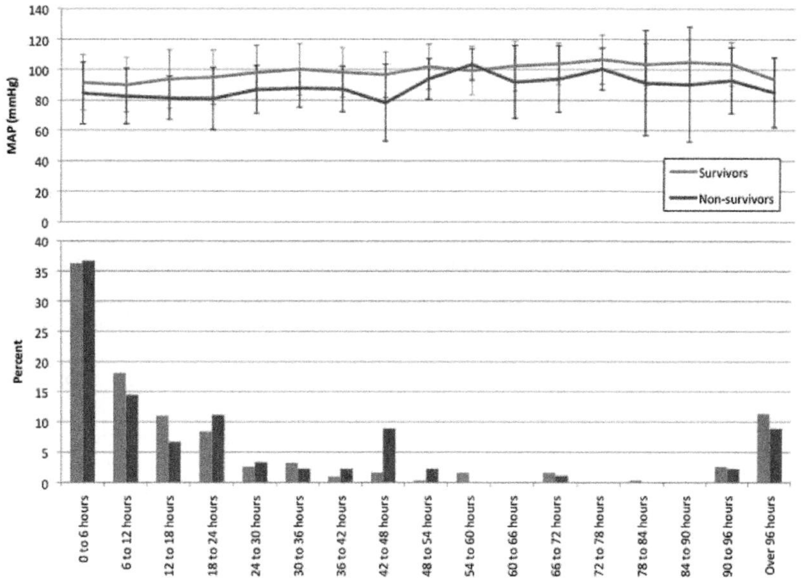

FIGURE 1.—Level and timing of lowest-recorded mean arterial blood pressure (*MAP*) in survivors vs. nonsurvivors. Regardless of mortality status, lowest-recorded blood pressure occurred most frequently within the first 6 hrs of admission. "Percent" in *bottom panel* refers to the % of dead or alive patients. (Reprinted from Mayer SA, on behalf of the STAT Investigators. Clinical practices, complications, and mortality in neurological patients with acute severe hypertension: the studying the treatment of acute hyperTension registry. *Crit Care Med.* 2011;39:2330-2336, with permission from the Society of Critical Care Medicine and Lippincott Williams & Wilkins.)

(CNS) insult. The most common diagnoses were subarachnoid hemorrhage (38%), intracerebral hemorrhage (31%), and acute ischemic stroke (18%), followed by traumatic brain injury (8%), hypertensive encephalopathy (4%), and status epilepticus (1%). Of patients with CNS insults, the mortality was 4 times as high, compared with patients with no CNS involvement. Interestingly, the median initial blood pressure was 183/95 mm Hg and did not differ between survivors and nonsurvivors; the time to achieve a target systolic blood pressure was 2 hours in survivors, and 1 hour in the nonsurvivors ($P = .005$). Although there was no difference in maximal levels of systolic or diastolic blood pressure, more nonsurvivors had lower systolic and diastolic blood pressures with the highest risk of hypotension within the first 6 hours of admission. The most commonly used first antihypertensive was labetalol (48%), followed by nicardipine (15%), hydralazine (15%), and sodium nitroprusside (13%). Nonsurvivors were more likely to have received nitroprusside, but this was not statistically significant. This study provides a contemporary interpretation of the practices, complications, and outcomes in neurological patients with hypertensive crisis and the effects of acute blood pressure lowering in 90-day mortality demonstrating the need for the development of strategies aimed at emphasizing rapid and precise blood pressure control while avoiding overtreatment in the context of more robust data emanated from clinical trials.

F. Rincon, MD

Management and outcome of mechanically ventilated neurological patients

Pelosi P, for the Ventila Study Group (Universita' degli Studi di Genova, Italy; et al)

Crit Care Med 39:1482-1492, 2011

Objective.—To describe and compare characteristics, ventilatory practices, and associated outcomes among mechanically ventilated patients with different types of brain injury and between neurologic and nonneurologic patients.

Design.—Secondary analysis of a prospective, observational, and multicenter study on mechanical ventilation.

Setting.—Three hundred forty-nine intensive care units from 23 countries.

Patients.—We included 552 mechanically ventilated neurologic patients (362 patients with stroke and 190 patients with brain trauma). For comparison we used a control group of 4030 mixed patients who were ventilated for nonneurologic reasons.

Interventions.—None.

Measurements and Main Results.—We collected demographics, ventilatory settings, organ failures, and complications arising during ventilation and outcomes. Multivariate logistic regression analysis was performed with intensive care unit mortality as the dependent variable. At admission, a Glasgow Coma Scale score ≤8 was observed in 68% of the stroke, 77% of the brain trauma, and 29% of the nonneurologic patients. Modes of ventilation and use of a lung-protective strategy within the first week of mechanical ventilation were similar between groups. In comparison with nonneurologic patients, patients with neurologic disease developed fewer complications over the course of mechanical ventilation with the exception of a higher rate of ventilator-associated pneumonia in the brain trauma cohort. Neurologic patients showed higher rates of tracheotomy and longer duration of mechanical ventilation. Mortality in the intensive care unit was significantly ($p < .001$) higher in patients with stroke (45%) than in brain trauma (29%) and nonneurologic disease (30%). Factors associated with mortality were: stroke (in comparison to brain trauma), Glasgow Coma Scale score on day 1, and severity at admission in the intensive care unit.

Conclusions.—In our study, one of every five mechanically ventilated patients received this therapy as a result of a neurologic disease. This cohort of patients showed a higher mortality rate than nonneurologic patients despite a lower incidence of extracerebral organ dysfunction.

▶ In this interesting retrospective multicenter cohort study from a prospective compiled and maintained registry, Pelosi et al studied the epidemiology, clinical characteristics, and clinical practices in relation to mechanical ventilation in a cohort of critically ill neurological patients. Although subarachnoid hemorrhage (SAH) patients were excluded, this study is an excellent description of day-to-day practices across different ICUs and confirms observations from prior cohorts. Not surprisingly, neurological patients had lower Glasgow Coma Scale (GCS) score on admission, more intensive care unit and ventilator days, more early tracheostomies, and more ventilator-associated pneumonias, but interestingly the rate of reintubation was similar to those of nonneurological patients. In this sense, this study provides support that mental status and GCS may not matter at the time of extubation and reintubation (GCS was higher in nonneurological patients, and the rate of reintubation was the same). Although the study is important, it doesn't answer the question of which neurological patients are more likely to get "stuck" on the ventilator or get reintubated.[1] The interaction with disease severity, age, neurological diagnosis, and important variables that make me worry at the time of extubating someone with brain injury such as characteristics and management of secretions, cranial nerve involvement (pupillary abnormalities, absence of gag, etc) are missing in this analysis.

F. Rincon, MD

Reference

1. Coplin WM, Pierson DJ, Cooley KD, Newell DW, Rubenfeld GD. Implications of extubation delay in brain-injured patients meeting standard weaning criteria. *Am J Respir Crit Care Med.* 2000;161:1530-1536.

Sedation for critically ill adults with severe traumatic brain injury: A systematic review of randomized controlled trials

Roberts DJ, Hall RI, Kramer AH, et al (Univ of Calgary and the Foothills Med Centre, Alberta, Canada; Dalhousie Univ and the Queen Elizabeth II Health Sciences Centre, Halifax, Nova Scotia, Canada)

Crit Care Med 39:2743-2751, 2011

Objectives.—To summarize randomized controlled trials on the effects of sedative agents on neurologic outcome, mortality, intracranial pressure, cerebral perfusion pressure, and adverse drug events in critically ill adults with severe traumatic brain injury.

Data Sources.—PubMed, MEDLINE, EMBASE, the Cochrane Database, Google Scholar, two clinical trials registries, personal files, and reference lists of included articles.

Study Selection.—Randomized controlled trials of propofol, ketamine, etomidate, and agents from the opioid, benzodiazepine, α-2 agonist, and antipsychotic drug classes for management of adult intensive care unit patients with severe traumatic brain injury.

Data Extraction.—In duplicate and independently, two investigators extracted data and evaluated methodologic quality and results.

Data Synthesis.—Among 1,892 citations, 13 randomized controlled trials enrolling 380 patients met inclusion criteria. Long-term sedation ($\geq$24 hrs) was addressed in six studies, whereas a bolus dose, short infusion, or doubling of plasma drug concentration was investigated in remaining trials. Most trials did not describe baseline traumatic brain injury prognostic factors or important cointerventions. Eight trials possibly or definitely concealed allocation and six were blinded. Insufficient data exist regarding the effects of sedative agents on neurologic outcome or mortality. Although their effects are likely transient, bolus doses of opioids may increase intracranial pressure and decrease cerebral perfusion pressure. In one study, a long-term infusion of propofol vs. morphine was associated with a reduced requirement for intracranial pressure-lowering cointerventions and a lower intracranial pressure on the third day. Trials of propofol vs. midazolam and ketamine vs. sufentanil found no difference between agents in intracranial pressure and cerebral perfusion pressure.

Conclusions.—This systematic review found no convincing evidence that one sedative agent is more efficacious than another for improvement of patient-centered outcomes, intracranial pressure, or cerebral perfusion pressure in critically ill adults with severe traumatic brain injury. High bolus doses of opioids, however, have potentially deleterious effects on intracranial pressure and cerebral perfusion pressure. Adequately powered, high-quality, randomized controlled trials are urgently warranted.

▶ Critical care specialists caring for patients with traumatic brain injury (TBI) often encounter the therapeutic dilemma of how to appropriately sedate patients in whom intracranial hypertension is suspected. This elegant systematic review by Roberts D et al summarizes the most important data on the topic. The authors did not find meta-analytic evidence that one sedative agent is more efficacious than another for improvement of patient-centered outcomes, intracranial pressure (ICP), or cerebral perfusion pressure (CPP, mean arterial pressure – ICP) in TBI patients. Importantly, the authors found that repeated boluses of opioids may be associated with drops in CPP and ICP crisis. This effect is mediated by reflex vasodilatation in the setting of impaired autoregulation. This observation is important and favors the use of lower but continuous infusions of analgesics or better CPP optimization when administering boluses of opioids (ie, fluid administration and maintenance of normovolemia). The use of novel agents such as dexmedetomidine, which has an intrinsic spinal analgesic effect, may be the goal of further studies.

F. Rincon, MD

Intracranial Hemorrhage, Outcome, and Mortality After Intra-Arterial Therapy for Acute Ischemic Stroke in Patients Under Oral Anticoagulants

De Marchis GM, Jung S, Colucci G, et al (Univ of Bern, Switzerland)
Stroke 42:3061-3066, 2011

Background and Purpose.—Use of intravenous tissue-type plasminogen activator (IV tPA) for acute ischemic stroke is restricted to patients with an international normalized ratio (INR) less than 1.7. However, a recent study showed increased risk of symptomatic intracranial hemorrhage after IV tPA use in patients with oral anticoagulants (OAC) even with an INR less than 1.7. The present study assessed the risk of symptomatic intracranial hemorrhage, clinical outcome, and mortality after intra-arterial therapy (IAT) in patients with and without previous use of OAC.

Methods.—Consecutive patients treated with IAT from December 1992 to October 2010 were included. Clinical outcome and mortality were assessed 90 days after stroke onset. Patients with and without previous use of OAC were compared.

Results.—Overall, 714 patients were treated with IAT. Twenty-eight patients (3.9%) were under OAC at time of symptom onset. Median INR in the OAC group was 1.79 (interquartile range [IQR], 1.41–2.3) and 1.01 (IQR, 1.0–1.09; $P<0.0001$) in the group without OAC. Patients treated with OAC at admission underwent more often mechanical-only IAT than did patients without OAC (46.4% versus 12.8%; $P<0.0001$). Comparing patients with and without previous use of OAC, we did not find any statistical difference in the rate of symptomatic intracranial hemorrhage (7.1% versus 6.0%; $P=0.80$), unfavorable outcome (modified Rankin Scale score, 3–6; 67.9% versus 50.9%; $P=0.11$), and mortality (17.9% versus 21.6%; $P=0.58$).

Conclusions.—Previous use of OAC did not significantly increase the risk of symptomatic intracranial hemorrhage after IAT or the risk of unfavorable outcome and mortality 90 days after IAT.

▶ In this interesting analysis, De Marchis et al tested the hypothesis that oral-anticoagulation (OAC) would be associated with poor outcome and more intracerebral hemorrhage (ICH) after ischemic stroke in patients receiving endovascular interventions (mechanical or intra-arterial thrombolytic) but not intravenous thrombolytics. The results reject their hypothesis, meaning OAC was not associated with more ICH or poorer outcomes and the conclusions are important because they support the results from other prospective but uncontrolled studies in which these interventions were safe in this patient subpopulation.[1,2] These conclusions favor the use of endovascular interventions in patients deemed not to be candidates for intravenous thrombolytics based on abnormal coagulation profiles.

F. Rincon, MD

References

1. Nogueira RG, Smith WS, MERCI and Multi MERCI Writing Committee. Safety and efficacy of endovascular thrombectomy in patients with abnormal hemostasis: pooled analysis of the MERCI and multi MERCI trials. *Stroke.* 2009;40:516-522.
2. Prabhakaran S, Rivolta J, Vieira JR, et al. Symptomatic intracerebral hemorrhage among eligible warfarin-treated patients receiving intravenous tissue plasminogen activator for acute ischemic stroke. *Arch Neurol.* 2010;67:559-563.

Intraventricular Fibrinolysis Versus External Ventricular Drainage Alone in Intraventricular Hemorrhage: A Meta-Analysis

Gaberel T, Magheru C, Parienti J-J, et al (Caen Univ Hosp, France; et al)

Stroke 42:2776-2781, 2011

Background and Purpose.—The purpose of this study was to analyze the effect of intraventricular fibrinolysis (IVF) compared with external ventricular drainage alone on mortality and functional outcome in the management of intraventricular hemorrhage secondary to spontaneous supratentorial intracerebral hemorrhage.

Methods.—The authors conducted a systematic review and performed a meta-analysis. They reviewed the PubMed, Cochrane Library, and Liliacs databases. In addition, they conducted a manual review of article bibliographies.

Results.—Using a prespecified search strategy, 4 randomized and 8 observational studies were included in a meta-analysis. These studies involved a total of 316 patients with intraventricular hemorrhage at baseline, of whom 167 had IVF (52·8%). Pooled odds ratios of the impact of IVF on patient mortality, functional outcomes, and complications were calculated. The overall mortality risk decreased from 46·7% in the external ventricular drainage alone group to 22.7% in the external ventricular drainage + IVF group, corresponding to an overall pooled Peto OR of 0.32 (95% CI, 0.19 to 0.52). This result was highly significant with urokinase, not with recombinant tissue-type plasminogen activator. IVF was also associated with an increase in good functional outcome. There was no difference between the 2 groups in terms of shunt dependence and complications.

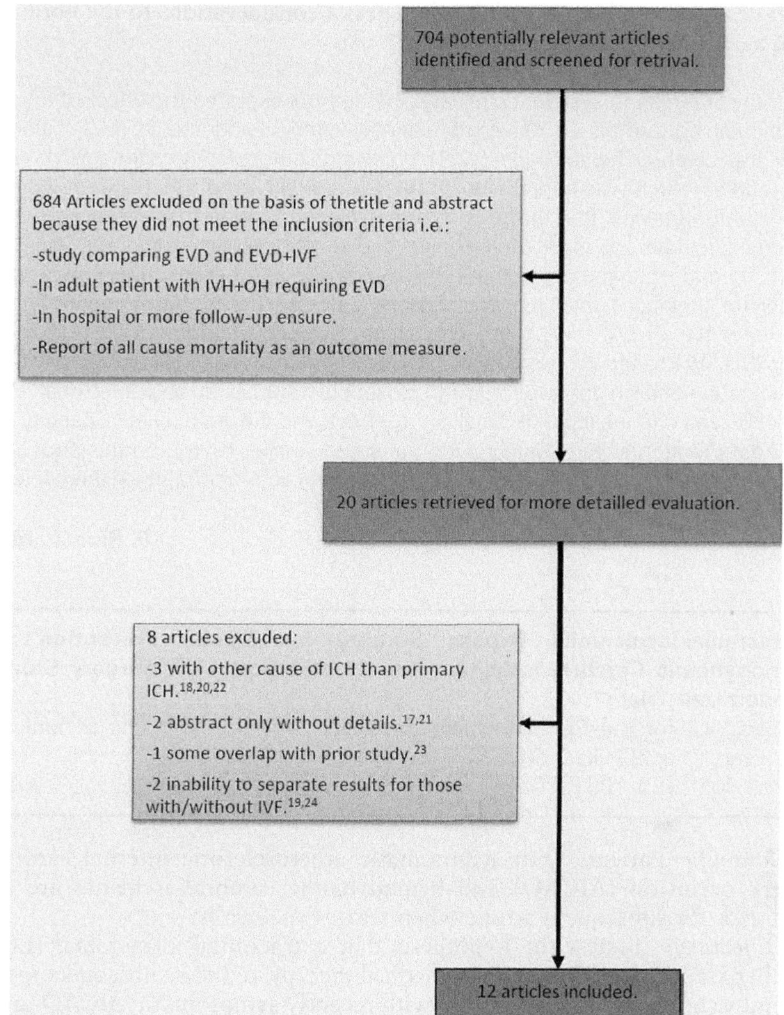

FIGURE 1.—Flow chart of the study selection process. EVD indicates extraventricular drainage; IVF, intraventricular fibrinolysis; OH, obstructive hydrocephalus; ICH, intracranial hemorrhage. (Reprinted from Gaberel T, Magheru C, Parienti J-J, et al. Intraventricular fibrinolysis versus external ventricular drainage alone in intraventricular hemorrhage: a meta-analysis. *Stroke*. 2011;42:2776-2781, with permission from American Heart Association, Inc.)

Conclusions.—The combination of IVF and external ventricular drainage in the management of severe intraventricular hemorrhage secondary to small intracerebral hemorrhage in young patients was associated with better survival and functional outcome results. Urokinase and recombinant tissue-type plasminogen activator could not have the same therapeutic effects.

Well-designed randomized trials with special considerations to the fibrinolytic agents are needed (Fig 1).

▶ In this interesting systematic review, the authors explored the effect of intraventricular fibrinolysis (IVF) versus external ventricular drainage (EVD) alone after intracerebral hemorrhage (ICH) plus intraventricular hemorrhage (IVH). The pooled effect was impressive for IVF for mortality and functional outcome at 1 month. It seems that at the end of day, clearing blood from the ventricular cisterns provides, at least biologically, a plausible explanation for improved mortality and outcomes after these devastating forms of stroke. The effect was better for urokinase than for recombinant activated tissue plasminogen. Until results of the CLEAR-IVH trial are available, we can't support the use of IVF after ICH/IVH based on these results, particularly because of issues such as the combination of both observational and prospective studies in the pooled analysis, selection and channeling bias, small study effect, and the limited heterogeneity of their data (patients were mainly young and had smaller ICHs). To this end, our institution participates in CLEAR-IVH, and we favor active enrolling in this clinical trial.

F. Rincon, MD

Extracranial-Intracranial Bypass Surgery for Stroke Prevention in Hemodynamic Cerebral Ischemia: The Carotid Occlusion Surgery Study Randomized Trial

Powers WJ, for the COSS Investigators (Univ of North Carolina School of Medicine, Chapel Hill; et al)

JAMA 306:1983-1992, 2011

Context.—Patients with symptomatic atherosclerotic internal carotid artery occlusion (AICAO) and hemodynamic cerebral ischemia are at high risk for subsequent stroke when treated medically.

Objective.—To test the hypothesis that extracranial-intracranial (EC-IC) bypass surgery, added to best medical therapy, reduces subsequent ipsilateral ischemic stroke in patients with recently symptomatic AICAO and hemodynamic cerebral ischemia.

Design.—Parallel-group, randomized, open-label, blinded-adjudication clinical treatment trial conducted from 2002 to 2010.

Setting.—Forty-nine clinical centers and 18 positron emission tomography (PET) centers in the United States and Canada. The majority were academic medical centers.

Participants.—Patients with arteriographically confirmed AICAO causing hemispheric symptoms within 120 days and hemodynamic cerebral ischemia identified by ipsilateral increased oxygen extraction fraction measured by PET. Of 195 patients who were randomized, 97 were randomized to receive surgery and 98 to no surgery. Follow-up for the primary end point until occurrence, 2 years, or termination of trial was 99% complete. No participant withdrew because of adverse events.

Interventions.—Anastomosis of superficial temporal artery branch to a middle cerebral artery cortical branch for the surgical group. Antithrombotic therapy and risk factor intervention were recommended for all participants.

Main Outcome Measure.—For all participants who were assigned to surgery and received surgery, the combination of (1) all stroke and death from surgery through 30 days after surgery and (2) ipsilateral ischemic stroke within 2 years of randomization. For the nonsurgical group and participants assigned to surgery who did not receive surgery, the combination of (1) all stroke and death from randomization to randomization plus 30 days and (2) ipsilateral ischemic stroke within 2 years of randomization.

Results.—The trial was terminated early for futility. Two-year rates for the primary end point were 21.0% (95% CI, 12.8% to 29.2%; 20 events) for the surgical group and 22.7% (95% CI, 13.9% to 31.6%; 20 events) for the nonsurgical group ($P = .78$, Z test), a difference of 1.7% (95% CI, −10.4% to 13.8%). Thirty-day rates for ipsilateral ischemic stroke were 14.4% (14/97) in the surgical group and 2.0% (2/98) in the nonsurgical group, a difference of 12.4% (95% CI, 4.9% to 19.9%).

Conclusion.—Among participants with recently symptomatic AICAO and hemodynamic cerebral ischemia, EC-IC bypass surgery plus medical therapy compared with medical therapy alone did not reduce the risk of recurrent ipsilateral ischemic stroke at 2 years.

Trial Registration.—clinicaltrials.gov Identifier: NCT00029146.

▶ What do we do for those patients with symptomatic atherosclerotic internal carotid occlusion? It seems that this question will need to be answered by a prospective and randomized clinical trial with different endpoint. The results of the Carotid Occlusion Surgery Study found no benefit from the provocative extracranial-intracranial bypass surgical option (Fig 3 in the original article). Despite graft patency being deemed excellent and the surgery clearly improving cerebral hemodynamics, the clinical outcomes were no different from the nonsurgical group. The study was closed prematurely based on the assumptions of futility. To this end, bypass surgery performed well in the short term, but in the long term was no different from medical therapy alone. The effect may have been attributed to optimization of medical therapies during the study (statin, antiplatelet, risk-factor modification, etc). The authors suggested that their results "reaffirm the hazard of using even the most carefully studied historical controls to infer therapeutic efficacy and the necessity of performing randomized controlled trials to establish clinical benefit."

F. Rincon, MD

Stenting versus Aggressive Medical Therapy for Intracranial Arterial Stenosis

Chimowitz MI, for the SAMMPRIS Trial Investigators (Med Univ of South Carolina, Charleston; et al)

N Engl J Med 365:993-1003, 2011

Background.—Atherosclerotic intracranial arterial stenosis is an important cause of stroke that is increasingly being treated with percutaneous transluminal angioplasty and stenting (PTAS) to prevent recurrent stroke. However, PTAS has not been compared with medical management in a randomized trial.

Methods.—We randomly assigned patients who had a recent transient ischemic attack or stroke attributed to stenosis of 70 to 99% of the diameter of a major intracranial artery to aggressive medical management alone or aggressive medical management plus PTAS with the use of the Wingspan stent system. The primary end point was stroke or death within 30 days after enrollment or after a revascularization procedure for the qualifying lesion during the follow-up period or stroke in the territory of the qualifying artery beyond 30 days.

Results.—Enrollment was stopped after 451 patients underwent randomization, because the 30-day rate of stroke or death was 14.7% in the PTAS group (nonfatal stroke, 12.5%; fatal stroke, 2.2%) and 5.8% in the medical-management group (nonfatal stroke, 5.3%; non–stroke-related death, 0.4%) (P = 0.002). Beyond 30 days, stroke in the same territory occurred in 13 patients in each group. Currently, the mean duration of followup, which is ongoing, is 11.9 months. The probability of the occurrence of a primary end-point event over time differed significantly between the two treatment groups (P = 0.009), with 1-year rates of the primary end point of 20.0% in the PTAS group and 12.2% in the medical-management group.

Conclusions.—In patients with intracranial arterial stenosis, aggressive medical management was superior to PTAS with the use of the Wingspan stent system, both because the risk of early stroke after PTAS was high and because the risk of stroke with aggressive medical therapy alone was lower than expected. (Funded by the National Institute of Neurological Disorders and Stroke and others; SAMMPRIS ClinicalTrials.gov number, NCT00576693.)

▶ Atherosclerotic intracranial arterial stenosis is one of the commonest causes of stroke, and those refractory to medical management are treated with percutaneous transluminal angioplasty and stenting (PTAS) to prevent recurrent stroke. This study involves a randomized controlled trial comparing aggressive medical management alone or aggressive medical management plus PTAS with the use of the Wingspan stent system in patients with 70% to 99% stenosis of the diameter of a major intracranial artery. The primary end point of the trial was stroke or death within 30 days after enrollment or after a revascularization procedure for the qualifying lesion during the follow-up period or stroke in the territory of the qualifying artery beyond 30 days. However, the enrollment had to be stopped midway after 451 patients because of the increased 30-day rate of stroke and death in the PTAS group compared with the medical-management group. However, beyond 30 days, stroke occurrence was similar for each group. The success of the medical regimen compared with prior medical trials (eg, the WASID trial) was attributed to the combination of aspirin and clopidogrel, as well as strict control of cholesterol levels and systolic blood pressure. Limitations of the trial include the halting of the enrollment midway, which hindered attainment of the ideal number of subjects as per the study design. Also because the study is ongoing, only about half the patients have undergone 1-year of follow-up, and the long-term assessments may bring different outcomes. The current results of this trial indicate that medical therapy is superior to PTAS, which is associated with a high risk of periprocedural stroke or death, and essential elements of the medical regimen used can readily be adopted in our clinical practice. At the end of the day, one should ask whether the natural course of the disease is better than the intervention or if we need better technologies to treat this disease endovascularly.

S. Dey, MD

Brain Hypoxia Is Associated With Short-term Outcome After Severe Traumatic Brain Injury Independently of Intracranial Hypertension and Low Cerebral Perfusion Pressure

Oddo M, Levine JM, MacKenzie L, et al (Univ of Pennsylvania Med Ctr, Philadelphia; et al)

Neurosurgery 69:1037-1045, 2011

Background.—Brain hypoxia (BH) can aggravate outcome after severe traumatic brain injury (TBI). Whether BH or reduced brain oxygen ($Pbto_2$) is an independent outcome predictor or a marker of disease severity is not fully elucidated.

Objective.—To analyze the relationship between $Pbto_2$, intracranial pressure (ICP), and cerebral perfusion pressure (CPP) and to examine whether BH correlates with worse outcome independently of ICP and CPP.

Methods.—We studied 103 patients monitored with ICP and $Pbto_2$ for >24 hours. Durations of BH ($Pbto_2 < 15$ mm Hg), ICP >20 mm Hg, and CPP <60 mm Hg were calculated with linear interpolation, and their associations with outcome within 30 days were analyzed.

Results.—Duration of BH was longer in patients with unfavorable (Glasgow Outcome Scale score, 1-3) than in those with favorable (Glasgow Outcome Scale, 4-5) outcome (8.3 ± 15.9 vs 1.7 ± 3.7 hours; $P < .01$). In patients with intracranial hypertension, those with BH had fewer favorable outcomes (46%) than those without (81%; $P < .01$); similarly, patients with low CPP and BH were less likely to have favorable outcome than those with low CPP but normal $Pbto_2$ (39% vs 83%; $P < .01$). After ICP, CPP, age, Glasgow Coma Scale score, Marshall computed tomography grade, and Acute Physiology and Chronic Health Evaluation II score were controlled for, BH was independently associated with poor prognosis (adjusted odds ratio for favorable outcome, 0.89 per hour of BH; 95% confidence interval, 0.79-0.99; $P = .04$).

Conclusion.—Brain hypoxia is associated with poor short-term outcome after severe traumatic brain injury independently of elevated ICP, low CPP, and injury severity. $Pbto_2$ may be an important therapeutic target after severe traumatic brain injury.

▶ Traumatic brain injury (TBI) is a leading cause of death and disability worldwide, and brain hypoxia is a common cause of secondary cerebral damage after severe TBI. In this study, Oddo et al have analyzed the relationship between $PbtO_2$, intracranial pressure (ICP), and cerebral perfusion pressure (CPP) and have examined whether brain hypoxia is an independent predictor of worse short-term outcome. One hundred three patients who were being monitored with ICP and $PbtO_2$ for 24 hours after severe TBI were retrospectively studied. Durations of hypoxia ($PbtO_2$ < 15 mm Hg), ICP greater than 20 mm Hg, and CPP less than 60 mm Hg were calculated with linear interpolation, and their associations with outcome within 30 days were analyzed. Although brain hypoxia along with poor Glasgow Coma Scale (GCS) scores (1–3), elevated ICP, and reduced CPP accounted for unfavorable outcome, $PbtO_2$ was also found to be associated with poor outcome independent of ICP, CPP, age, GCS score, Marshall CT grade, and Acute Physiology and Chronic Health Evaluation (APACHE) II score. Limitations of this trial include a small sample size from a single academic center, which can limit the generalization of results, the fact that treatment intensity was not clarified, and that the ability to identify responders versus not responders is not elucidated from the analysis. This is important because at the end of the day, one wants to see whether response to treatment is really associated with improved outcomes.

S. Ghosh, MBBS

11 Ethics/Socioeconomic/ Administrative Issues

Other

Return to work after burn—A prospective study
Öster C, Ekselius L (Uppsala Univ, Sweden)
Burns 37:1117-1124, 2011

Return to work (RTW) is one of the most important objectives to strive for in burn rehabilitation. Most individuals do return to work after burn but there is a subgroup that does not. Prospective long-time follow-up studies focusing on RTW after burn are scarce. Consecutive adult burn patients employed before injury ($n = 58$) were included in the present study during hospitalization and subsequently followed up for 12 months. In addition, a structured interview was performed at 2–7 years after burn. At that time; mean 4.5 years (SD 2.0) after burn; 67% of the participants had returned to their work. Predictive variables for time to RTW were length of stay (LOS) at the burn center and fulfilling criteria for Any personality disorder. No RTW was predicted by LOS and having Any anxiety disorder or Any substance use disorder prior to the burn. The non-working group reported lower generic (EQ-5D) and burn-specific (BSHS-B) HRQoL than the working group at every time point. Identification of risk factors associated with difficulties in RTW is required in order to execute individualized vocational rehabilitation.

▶ In the "old days," burn survival in patients with large burns was really the only statistic that mattered. Since the 1970s, burn care has evolved to such a degree in burn centers in high-income countries that comparing survival rates between burn centers is a fairly meaningless activity. So what are the relevant outcome variables? Currently, cosmesis, functionality, and return to the previous or highest level of wellness possible (eg, quality of life) are relevant indicators. One of the biggest pieces of the quality-of-life metric is the work factor. It makes sense that patients with larger burns stay longer in burn centers. Patients who are underresourced may represent a group of patients who have the greatest financial need to return to work as quickly as possible. Sadly, patients with psychiatric comorbidities are often the least able to afford a situation in which they are unable to return to work, and this ability is often compromised. Patients with a personality disorder are overrepresented in the burn patient population, making it even more of a problem in this particular group of patients. Rehabilitation efforts for burn patients must meet the global requirements of these patients to prevent them from needlessly joining the rolls (and roles) of the disabled.

B. A. Latenser, MD, FACS

Developing clinical quality indicators for a Bi-National Burn Registry

Watterson D, Cleland H, Darton A, et al (Monash Univ, Melbourne, Australia; Royal North Shore Hosp, Sydney, Australia; et al)

Burns 37:1296-1308, 2011

Background.—Clinical quality indicators are routinely used to benchmark and drive improvements in healthcare. There is a dearth of standardised clinical quality indicators established for management of burns that allow quality of care to be monitored and benchmarked across Australia and New Zealand.

Method.—Using published quality indicator development processes and clinician experience, the Bi-National Burn Registry (Bi-NBR) working party developed quality indicators for burn care to be included as routine data items in the Bi-NBR.

Results.—Twenty indicators covering structure, process and outcome measures were identified. Preliminary testing resulted in further revision to the quality indicators to increase validity, reliability and improve data quality. The quality indicators are routinely collected in the Bi-NBR and reported quarterly.

Conclusion.—This is the first published account of the development and testing of standardised Bi-National clinical quality indicators for burns. The Bi-NBR quality indicators project remains a work in progress and it is hoped that further refinement of the indicators, in conjunction with international collaborators will assist in driving improvements in burn care.

▶ The authors have presented an easy-to-follow, step-by-step guide for developing a way to benchmark and monitor burn quality indicators. The story they tell describes how, over a several-year period, they were able to take standard quality indicators that had been established at individual burn centers in Australia and New Zealand, get agreement on some of those indicators, and then put them into place using test cases. Changes were made by the working group, and the improved quality indicators had a revised launch a year later. The difficulties of this task are nicely outlined in this review. The importance of this work for burn-specific quality indicators underscores the importance of being able to compare quality of burn care between institutions and regions.

Currently, it is completely unrealistic to think that one world standard for burn care, as epitomized by burn care in most high-income countries, is applicable and appropriate for low-income countries where the government spends just a few dollars per person per year on medical care. The American Burn

Association has spent a decade working on the National Burn Repository, a descendant of the National Burn Information Exchange of the early 1970s. It represents a collection of some of the clinical characteristics and course for burn treatment from specialized burn centers in the United States and Canada over the previous decade and is updated annually. The work is published by the American Burn Association, and copies may be obtained from them at www.ameriburn.org. This is an invaluable source for research projects, making it clear that it really is possible to compare like events.

The process and methods described in this article could well be adapted to middle-income countries and, in the future, perhaps burn care providers in low-income countries. Although the burden of burn injury is thought to be much higher than reported in low-income countries that bear some of the highest burn burdens, burn data from these underrepresented countries might be a great step in getting the world's attention to this killer of predominantly children under the age of 5 years.

B. A. Latenser, MD, FACS

Optimizing Advanced Practitioner Charge Capture in High-Acuity Surgical Intensive Care Units

Butler KL, Calabrese R, Tandon M, et al (Hartford Hosp, CT)
Arch Surg 146:552-555, 2011

Objective.—To determine the impact of standardized critical care documentation tools on charge capture by intensive care unit (ICU) advanced practitioners (APs).

Design.—Prospective charge capture analysis of AP critical care charges (*Current Procedural Terminology* codes 99291 or 99292).

Setting.—Neurosurgical, general surgical, and cardio-thoracic ICUs in a level I, 800-bed hospital. The AP provider to patient ratio was 1:6, with 24-hour surgical intensivist oversight.

Participants.—Advanced practice registered nurses and physician assistants in the ICU.

Interventions.—Standardized templates were developed to simplify documentation and optimize billing of critical care. All APs participated in comprehensive educational sessions on billing compliance and documentation.

Main Outcome Measures.—Charge capture was collected for 3 years, and comparisons were made between the first quarter before (fiscal year [FY] 2008), during (FY 2009) and after (FY 2010) implementation. The number of ICU patient-days, length of stay, and of beds was collected.

Results.—During the implementation/education phase (FY 2009), there were no differences in charge capture compared with FY 2008. Each unit demonstrated an increase in charge capture after implementation, and an overall increase of 48% for all 3 ICUs was seen. The number of admissions and length of stay were not statistically different. The total number of ICU beds increased from 42 to 45 during the evaluation period. The salary offset for APs increased from 62% to 80%.

Conclusions.—Advanced practitioners represent an important component of the critical care services provided to patients in high-acuity surgical ICUs. Standardized critical care documentation and comprehensive education on evaluation and management guidelines significantly increased charge capture.

▶ As more organizations are making meaningful use of the electronic medical record (EMR), the ability to leverage the technical capabilities to create standardized documentation and order set templates is being explored. Dr Butler and colleagues attempted to determine the financial impact that an EMR-designed documentation tool may have in terms of charge capture rates in a surgical intensive care unit. The study was prospective and involved advanced practitioners with intensivist supervision. After successful implementation of a critical care standardized documentation tool, net revenue and charge capture significantly increased with stable volumes.

This article demonstrates how systems can use EMR to reliably and accurately document the care that is provided to critically ill patients. When done consistently, the process can add to the bottom line. This revenue increase offsets the expense of the EMR itself, the costs of allied health providers, and the reimbursement cuts that many systems are feeling. The article does not address the specifics of the auditing process and whether there was a need for any reeducation or ongoing provider evaluation. A common concern when designing a standardized template for documentation of review of systems, physical exam, and assessment/plan is the risk for "cut-and-paste" that can occur unknowingly. Given the sheer volume of information that is transferred across components of a critically ill patient's chart by multiple providers and ancillary support staff, inadvertent mistakes can and do occur. Although this poses a risk from a compliance standpoint with reimbursement, delays and medical errors based on inaccurately cut-and-pasted notes could be disastrous for the patient.

Examining revenue increases with EMR-designed systems must also simultaneously include ways to cut overall system costs. Increasing efficiency, quality, and reliability, while maintaining affordability, allows providers to deliver the best care possible. By leveraging EMRs to provide safer care, improve discharge processes, and reduce readmission rates, value improves, and we will ultimately decrease the total cost of care.

G. B. Collins, MD

Impact of Nonphysician Staffing on Outcomes in a Medical ICU

Gershengorn HB, Wunsch H, Wahab R, et al (Beth Israel Med Ctr, NY; New York Presbyterian Hosp-Columbia)

Chest 139:1347-1353, 2011

Background.—As the number of ICU beds and demand for intensivists increase, alternative solutions are needed to provide coverage for critically ill patients. The impact of different staffing models on the outcomes of patients in the medical ICU (MICU) remains unknown. In our study, we compare outcomes of nonphysician provider-based teams to those of medical house staff-based teams in the MICU.

Methods.—We conducted a retrospective review of 590 daytime (7:00 AM-7:00 PM) admissions to two MICUs at one hospital. In one MICU staffed by nurse practitioners and physician assistants (MICU-NP/PA) there were nonphysicians (nurse practitioners and physicians assistants) during the day (7:00 AM-7:00 PM) with attending physician coverage overnight. In the other MICU, there were medicine residents (MICU-RES) (24 h/d). The outcomes investigated were hospital mortality, length of stay (LOS) (ICU, hospital), and posthospital discharge destination.

Results.—Three hundred two patients were admitted to the MICU-NP/PA and 288 to the MICU-RES. Mortality probability model III (MPM_0-III) predicted mortality was similar ($P=.14$). There was no significant difference in hospital mortality (32.1% for MICU-NP/PA vs 32.3% for MICU-RES, $P=.96$), MICU LOS (4.22 ± 2.51 days for MICU-NP/PA vs 4.44 ± 3.10 days for MICU-RES, $P=.59$), or hospital LOS (14.01 ± 2.92 days for MICU-NP/PA vs 13.74 ± 2.94 days for MICU-RES, $P=.86$). Discharge to a skilled care facility (vs home) was similar (37.1% for MICU-NP/PA vs 32.5% for MICU-RES, $P=.34$). After multivariate adjustment, MICU staffing type was not associated with hospital mortality ($P=.26$), MICU LOS ($P=.29$), hospital LOS ($P=.19$), or posthospital discharge destination ($P=.90$).

Conclusions.—Staffing models including daytime use of nonphysician providers appear to be a safe and effective alternative to the traditional house staff-based team in a high-acuity, adult ICU.

▶ This article examines alternative staffing models in a medical intensive care unit using nonphysician providers. A retrospective look at 590 daytime admissions (7 AM–7 PM) demonstrated no difference in hospital mortality, hospital and intensive care unit (ICU) length of stay, or percentage of patients discharged to a skilled nursing facility compared with a resident-staffed model.

The major strength of the article is that the authors are working to identify solutions to problems that many ICUs face: physician shortage, expectation of 24-hour intensivist coverage, resident duty hour restrictions, and economic constraints. Many ICUs use nurse practitioners, physician assistants, and residents as part of the provider team, but few look back at patient outcomes. A prospective study, possibly involving telemedicine models, may ultimately answer more specific questions about patient outcomes, resource utilization, decision-making skills, and the true need for a board-certified intensivist close to the bedside 24 hours per day.

Systems are continually being asked to provide the highest quality care while being as cost-effective as possible. Patients expect value and reliability regardless of the staffing models used. As providers, it is crucial that outcomes are closely tracked when unique processes are changed as they relate to the critically ill or injured.

G. B. Collins, MD

Qualitative analysis of an intensive care unit family satisfaction survey

Henrich NJ, Dodek P, Heyland D, et al (St Paul's Hosp, Vancouver, British Columbia, Canada; St Paul's Hosp and Univ of British Columbia, Vancouver, Canada; Queens Univ, Kingston, Ontario, Canada; et al)

Crit Care Med 39:1000-1005, 2011

Objectives.—To describe the qualitative findings from a family satisfaction survey to identify and describe the themes that characterize family members' intensive care unit experiences.

Design.—As part of a larger mixed-methods study to determine the relationship between organizational culture and family satisfaction in critical care, family members of eligible patients in intensive care units completed a Family Satisfaction Survey (FS-ICU 24), which included three open-ended questions about strengths and weaknesses of the intensive care unit based on the family members' experiences and perspectives. Responses to these questions were coded and analyzed to identify key themes.

Setting.—Surveys were administered in 23 intensive care units from across Canada.

Participants.—Surveys were completed by family members of patients who were in the intensive care unit for >48 hrs and who had been visited by the family member at least once during their intensive care unit stay.

Interventions.—None.

Measurements and Main Results.—A total of 1381 surveys were distributed and 880 responses were received. Intensive care unit experiences were found to be variable within and among intensive care units. Six themes emerged as central to respondents' satisfaction: quality of staff, overall quality of medical care, compassion and respect shown to the patient and family, communication with doctors, waiting room, and patient room. Within three themes, positive comments were more common than negative comments: quality of the staff (66% vs. 23%), overall quality of medical care provided (33% vs. 2%), and compassion and respect shown to the patient and family (29% vs. 12%). Within the other three themes, positive comments were less common than negative comments: communication with doctors (18% vs. 20%), waiting room (1% vs. 8%), and patient rooms (0.4% vs. 5%).

Conclusions.—The study provided improved understanding of why family members are satisfied or dissatisfied with particular elements of the intensive care unit and this knowledge can be used to modify intensive care units to better meet the physical and emotional needs of the families of intensive care unit patients.

▶ Examining family satisfaction surveys in the intensive care unit (ICU) provides valuable information that facilitates improvements in the delivery of patient-centered care. Dr Henrich and colleagues set out to better characterize family experience in the critical care setting. Multiple themes emerged, including families' perceived quality of staff and care, compassion and respect, environmental factors, and communication with physicians. From 880 respondents, the team learned that the main areas for improvement were communication with physicians and the state of patient and waiting rooms. The remaining themes had a majority of positive comments, thus directing this critical care unit where to strategically focus energy.

One of the important findings from this study was the need for improved communication with physician in terms of frequency, inclusion of family in daily discussions, and the level of directness used. A key factor in building strong relationships is establishing expectations early on. For some families, a daily update is sufficient, but in other cases, touching base multiple times with any clinical changes is the expectation. This information can be gleaned at the time of admission or throughout the stay by providers, chaplains, and bedside staff. It is important to meet or exceed reasonable patient and family expectations because this is, by definition, a positive experience in any industry. Subjective and variable expectations that are clearly delineated are more likely to be satisfied. A team approach is therefore crucial.

As value-based purchasing becomes a more common reimbursement model, there will be increasingly more experience measures that are important for health care consumers, payers, and regulatory agencies. Providers and organizations that proactively identify areas requiring technical and adaptive change to make improvements will be better prepared for future market shifts and landscape changes. Dr Henrich and her colleagues have made family satisfaction in the ICU a priority a part of an overall assessment of organizational culture. More such surveys will continue to provide the necessary data required to improve overall care and patient experience.

G. B. Collins, MD

Quality of Life/End of Life/Outcome Prediction

Selection of intensive care unit admission criteria for patients aged 80 years and over and compliance of emergency and intensive care unit physicians with the selected criteria: An observational, multicenter, prospective study

Garrouste-Orgeas M, on behalf of the ICE-CUB Group (Saint Joseph Hosp Network, Paris, France; et al)

Crit Care Med 37:2919-2928, 2009

Objective.—To describe intensive care unit referral decisions by emergency room physicians in patients aged ≥80 yrs.

Design.—Prospective, observational cohort study of patients aged ≥80 yrs who were triaged in the emergency room, using a list of intensive care unit admission criteria selected by emergency physicians among 76 preliminary criteria adapted from the 1999 Society of Critical Care Medicine guidelines. The Delphi method was used to select the criteria.

Setting.—Fifteen French hospitals.

Patients.—A total of 2646 patients aged ≥80 yrs with at least one criterion.

Interventions.—None.

Measurements and Main Results.—In the Delphi process, level of agreement was assessed as follows: when all answers fell within a single interval

(7–9 = definite admission criteria; 4–6 = equivocal admission criteria or 1–3 = inappropriate admission), agreement was strong; when answers spanned two intervals, agreement was fair; and when answers spanned all three intervals, agreement was poor. Of the 76 preliminary criteria, two were removed; 44 were selected as definite intensive care unit admission criteria; and 30 were selected as equivocal intensive care unit admission criteria. Of the 1426 patients meeting definite admission criteria, 441 (30.9%) were referred for intensive care unit admission and 231 of 441 (52.4%) were admitted to the intensive care unit. Of the 1041 patients with equivocal admission criteria, 181 (17.3%) were referred for intensive care unit admission; and, of these, 79 (43.6%) were admitted to the intensive care unit. Factors associated independently with no intensive care unit referral were age odds ratio [OR], 1.04; 95% confidence interval [CI], 1.04–1.07), active cancer (OR, 1.61; 95% CI, 1.09–1.38), unknown hospitalization status (OR, 1.53; 95% CI, 1.11–2.11), unknown living arrangements (OR, 1.69; 95% CI, 1.19–2.42), regular psychotropic medications (OR, 1.42; 95% CI, 1.10–1.81), low severity at referral (OR, 0.60; 95% CI, 0.53–0.68), low activity in daily living score (OR, 0.93; 95% CI, 0.88–0.99).

Conclusions.—Emergency and intensive care unit physicians were extremely reluctant to consider intensive care unit admission of patients aged ≥80 yrs, despite the presence of criteria indicating that intensive care unit admission was certainly or possibly appropriate.

▶ Merriam-Webster defines intensive care as having special medical facilities, services, and monitoring devices to meet the needs of gravely ill patients. Although easily defined in theory, the reality is that the decision of who should receive intensive care is not always clear-cut. This is further complicated when age is considered as an admission criterion for intensive care unit (ICU) admission. The prior studies have shown that even after adjusting for disease severity, elderly patients have higher ICU and post-ICU mortality rates.[1] The United Nations projects that 4.1% of the world's population will be older than 80 years in 2050, a number expected to be approximately 379 million people.[2] Therefore, the decision on who is or is not admitted to the ICU will continue to be an evolving process for intensivists and other clinicians who will be taking care of this elderly population.

This study sought to investigate the compliance of emergency care physicians and intensivists regarding the admission of patients older than 80 years to the ICU in Paris metropolis, France. Given that very few studies have evaluated clinical outcomes in this patient group, this study may inspire further investigation in this complex subject.[3] It was revealed that emergency physicians were unlikely to refer patients older than 80 years to the ICU. Likewise, when receiving referrals from their emergency physician counterparts, ICU physicians were not likely to admit patients older than 80 years to the ICU even when criteria on admission supported a referral to the ICU. Nonreferral to the ICU was associated with increased age, poor functional status, and the specific diagnosis for which the person was admitted. These findings raise many questions about health care for the elderly population. including potential biases and subjective factors that may influence physicians' decisions. How does clinical judgment play a role? As described in the article, there is no straightforward clear-cut algorithm that physicians can follow to make the right decisions regarding elevation of the level of care. Doctors still have to eyeball the patient and make sound clinical decisions, that is, practice the art of medicine. All patients are not created equal, and although 2 patients may both have renal failure, their over all clinical picture may differ greatly. Performance status, even presumed performance status, might influence decisions.

In the United States, studies have shown mixed results when evaluating whether elderly patients were less likely to be admitted to an ICU.[4,5] Unfortunately, we lack the tools or fail to implement their uses regarding admissions of the elderly to the ICU (eg, APACHE II score). What remains important is that physicians continue to evaluate patients with an open mind and try to provide the appropriate care for each individual patient's needs.

T. Cartwright, MD
V. Rajput, MD

References

1. Boumendil A, Somme D, Garrouste-Orgeas M, Guidet B. Should elderly patients be admitted to the intensive care unit? *Intensive Care Med.* 2007;33:1252-1262.
2. United Nations: World Population Ageing 1950-2050 http://www.un.org/esa/population/publications/worldageing19502050. Actual: http://www.un.org/esa/population/publications/worldageing19502050/pdf/90chapteriv.pdf. Accessed January 6, 2011.
3. Somme D, Maillet JM, Gisselbrecht M, Novara A, Ract C, Fagon JY. Critically ill old and the oldest-old patients in intensive care: short- and long-term outcomes. *Intensive Care Med.* 2003;29:2137-2143.
4. Yu W, Ash AS, Levinsky NG, Moskowitz MA. Intensive care unit use and mortality in the elderly. *J Gen Intern Med.* 2000;15:97-102.
5. Wunsch H, Harrison D, Linde-Zwirble W, Agnus D, Rowan K. Differences for ICU admissions in the elderly between the United States and the United Kingdom. *Critical Care.* 2006;10:S179 [abstract P429].

The delivery of futile care is harmful to other patients

Niederman MS, Berger JT (Winthrop-Univ Hosp, Mineola, NY; SUNY at Stony Brook, NY)
Crit Care Med 38:S518-S522, 2010

Objective.—Intensive care units (ICUs) in different parts of the world provide care to patients with advanced age and terminal illness at different rates and in different patterns. In the United States, ICU beds make up a disproportionate number of acute care beds. Nearly half of all patients who die in U.S. hospitals have received ICU, some of which may be futile. The objective of this study was to examine ways in which the delivery of futile care in the ICU can cause harm to patients other than those receiving the futile care.

Design.—Review of available studies of patient and family attitudes about cardiopulmonary resuscitation and other supportive modalities, including antibiotic therapy, and the relationship of the delivery of such care to the outcomes of others treated in the ICU.

Patients.—Those treated in ICUs and those receiving futile care.

Measurements and Main Results.—Compared with younger patients, the elderly in the United States use more ICU care, at higher cost, have more serious comorbidities, and have a higher mortality rate. Certain populations demand ICU care more than others and often with less benefit than less-demanding populations. In a situation of unlimited resources, the provision of ICU care, even when futile, has been viewed as an individual patient decision with no harm to others within the hospital. However, even with unlimited resources, the use of antibiotics for those who are receiving futile care can be considered unethical by egalitarian theory because it can lead to antibiotic resistance that may make the treatment of other patients impossible. In the setting of limited resources, like in pandemic influenza, or with the potential limiting of resources, in a pay-for-performance environment, the provision of futile care can also harm the hospital population as a whole.

Conclusions.—The delivery of futile care is not only an individual patient decision, but must be viewed in a broader context. Societal awareness of this problem is necessary, and better scoring systems to identify when ICU care has limited benefit are needed to address these difficult and challenging realities.

▶ The majority of health care monies in the United States are spent on elderly patients who have been admitted to the intensive care unit (ICU) where they remain until death. These hospital stays can sometimes amount to hundreds of days, during which time patients often remain on life support. These individuals usually suffer from a number of complex medical conditions; as the age of these patients increases, the mortality rate does as well. Compared with European countries, the United States has more hospital beds dedicated for ICU rather than acute care use.

Neiderman and Berger argue that this is unethical on 2 accounts. First, some treatments, such as the use of antibiotics in a patient that will receive no benefit, should not be permitted; if resistance occurs, this treatment would prove to be harmful to others through indirect means. Second, they hold that physicians are obliged to withhold treatments that are for symbolic use and do not serve a beneficial medical purpose. These claims are based on communitarian and egalitarian theories, which arise from the notions of interaction with others, the distribution of resources, and fair opportunities to equalize potential benefits. Important to make clear is the distinction between medical treatment and medical care, as it is ethical to declare medical treatments futile and, therefore, remove such measures; however, medical care for a patient can never ethically be stopped. Medical treatments are aimed at combating a particular pathology or curing a condition and are thought to be futile when a patient is no longer gaining benefit; whereas medical care involves keeping a patient comfortable by treating a patient's symptoms and providing the necessary support to ensure that a patient is not suffering (comfort care).

Futility can occur under circumstances in which there are unlimited resources or limited resources. Using antibiotics to treat a patient who has no chance of recovery is an example of futile care when ample resources are available; however, providing futile care via a ventilator during an influenza epidemic or continuing futile care in a hospital that is held under pay-for-performance standards are such examples in which the opposite is true. Overall, it was concluded that a system must be implemented that will limit certain therapies in elderly/terminal patients and that a definition of futile care must be established.

In analyzing this article, a principalistic approach to ethics can be utilized. Under the principle of autonomy and respect for persons, the patient or his proxy must be involved in determining the treatment course that he will receive. Beneficence and nonmaleficence hold that good should be done and harm should be avoided, respectively. In this case, beneficence is observed if the treatment that a patient is receiving provides true benefit to the patient. On the other hand, if it provides greater stress than benefit, then nonmaleficence is being disregarded. Additionally, nonmaleficence can be applied to a closed community, such as to patients admitted to the ICU when discussing the ethics of futile administration of antibiotics. If such drugs are continuously given to a patient who is gaining no benefit, the potential exists for resistant bacteria to develop that could consequently infect the remainder of patients in the ICU. Some may argue that autonomy is being undermined in this particular situation. Futility occurs not only when a physician determines a treatment to be of no benefit or even harm a patient but also when providing a treatment causes harm to other patients.[1] Finally, justice, which states that each should be given his due, supports the idea that treatments should be administered to patients if they are available; nonetheless, in accordance with distributive justice, resources are limited and must be shared equitably.

In an article by Robert Sibbald and colleagues, a definition of "futile care" was formulated and published after researchers conducted interviews with ICU patients' caregivers to determine their perceptions of this term. They determined the phrase "futile care" to mean the following: "the use of considerable resources without a reasonable hope that the patient would recover to a state of relative independence or be interactive with their environment." The point being made here is that although it may be possible to keep a patient alive via extraordinary means, such as with a ventilator, the patient may never regain any reasonable quality of life. These researchers also found that many caregivers would prefer that there be more concrete ethical and legal standards implemented to decide whether care given to a patient would be nonbeneficial.[2]

This article makes many valid points, especially as it pertains to antibiotic use that has become futile, because of the potential for other individuals to be harmed. As more resistance is developed, the chance of infection increases and consequences of contraction of the organism worsen. Moreover, although defining "futile care" would provide a more objective approach to patient treatment, each patient has different needs and circumstances; therefore, all cases must be addressed individually.

V. Rajput, MD
K. Contino, BS

References

1. Wilkinson DJ, Savulescu J. Knowing when to stop: futility in the ICU. *Curr Opin Anaesthesiol.* 2011;24:160-165.
2. Sibbald R, Downar J, Hawryluck L. Perceptions of "futile care" among caregivers in intensive care units. *CMAJ.* 2007;177:1201-1208.

An Empirical Study of Surrogates' Preferred Level of Control over Value-laden Life Support Decisions in Intensive Care Units

Johnson SK, Bautista CA, Hong SY, et al (Univ of California San Francisco; Univ of Pittsburgh, PA; et al)
Am J Respir Crit Care Med 183:915-921, 2011

Rationale.—Despite ongoing ethical debate concerning who should control decisions to discontinue life support for incapacitated, critically ill patients, the perspectives of surrogate decision makers are poorly understood.

Objectives.—To determine (*1*) what degree of decisional authority surrogates prefer for value-sensitive life support decisions compared with more technical biomedical decisions, and (*2*) what predicts surrogates' preferences for more control over life support decisions.

Methods.—This was a prospective study of 230 surrogate decision makers for incapacitated, mechanically ventilated patients at high risk of death. Surrogates reported their preferred degree of decisional authority using the Degner Control Preferences Scale for two types of decisions: a value-sensitive decision about whether to discontinue life support and a decision regarding which antibiotic to prescribe for an infection.

Measurements and Main Results.—The majority of surrogates (55%, 127/230; 95% confidence interval, 49–62%) preferred to have final control over the value-sensitive life support decision; 40% (91/230) wished to share control equally with the physician; 5% (12/230) of surrogates wanted the physician to make the decision. Surrogates preferred significantly more control over the value-sensitive life support decision compared with the technical decision about choice of antibiotics ($P < 0.0001$). Factors independently associated with surrogates' preference for more control over the life support decision were: less trust in the intensive care unit physician, male sex, and non-Catholic religious affiliation.

Conclusions.—Surrogates vary in their desire for decisional authority for value-sensitive life support decisions, but prefer substantially more authority for this type of decision compared with technical, medical

judgments. Low trust in physicians is associated with surrogates preferring more control of life support decisions.

▶ Varying opinions exist as to the role and extent of surrogates' decision-making involvement in end-of-life care for patients in intensive care units (ICUs). Whether a patient assigns a durable power of attorney or his next of kin serves as a substitute decision maker, the hope is that the individual offering substituted judgment will provide a philosophical view into life and death decisions and give insight into the treatment and care options the patient would have chosen if he or she was capable of doing so on his or her own. Extensive research has been performed with the intent of defining the depth to which surrogates should be involved in making medical choices.

Specifically, this article questions the difference between value judgments and decisions of complex and specific medical care as it pertains to life support and complicated medical treatments. In implementing a principalistic ethical approach and analysis to the question, the patient's autonomy, under the principle of respect for persons, has been transferred to his assigned proxy; therefore, his substituted judgment should represent the patient's beliefs and values. One must consider whether a patient, in his or her own functional baseline mental state, would be involved in making decisions specific to treatment, such as antibiotic choice when all options provide the same efficacy. Beneficence and nonmaleficence, defined as doing good and avoiding harm, respectively, hold that whatever is in the best interest of the patient should be done. In this case, the value judgment, being whether the patient would desire to be sustained on life support measures, should be left to the proxy to decide after he or she has been educated by the physician on the patient's state and prognosis; whereas, complex medical treatment decisions should likely be left to the medical professionals. Finally, in accordance with justice, all persons should be treated equally and be given their due; when these patients are unable to make decisions for themselves, specifically as they relate to personal values, substituted judgment must be utilized.

Two important points were made in this article. Unlike the results of most other studies, these researchers found that some of the participating surrogates wished to have the authority in making final medical decisions for the patient for whom they provide substituted judgment, which was the first time that these results were found. Second, the overall conclusion, which is consistent with that of many other researchers, is that even with value decisions, surrogates did not wish to have complete authority in the decision-making process; rather, they prefer that physicians provide the appropriate counsel and assistance and be truthful in their assessment of prognosis and realistic potential for recovery. Therefore, because of the vast range of surrogates' desired involvement, physicians must adapt to each case accordingly.

A 2011 article by Billings and Krakauer states that in withholding knowledge and expertise, a physician is, in essence, undermining patient autonomy by preventing the proxy from making an informed decision for the patient, which could ultimately cause harm to the patient. Consequently, the surrogate, acting in the best interest of the patient, should be provided with adequate information to make reasonable decisions.[1]

Another article published in 2010 by Curtis and Vincent found that there is great variation in the amount of involvement surrogates and patients desire in making decisions regarding patient treatments and end-of-life care. Ultimately, they concluded that communication with the family regarding goals of care and realistic assessment of prognosis in spite of uncertainty is key, so that which is in the best interest of the patient is done. Some suggestions made to assist in implementation of this process include involvement of the family in ICU rounds and patient inclusion in interdisciplinary rounds.[2]

Surrogate involvement in end-of-life care has remained one of the most controversial issues in health care as medicine advances and the cost of keeping patients on life support for prolonged periods continues to arise. The findings presented in the article by Sara Johnson and colleagues should be used in conjunction with those of other studies, which generally conclude that surrogates should be adequately informed to make appropriate value judgments and provide a better understanding of the goals of care the patient may have preferred for treatment in that particular situation. Because of the lack of evidence behind surrogate involvement in technical medical treatment decisions, more research is needed in this area.

K. Contino, BS
V. Rajput, MD

References

1. Billings JA, Krakauer EL. On patient autonomy and physician responsibility in end-of-life care. *Arch Intern Med.* 2011;171:849-853.
2. Curtis JR, Vincent JL. Ethics and end-of-life care for adults in the intensive care unit. *Lancet.* 2010;376:1347-1353.

Power and limitations of daily prognostications of death in the medical Intensive care unit

Meadow W, Pohlman A, Frain L, et al (The Univ of Chicago, IL)
Crit Care Med 39:474-479, 2011

Objective.—We tested the accuracy of predictions of impending death for medical intensive care unit patients, offered daily by their professional medical caretakers.

Design.—For 560 medical intensive care unit patients, on each medical intensive care unit day, we asked their attending physicians, fellows, residents, and registered nurses one question: "Do you think this patient will die in the hospital or survive to be discharged?"

Results.—We obtained >6,000 predictions on 2018 medical intensive care unit patient days. Seventy-five percent of MICU patients who stayed ≥4 days had discordant predictions; that is, at least one caretaker predicted survival, whereas others predicted death before discharge. Only

107 of 206 (52%) patients with a prediction of "death before discharge" actually died in hospital. This number rose to 66% (96 of 145) for patients with 1 day of corroborated (i.e., >1) prediction of "death," and to 84% (79 of 94) with at least 1 unanimous day of predictions of death. However, although positive predictive value rose with increasingly stringent prediction criteria, sensitivity fell so that the area under the receiver-operator characteristic curve did not differ for single, corroborated, or unanimous predictions of death. Subsets of older (>65 yrs) and ventilated medical intensive care unit patients revealed parallel findings.

Conclusions.—1) Roughly half of all medical intensive care unit patients predicted to die in hospital survived to discharge nonetheless. 2) More highly corroborated predictions had better predictive value; although, approximately 15% of patients survived unexpectedly, even when predicted to die by all medical caretakers.

▶ Patients' treatments in the intensive care unit are costly, requiring expensive and limited resources. Many of these patients have poor prognosis for survival. The patients with the worst prognosis are often targeted for rationing. However, an accurate predictor death does not exist. Although multiple studies have attempted to assess clinical predictions of survival of medical intensive care unit (MICU) patients, these studies have failed to look longitudinally or as continuum at individual patients and instead assess prognosis at a single point during the admission to the intensive care unit (ICU). The authors believe that serial predictions obtained daily from clinical caretakers would be more effective in determining clinical prognosis.

In this study, the authors followed up with 560 ICU patients over a period of 7 months. The patients' caretakers (physicians, fellows, residents, and nurses) were asked daily "Do you think this patient will die in the hospital or survive to be discharged?" Each caretaker was asked individually to minimize influence of one opinion over another.

It was found that over time, outcomes for ICU patients become progressively less clear. Only 27% of patients who left the ICU within the first 3 days had disagreement about their prognosis among their caretakers. For those who remained in the ICU for more than 3 days, caretaker disagreement increased to 75%. Additionally in the patients who remained in the ICU for more than 3 days, it was determined that likelihood of survival decreased each subsequent day. Most importantly, it was found that almost half of ICU patients predicted to die in the hospital survived to discharge. Although more highly corroborated predictions had better predictive value, 12% of patients who were unanimously predicted to die by all caretakers actually survived.

A separate study investigated the diagnostic role of gut feelings in general practice. Some physicians base clinical decisions on gut feeling alone, whether it is a sense of reassurance or a sense of alarm, despite actual medical evidence. The physicians may not even be aware that their own intuition may be acting as a diagnostic instrument. Similar situations can arise when looking at the decision to withhold or continue life-sustaining treatment in the ICU, as gut feelings can potentially increase subjectivity unknowingly.[1]

Despite the many studies aimed to assess patients' prognoses and likelihood of death in the ICU, there is still no sufficient manner to accurately determine an ICU patient's clinical outcome. The authors determined that even serial clinical predictions are imperfect predictors of outcome evidenced by the fact that nearly half of all patients predicted to die survived to discharge.

C. Mannino, MD
V. Rajput, MD

Reference

1. Stolper E, van Bokhoven M, Houben P, et al. The diagnostic role of gut feelings in general practice. A focus group study of the concept and its determinants. *BMC Fam Pract.* 2009;10:17.

What to do when a competent ICU patient does not want to live anymore but is dependent on life-sustaining treatment? Experience from The Netherlands

van der Hoven B, de Groot YJ, Thijsse WJ, et al (Erasmus MC Univ Med Ctr, Rotterdam, The Netherlands)
Intensive Care Med 36:2145-2148, 2010

If patients on the intensive care unit (ICU) are awake and life-sustaining treatment is suspended because of the patients' request, because of recovering from the disease, or because independence from organ function supportive or replacement therapy outside the ICU can no longer be achieved, these patients can suffer before they inevitably die. In The Netherlands, two scenarios are possible for these patients: (1) deep palliative (terminal) sedation through ongoing administration of barbiturates or benzodiazepines before withdrawal of treatment, or (2) deliberate termination of life (euthanasia) before termination of treatment. In this article we describe two awake patients who asked for withdrawal of life-sustaining measures, but who were dependent on mechanical ventilation. We discuss the doctrine of double effect in relation to palliative sedation on the ICU. Administration of sedatives and analgesics before withdrawal of treatment is seen as normal palliative care. We conclude that the doctrine of the double effect is not applicable in this situation, and mentioning it criminalised the practice unnecessarily and wrongfully.

▶ There has been increased discussion regarding the ethical nature of providing palliative sedation to patients who are dependent on life support when such measures are removed. The main issue lies in delineating euthanasia from palliative care. Because of the advancements in medical technology, it is possible to keep patients alive for prolonged periods of time by unnatural means, such as mechanical ventilation. Patients retain the autonomy to request that these means of sustaining life be removed to allow the pathology to run its course if they do not wish to continue living in this manner; however, if this course is taken, the patient must also be kept comfortable, so that he or she may die with dignity.

The purpose of the article by Ben van der Hoven and colleagues was to determine whether terminal sedation before the removal of life-sustaining support is ethical or if it is, in actuality, synonymous with euthanasia. Per the doctrine of double effect, euthanasia is unethical because the intention of administering specific drugs is to directly take the patient's life. Palliative sedation is more controversial depending on the circumstances and the timing of medication administration. Sedation given to control anxiety, suffering, respiratory distress, and pain after a patient is removed from life support is, in fact, permissive and in accordance with the doctrine of double effect; however, giving enough drugs to render a patient unconscious before discontinuing such life-sustaining means is unethical. Moreover, no further distinction between terminal sedation and euthanasia can be made.

Numerous articles have been published on palliative sedation that support its use in relieving pain and other distressing symptoms. According to Dr. Timothy Quill and colleagues, palliative sedation exists within 3 distinct categories: ordinary sedation, which relieves symptoms while altering the patient's state of consciousness; proportionate palliative sedation (PPS), which uses benzodiazepines and analgesics, resulting in both symptom relief and waking/sleeping sedation; and palliative sedation to unconscious (PSU) in which the ultimate intention is sedation. Authors argue that strict guidelines should be put into place to ensure that the intent of sedating the patient, especially as it pertains to PSU, is to minimize and relieve patient suffering, rather than to cause death. The ethics and practice of PSU are further likened to that of withholding artificial hydration and nutrition in that the physician's intent in doing so must be to carry out the patient's wishes. In both cases, the goal is different from that in euthanasia, which is to directly terminate a patient's life.[1]

Susan Bruce and colleagues,[2] palliative care nurses, uphold the position that supportive, palliative care and even sedation given to make the patient comfortable and provide relief from the pathology running its course is ethical and must be used with the purpose and intention of helping the patient to die with dignity. Not only do they hold that this is true under the doctrine of double effect, they also provide evidence that the ethical principles of beneficence, autonomy, and the principle of proportionality can also be applied.[2] Mohamed Rady and Joseph Verheijde[3] presented an article in 2009 further confirming that terminal sedation contradicts the premise behind the doctrine of double effect for 2 reasons. First, it induces a coma to relieve suffering and socially isolate the patient. Second, it is known to shorten one's life, which is an intentional result of this practice.

Although the geographic focus of this article was the Netherlands, a country in which it is legal for physicians to participate in the practice of euthanasia, their conclusion that palliative sedation given to initiate a state of unconsciousness before the removal of life support can be effectively applied to the patient population within the United States. Patients in the intensive care unit should be treated with medications to help relieve their symptoms and remain comfortable, as they are dying to ensure that they are able to die with dignity without implementing means that can be mistaken for euthanasia.

K. Contino, BS
V. Rajput, MD

References

1. Quill TE, Lo B, Brick DW, Meisel A. Last-resort options for palliative sedation. *Ann Intern Med.* 2009;151:421-424.
2. Bruce SD, Hendrix CC, Gentry JH. Palliative sedation in end-of-life care. *J Hosp Palliat Nurs.* 2006;8:320-327.
3. Rady MY, Verheijde JL. Continuous deep sedation until death: palliation or physician-assisted death? *Am J Hosp Palliat Care.* 2010;27:205-214.

Knowing when to stop: futility in the ICU

Wilkinson DJC, Savulescu J (Univ of Oxford, UK)
Curr Opin Anaesthesiol 24:160-165, 2011

Purpose of Review.—Decisions to withdraw or withhold potentially life-sustaining treatment are common in intensive care and precede the majority of deaths. When families resist or oppose doctors' suggestions that it is time to stop treatment, it is often unclear what should be done. This review will summarize recent literature around futility judgements in intensive care emphasising ethical and practical questions.

Recent Findings.—There has been a shift in the language of futility. Patients' families often do not believe medical assessments that further treatment would be unsuccessful. Attempts to determine through data collection which patients have a low or zero chance of survival have been largely unsuccessful, and are hampered by varying definitions of futility. A due-process model for adjudicating futility disputes has been developed, and may provide a better solution to futility disputes than previous futility statutes.

Summary.—Specific criteria for unilateral withdrawal of treatment have proved hard to define or defend. However, it is ethical for doctors to decline to provide treatment that is medically inappropriate or futile. Understanding the justification for a futility judgement may be relevant to deciding the most appropriate way to resolve futility disputes.

▶ The decision to withdraw or withhold intensive care treatment precedes the majority of deaths in emergency departments and intensive care units. When an agreement between doctors and patients' families can be made, the plan to withhold life-sustaining treatment is rather straightforward. On the other hand, there is often opposition from families who disagree on whether life-sustaining treatment should be withheld despite low or zero chance of survival. Such disagreement brings up the concept of "futility," interventions that are unlikely to produce significant benefit for the patient. In this article, the authors discuss the most recent literature and aim to answer ethical questions surrounding the issue of futility.

Recent literature shows the most frequent criticism surrounding the issue of futility is the presence of subjectivity that comes with a doctor's decision that treatment is no longer appropriate. To a physician, a chance of recovery less than 0.5% is small; yet some patients or their families can justify continuing treatment despite the minimal chance for recovery. Many times, surrogates would continue treatment for a family member despite minimal chance for survival. Although this is a small step in the futility debate, the authors suggest that consistent terminology among physicians can help families reach an understanding. The term "medically inappropriate" is preferred to "futile" because it removes some of the objectivity implied by the term "futile" and highlights that these are judgments made by medical professionals.

Another important step suggested by the authors is to be honest with families about why treatment is deemed medically inappropriate. Ultimately only 2 ethical justifications for refusing treatment to a patient can be made, the first being when a physician believes that further treatment would provide more harm to the patient than benefit. The second justification, although more controversial, is that in the setting of limited resources, providing treatment to a patient with a minute chance of survival takes away resources to other patients who could significantly benefit from them.

Thus far, it has not been possible to generate specific criteria for if and when to withdraw or withhold life-sustaining or intensive care treatment. Regardless, it is believed that declining to provide medically inappropriate treatment is ethical. Despite the Hippocratic Oath promising not to treat patients who were "overmastered by their disease," it is still at times difficult to reach an agreement with those who wish to continue intensive care deemed futile by physicians. Continuous dialogue and mutual agreement on goals of care with families and better use of advanced directives and living wills may help in this difficult cliental-ethical dilemma.

C. Mannino, BS
V. Rajput, MD

Informed consent in research to improve the number and quality of deceased donor organs

Rey MM, Ware LB, Matthay MA, et al (Univ of Pennsylvania School of Medicine, Philadelphia; Vanderbilt Univ School of Medicine, Nashville, TN; Univ of California San Francisco; et al)

Crit Care Med 39:280-283, 2011

Improving the management of potential organ donors in the intensive care unit could meet an important public health goal by increasing the number and quality of transplantable organs. However, randomized clinical trials are needed to quantify the extent to which specific interventions might enhance organ recovery and outcomes among transplant recipients. Among several barriers to conducting such studies are the absence of guidelines for obtaining informed consent for such studies and the fact that deceased organ donors are not covered by extant federal regulations governing oversight of research with human subjects. This article explores the underexamined ethical issues that arise in the context of donor management studies and provides ethical guidelines and suggested regulatory oversight mechanisms to enable such studies to be conducted ethically. We conclude that both the respect that is traditionally accorded to the prior wishes of the dead and the possibility of postmortem harm support a role for surrogate consent of donors in such randomized controlled trials. Furthermore, although recipients will often be considered human subjects under federal regulations, several ethical arguments support waiving requirements for recipient consent in donor management randomized controlled trials. Finally, we suggest that new regulatory mechanisms, perhaps linked to existing regional and national organ donation and transplantation infrastructures, must be established to protect patients in donor management studies while limiting unnecessary barriers to the conduct of this important research.

▶ There is a growing need for research into the management of deceased donor organs and its effect on organ viability. Given the need for rigorous studies such as randomized clinical trials (RCT), the authors questioned what consent, and from which parties, would be required by ethical and regulatory guidelines. The authors draw from their own experience in leading a recent placebo-controlled study, the BOLD trial, which tested nebulized albuterol's effect on the deceased donor's lung function. Because the donor subjects in management studies are declared dead by brain-death criteria, they are not considered human subjects by federal regulations, and thus consent is not required. Rey and colleagues assessed the 5 donor management RCTs published to date and whether they obtained consent from a surrogate. Only 3 of the 5 RCTs published described a surrogate consent process. To ensure that donor management studies are in concordance with biomedical ethics, the authors begin an important discussion.

The authors argue that because our society grants the deceased some form of autonomy and protection of harm (such as of reputation or privacy), informed consent through surrogates, or less often though a living will, is required. However, the authors grapple more with the question of whether recipients in donor management trials must consent to these trials. Whether recipients in such trials would be considered human subjects is a vexing issue. Before transplant, do intended recipients have to be consented for research therapies intended to extend and improve viability? The authors argue because it is unknowable when an organ will become available, and because there would be limited time to obtain consent, the emergency waiver may apply. Rey et al also describe donor management research as "minimal risk" and therefore feel confident that this waiver could be used as well. Their most compelling argument for waiving recipient consent is that any requirement for consent would coerce recipients to acquiesce or else refuse life-saving treatment. However, it is questionable to what ease such waivers may be obtained. To reduce obstacles for these important trials, Rey and others implore the organ transplant society to continue this discussion and formalize ethical guidelines into regulations, so that researchers and institutions may move swiftly on important research.

Indeed, the area of donor management research is not a theoretical discussion but an area of work that can save lives. In one highly cited randomized controlled trial, hormonal resuscitation of the donor leads to a 22.5% increase in the number of viable organs.[1] In another influential RCT, the effect of steroids on a donor lung was found to statistically and significantly increase the yield of viable organs.[2] Although these studies exemplify the benefit of waiving consent from recipients, negative studies or studies showing harm from intervention will show the ethical tension between discovery and protection of research subjects.

Although a growing area of research, donor management studies play an important role in teaching us how to increase the supply of viable organs. With ethical guidelines, the transplant community can continue to show respect to the invaluable gift that these donors have given and uphold the trust of their families and society.

W. Rafelson, MBA
V. Rajput, MD

References

1. Rosendale JD, Kauffman HM, McBride MA, et al. Aggressive pharmacologic donor management results in more transplanted organs. *Transplantation*. 2003; 75:482-487.
2. Venkateswaran RV, Patchell VB, Wilson IC, et al. Early donor management increases the retrieval rate of lungs for transplantation. *Ann Thorac Surg*. 2008; 85:278-286.

Patient and healthcare professional factors influencing end-of-life decision-making during critical illness: A systematic review

Frost DW, Cook DJ, Heyland DK, et al (Univ of Toronto, Ontario, Canada; McMaster Univ, Hamilton, Ontario, Canada; Queens Univ, Kingston, Ontario, Canada; et al)

Crit Care Med 39:1174-1189, 2011

Objectives.—The need for better understanding of end-of-life care has never been greater. Debate about recent U.S. healthcare system reforms has highlighted that end-of-life decision-making is contentious. Providing compassionate end-of-life care that is appropriate and in accordance with patient wishes is an essential component of critical care. Because discord can undermine optimal end-of-life care, knowledge of factors that influence decision-making is important. We performed a systematic review to determine which factors are known to influence end-of-life decision-making among patients and healthcare providers.

Data Sources, Selection, and Abstraction.—We conducted a structured search of Ovid Medline for interventional and observational research articles incorporating critical care and end-of life decision-making terms.

Data Synthesis.—Of 6259 publications, 102 were relevant to our review question. Patient factors predicting less intensive end-of life care include increasing age, comorbidity, and limited functional status; these factors appear to be influential for both clinicians and patients. Patient and clinician race, ethnicity, and nationality also appear to influence the technological intensity of end-of-life care. In general, white patients and those in North America and Northern Europe may be less likely to desire intensive end-of-life care than others. Physicians of similar geo-ethnic origin to patients appear less likely to prescribe such therapy. Physicians with more clinical experience and those routinely working in the intensive care unit are less likely than other physicians to recommend technologically intense care for critically ill patients at the end-of-life.

Conclusions.—Patients and clinicians may approach end-of-life discussions with different expectations and preferences, influenced by religion, race, culture, and geography. Appreciation of those factors associated with more and less technologically intense care may raise awareness, aid communication, and guide clinicians in end-of-life discussions.

▶ Providing appropriate, compassionate, and culturally competent end-of-life care is essential in our ever-changing health care system. Numerous studies and surveys have been done over the years to look at various influences on end-of-life decision making, including regional culture, family influence, and numerous patient and physician demographics. As life expectancy increases and technology improves, older literature and previous practices may be less valuable in helping to establish meaningful decision algorithms for the care of critically ill patients. However, review the literature can be used to get a better understanding of which factors are consistently influential in end-of-life care.

This work was a systematic review of observational and interventional research articles (between 1950 and 2010) relating to critical care, end-of-life decision making. The authors were specifically interested in patient and health care professional factors influencing decision making. Although more than 6000 citations were initially retrieved, only 102 articles had appropriate data for review in this study. Because of considerable differences in study design, meta-analysis could not be used. Instead, findings were summarized as narrative systematic review with qualitative descriptions. Age, comorbidity, functional status, severity of present illness, and patient gender, race, and ethnicity all emerged as consistent influences. Yet depending on the type of study, different conclusions might be reached. For example, in several cohort studies, patient age was shown to be an independent predictor of intensity of care, but in studies using scenario-type surveys, physicians considered severity of illness and medical history more important than age. Of particular note, female gender was identified in cohort studies as being independently associated with do not resuscitate (DNR) orders and less likelihood of receiving cardiopulmonary resuscitation even in the case of absent DNR orders. The question then arises, are physicians more comfortable addressing end-of-life care with female patients, or are they subconsciously treating this population under a different, perhaps lower, standard of care? Similarly, review of retrospective studies showed differences in DNR orders in white and nonwhite patients, with nonwhite patients less likely to have a DNR order. Again, we must consider whether there are barriers such as health literacy, cultural competency, or distrust that play into these differences.

Although this review included articles with the objective of looking at health care provider influences, the authors acknowledge the paucity of studies, although they were able to summarize some observations. Cohort studies showed (1) forgoing intense therapy was associated more with increased seniority and experience and (2) physicians in North America and northern European countries are more likely to carry out DNR orders than those in the Middle East or southern Europe. Survey studies regarding physicians' desire for their own personal care showed black physicians more likely to want life-supportive measures and women in general were less likely than men to accept less intense treatment.

This review is an interesting one, primarily because it reveals a number of factors that seem to have persisted over the years in influencing end-of-life care. The downside is that there is no real consistency in how these factors are assessed. As the demographics in the United States continue to change, it is crucial to take pause and consider the cultural and socioeconomic influences that may play a role in the decision making of a critically ill patient. Not only do clinicians need to consider the patient's cultural and religious beliefs, they also need to be objective enough to see how their own beliefs weigh in on the decision-making process. As shown in another recent study, religious faith and ethnicity is influential in physician use of continuous deep sedation and support of assisted dying.[1] This current review certainly provides its readers with a broad overview of the many factors that contribute to the increasingly complex process of end-of-life care. More effort needs to be made to achieve high-quality, compassionate care. With so many influential and often conflicting influences affecting care management, perhaps we need to focus more on patient-directed care and increase our efforts of encouraging completion of advanced directives before the point of critical need.

J. Mitchell-Williams, MD, PhD
V. Rajput, MD

Reference

1. Seale C. The role of doctors' religious faith and ethnicity in taking ethically controversial decisions during end-of-life care. *J Med Ethics*. 2010;36:677-682.

The Impact of Country and Culture on End-of-Life Care for Injured Patients: Results From an International Survey

Ball CG, Navsaria P, Kirkpatrick AW, et al (Emory Univ, Atlanta, GA; Univ of Cape Town, South Africa; Univ of Calgary, Calgary, Canada; et al)
J Trauma 69:1323-1334, 2010

Background.—Up to 20% of all trauma patients admitted to an intensive care unit die from their injuries. End-of-life decision making is a variable process that involves prognosis, predicted functional outcomes, personal beliefs, institutional resources, societal norms, and clinician experience. The goal of this study was to better understand end-of-life processes after major injury by comparing clinician viewpoints from various countries and cultures.

Methods.—A clinician-based, 38-question international survey was used to characterize the impacts of medical, religious, social, and system factors on end-of-life care after trauma.

Results.—A total of 419 clinicians from the United States (49%), Canada (19%), South Africa (11%), Europe (9%), Asia (8%), and Australasia (4%) completed the survey. In America, the admitting surgeon guided most end-of-life decisions (51%), when compared with all other countries (0–27%). The practice structure of American respondents also varied from other regions. Formal medical futility laws are rarely available (14–38%). Ethical consultation services are often accessible (29–98%), but rarely used (0–29%), and typically unhelpful (<30%). End-of-life decision making for patients with traumatic brain injuries varied extensively across regions with regard to the impact of patient age, Glasgow Coma Scale score, and clinician philosophy. Similar differences were observed for spinal cord injuries (age and functional level). The availability and use of "donation after cardiac death" also varied substantially between countries.

Conclusions.—In this unique study, geographic differences in religion, practice composition, decision-maker viewpoint, and institutional resources resulted in significant variation in end-of-life care after injury. These disparities reflect competing concepts (patient autonomy, distributive justice, and religion).

▶ The end-of-life decision-making process is extremely complex, especially in patients suffering from traumatic injuries. There are many factors to take into account, including expected level of recovery and function, availability of essential support services and care providers, and personal beliefs. An important area of consideration is whether the physician's own personal beliefs effect decision making. Individual nations or geographic regions may have adopted certain standards for such end-of-life decisions. With many countries undergoing significant demographic changes, it is important to understand practices from a wide variety of areas. Identifying common practices, understanding cultural beliefs, and evaluating differences may be helpful in the establishment of best practices.

The investigators of this study used an online questionnaire to survey clinicians from several geographic regions about their end-of-life practices. The 38-question survey targeted trauma surgeons and critical care intensivists. The clinicians were queried about their years of experience, percentage of time spent in the intensive care unit (ICU), and their religious declaration. Additionally, they were asked to provide information about their institutions end-of-life procedures and ethics consultation services. Of particular interest in this study was the comparison of practices across regions of patients with traumatic brain injury (TBI) versus spinal cord injury (SCI) and the level of organ donation.

Data were collected from six geographic regions with the largest number of respondents from the United States. US clinicians were more likely to serve as both trauma surgeon and intensivist than others in the study. The highest represented religious declaration was Christian, followed by agnostic/atheist; however, religion was not found to be a relevant factor in end-of-life decision making. These decisions were generally made by the attending critical care physician. Many sites lacked ethics consultation services, but many with access to these services did not find them helpful. For both TBI and SCI, patient age did seem to play a role in decision making. For TBI, most clinicians indicated that the Glasgow Coma Score (GCS) did not influence their decisions, yet when asked in a cased-based manner, with GCS less than 3, the data suggested otherwise for some regions, especially Asia (97%). American respondents were much less likely to withdraw care with low GCS and TBI. Losing diaphragmatic function, however, had an influential effect across all regions.

The variability of organ donation after cardiac death across regions was particularly interesting. Participants who did not have donation options available indicated that they would use it if it became available. In the areas in which it was available, it was not used by a significant number of survey respondents. One would question whether physician discomfort in having the discussion of donation is in part responsible for the underutilization of organ harvesting. End-of-life discussion are never easy and are even more complex in the case of traumatic injuries. Family members may already be struggling to accept the seriousness of their loved one's injury. Discussion of organ donation may cause further family distress, anger, and even distrust because of lack education or misunderstanding. The caregiver may not be willing to broach the subject because of increased time commitment, inexperience with these types of discussions, or fear of litigation.

Having a more uniform algorithm for decisions during end-of-life care in trauma patients would have many benefits. It would help guide less experienced physicians, and by using a "standard" of care approach, it could improve the level of trust with family members. It seems illogical that the use of ethics consultation services were not found to be useful. Perhaps further evaluation of the structure and content of those services should be done because they should be able to ensure legality of decision making and cultural competency of care.

J. Mitchell-Williams, MD, PhD
V. Rajput, MD

Ethics and end-of-life care for adults in the intensive care unit

Curtis JR, Vincent J-L (Univ of Washington, Seattle, WA; Université Libre de Bruxelles, Brussels, Belgium)
Lancet 375:1347-1353, 2010

The intensive care unit (ICU) is where patients are given some of the most technologically advanced life-sustaining treatments, and where difficult decisions are made about the usefulness of such treatments. The substantial regional variability in these ethical decisions is a result of many factors, including religious and cultural beliefs. Because most critically ill patients lack the capacity to make decisions, family and other individuals often act as the surrogate decision makers, and in many regions communication between the clinician and family is central to decision making in the ICU. Elsewhere, involvement of the family is reduced and that of the physicians is increased. End-of-life care is associated with increased burnout and distress among clinicians working in the ICU. Since many deaths in the ICU are preceded by a decision to withhold or withdraw life support, high-quality decision making and end-of-life care are essential in all regions, and can improve patient and family outcomes, and also retention of clinicians working in the ICU. To make such a decision requires adequate training, good communication between the clinician and family, and the collaboration of a well functioning interdisciplinary team.

▶ How can we identify and categorize all the major ethical issues that arise in the intensive care unit (ICU)? Curtis and Vincent[1] take on this daunting task in their article in a journal with a generalist audience. They begin by searching major literature databases in the past 15 years for relevant articles. An important initial finding, they note, is the variability in end-of-life care that varies not only by country but also by region, hospital, and physician. The authors created 4 broad categories for ethics and end-of-life issues in the ICU: explicit policies, interdisciplinary communication, communication with families, and withholding or withdrawing life support. Their goal was to identify global similarities and differences in practice; what techniques work better than others; and, ultimately, what changes need to be made to improve the outcomes in end-of-life care in ICUs around the world.

The ethical principles should always apply, regardless of the location and resources available to an ICU. A summary of these principles, as outlined by the American Thoracic Society, is as follows:

- The equal value of every individual's life
- The respect for a patient's autonomy, demonstrated by informed consent
- The provision of resources that meet an individual's medical needs and enhance their welfare
- ICU care is a basic component to health care services that should be available to all patients
- The only limitation to providing health care to a patient is when doing so unfairly compromises the resources needed by other patients[2]

Unfortunately, the Curtis review noted that most intensivists did not use these criteria on a regular basis. Given that the criteria are highly generalized, many intensivists felt that applying them to an individual patient's case was often difficult.[3] The authors point the reader to important work by researchers in ICU ethics. A 2003 randomized controlled trial by Schneiderman et al[4] found that ethics consultations in ICUs reduced ICU and hospital days and days of life-sustaining treatments, without increasing mortality. This replicated similar findings in a 2000 study by Schneiderman et al[5]; in both studies, participants reported a high rate of satisfaction with the ethics consultation process.

A number of studies reviewed in this article concluded that early discussion about end-of-life care, advance directives, and other concerns resulted in decreased admissions to the ICU, better family evaluations of end-of-life care, less aggressive care, and decreased health care costs overall. Most critical care societies agree that medical decision making should be shared among the doctor, the patient, and, if possible, the patient's family.[6] This review distills the shared decision-making process down to 3 steps: (1) the physician's control of the decision-making process should increase as the prognosis worsens and the certainty of the prognosis increases, (2) the physician must assess the preferred decision-making role of the family, and (3) the final approach should be adapted to match the patient's and family's needs identified in the first 2 steps.[7]

Curtis and Vincent indicate that these meetings should be conducted in 3 stages. First, a private and quiet location should be identified and reserved ahead of time. The clinicians involved in the patient's care should ideally reach a consensus before this time, so that the information provided is consistent. Second, the physician should use active listening and provide adequate time for the family to voice all concerns. Third, at the end of the meeting, the physician should summarize the information given and the decisions made.[1]

The Curtis review indicates that for this kind of family meeting to be successful, it is helpful to have a number of other professionals involved. The presence of a professional medical interpreter or specific religious or community leaders often leads to significant improvements in patient and family satisfaction with end-of-life care.[8]

A collaborative approach with nurses and other health professionals has been shown to benefit all parties in end-of-life communication. This approach was also shown to prevent physician conflict, decrease job stress, and improve quality of care for patients overall.[9] Despite this finding, the Curtis and Vincent study indicates that interdisciplinary collaboration concerning end-of-life care in the ICU varies greatly across countries. Collaboration was most common in northern and central Europe, followed by Japan, Brazil, southern Europe, and the United States.[10]

Curtis and Vincent noted similar international variation in the practice of withdrawing and withholding life support in ICUs. The physician's religion, often reflected by the dominant religion in a given country, appeared to be a key factor in this decision. The Ethicus study demonstrated that physicians who are Jewish, Greek orthodox, or Muslim are significantly more likely to withhold life support, whereas Catholic, Protestant, or nonreligious physicians are more likely to withdraw.[11] The Curtis review concluded that the successful withdrawing or withholding of treatment required the same high level of training and best-practice guidelines as any other procedure in the ICU. The review also indicates the importance of having a discussion with the patient's family that addresses the predicted time course, a regular assessment of the patient's comfort, and a treatment plan for any presenting symptoms. The details and rationale for treatment withdrawal should also be carefully documented in the medical record.[12]

The Curtis and Vincent review of end-of-life care in the ICU demonstrates significant international differences in practice among critical care physicians. These differences are in part because of variable religious and cultural beliefs about end-of-life care and also because of the significant lack of ICU resources in some countries. Lack of resources includes minimal access to the literature that has proven certain practices are universally applicable. This article demonstrates the need for an open and continuous global forum to determine a consensus about end-of-life care. As global medicine becomes more and more of a reality, it is increasingly important for physicians to be aware of all the cultural differences that exist. This study aptly concludes that high-quality end-of-life care should always emphasize ethical decision making, constant communication between physicians, patients, and families, collaboration of the entire interdisciplinary team, and a constant re-evaluation of best practices, based on both the individual needs of each patient and family and on the evolving global consensus.

W. Rafelson, MBA
V. Rajput, MD

References

1. Curtis JR, Vincent JL. Ethics and end-of-life care for adults in the intensive care unit. *Lancet.* 2010;376:1347-1353.
2. Fair allocation of intensive care unit resources. American Thoracic Society. *Am J Respir Crit Care Med.* 1997;156:1282-1301.
3. Wunsch H, Angus DC, Harrison DA, et al. Variation in critical care services across North America and Western Europe. *Crit Care Med.* 2008;36:2787-2793.
4. Schneiderman LJ, Gilmer T, Teetzel HD, et al. Effect of ethics consultations on nonbeneficial life-sustaining treatments in the intensive care setting: a randomized controlled trial. *JAMA.* 2003;290:1166-1172.
5. Schneiderman LJ, Gilmer T, Teetzel HD. Impact of ethics consultations in the intensive care setting: a randomized, controlled trial. *Crit Care Med.* 2000;28: 3920-3924.
6. Troug RD, Campbell ML, Curtis JR, et al. Recommendations for end-of-life care in the intensive care unit: a consensus statement by the American College [corrected] of Critical Care Medicine. *Crit Care Med.* 2008;36:953-963.
7. Curtis JR, White DB. Practical guidance for evidence-based ICU family conferences. *Chest.* 2008;134:835-843.
8. Gries CJ, Curtis JR, Wall RJ, Engelberg RA. Family member satisfaction with end-of-life decision making in the ICU. *Chest.* 2008;133:704-712.
9. Studdert DM, Mello MM, Burns JP, et al. Conflict in the care of patients with prolonged stay in the ICU: types, sources, and predictors. *Intensive Care Med.* 2003;29:1489-1497.
10. Yaguchi A, Truog RD, Curtis JR, et al. International differences in end-of-life attitudes in the intensive care unit: results of a survey. *Arch Intern Med.* 2005; 165:1970-1975.
11. Sprung CL, Maia P, Bulow HH, et al. The importance of religious affiliation and culture on end-of-life decisions in European intensive care units. *Intensive Care Med.* 2007;33:1732-1739.
12. Kompanje EJ, van der Hoven B, Bakker J. Anticipation of distress after discontinuation of mechanical ventilation in the ICU at the end of life. *Intensive Care Med.* 2008;34:1593-1599.

End-of-life attitudes of intensive care physicians in Poland: results of a national survey

Kübler A, Adamik B, Lipinska-Gediga M, et al (Wroclaw Med Univ, Poland)

Intensive Care Med 37:1290-1296, 2011

Purpose.—This study was designed to assess the ethical attitudes and practices of intensive care physicians regarding life-sustaining treatment in intensive care units (ICUs) in Poland.

Methods.—A questionnaire was distributed to intensive care physicians taking part in a national medical congress. Participation in the study was voluntary and anonymous.

Results.—A total of 400 questionnaires were distributed, of which 217 (54%) were returned completed. Almost all respondents (93%) reported having withheld therapy, and 75% of respondents reported withdrawing therapy. Physicians aged 40 years and over who had no religious affiliation more frequently reported withholding treatment. Only 5% of physicians reported deliberately administering drugs until death ensued. Respondents from large hospitals (more than 400 beds) more easily accepted foregoing life-sustaining therapy in ICU patients. In clinical scenario in which the family demanded the maximum available treatment, physicians reported that they were considerably influenced to modify decisions concerning life-sustaining therapy.

Conclusions.—The ethical attitudes of intensive care physicians regarding end-of-life decisions are similar to the opinion presented in other European survey studies. The practice of withholding and withdrawing therapy in ICU patients is common in Poland. Actively shortening life is considered unacceptable. The request of the family even without legal consultation can influence physicians' decisions.

▶ Kubler et al surveyed Polish intensive care physicians on their attitudes and practices regarding end-of-life care. A questionnaire was adapted from a similar study looking at ethical issues in intensive care units (ICUs) throughout Europe. Kubler group concluded that Polish intensive care physicians think and behave similarly to their counterparts in other European countries. To that end, they demonstrated that withholding and withdrawing therapy is a common practice among the intensivists in Poland. Unlike the European study, the deliberate administration of drugs to accelerate death was shown to be rare. The survey data also demonstrated that withholding treatment was more common among physicians who were older, without religious affiliation, and who were working in a large hospital. In addition, this study found that the majority of intensivists reported that their decisions about end-of-life care were influenced by the wishes of the patient's family. These conclusions have been echoed in a number of similar questionnaire-based studies throughout Europe and Asia[1].

A comparable study with many of the same endpoints was recently completed in Brazil. Gaudencia et al[2] found that the majority of intensive care physicians admitted to withdrawing and/or withholding life-staining treatment to critically ill patients. Treatment withdrawal was shown to be more common among physicians with a religious affiliation. Catholic physicians were isolated as the group least likely to withdraw therapy. The Kubler group also noted that Catholic physicians in Poland were significantly less likely to withdraw or withhold life-sustaining treatment. The comparison is somewhat limited because Catholic physicians represented the majority of study participants in both studies. The Gaudencia study concluded that the majority of physicians were against active administration of medications that would accelerate death. Interestingly, the percentage of physicians in favor of euthanasia in the Brazilian study was 32.9%, whereas only 1.5% of Polish intensivists surveyed favored deliberate shortening of life with sedatives or analgesics. Both studies demonstrated that the majority of ICU physicians modify their decisions based on decisions made by the patient's family.

The Solarino group[3] used a similar questionnaire to survey physicians in Italy who were treating patients in a persistent vegetative state (PVS). Unlike the Kubler study, this questionnaire focused on Italian physicians' opinions in the context of a single, real-life scenario involving a woman in a PVS. The case was widely covered in the national media and brought to light numerous comparisons to the Terry Schiavo and Nancy Cruzan cases in the United States. The Solarino study not only affirmed the conclusions of the Kubler and Gaudencia studies but did so on a much larger scale; 22 219 Italian physicians submitted questionnaires. This study population was somewhat different from the Kubler and Gaudencia studies in that the physicians surveyed were from all medical specialties. That being said, more than 60% of these physicians indicated that withdrawal of assisted nutrition and hydration, which were considered life-sustaining therapies, is an appropriate measure as long as it is in accordance with the patient's wishes. This study also demonstrated that a significant number (42%) of Italian physicians are in favor of euthanasia in the setting of PVS. This result is surprising because the Italian constitution effectively deems withdrawal, withholding, and euthanasia by a physician to be illegal. The Solarino group points out that this law has been recently challenged by the Italian Supreme Court ruling that granted the father of a patient in a PVS the right to terminate life-sustaining therapy for his daughter.

Looking at these studies as a group, it becomes clear that the attitude and behavior of intensive care physicians toward end-of-life care is largely similar around the world. From these studies, it appears that most physicians agree that withholding or withdrawing life-sustaining treatment is an acceptable practice in certain critical scenarios. It is the details of these scenarios, however, that remain unclear for most physicians. Furthermore, there appears to be a disagreement among physicians on the use of medication to deliberately accelerate death. One underlying theme in all of these studies is a concern for the lack of formal guidelines regarding end-of-life decision making and best practices. Each study calls for more large-scale research on this topic in addition to a push for national medical societies to produce consensus guidelines. The hope is that these research-based guidelines would offer a defined set of recommendations that physicians could readily reference. In the past 5 years, there has been some effort by national medical societies to produce this kind of end-of-life decision-making guideline. This is the case in Italy and in the United States.[4,5] As noted in the Kubler and Gaudencia articles, countries like

Brazil and Poland lag behind in this arena. It is important to note that the mere presence of a medical society guideline does require recognition by the country's legal system.

L. Irwin, BS
V. Rajput, MD

References

1. Kübler A, Adamik B, Lipinska-Gediga M, Kedziora J, Strozecki L. End-of-life attitudes of intensive care physicians of Poland: results of a national survey. *Intensive Care Medicine.* 2011;37:1290-1296.
2. Gaudencio D, Messeder O. Dilemmas of the end of life: information about medical practice in the ICUs. *Cien Saude Colet.* 2011;16:813-820.
3. Solarino B, Bruno F, Frati G, Dell'Erba A, Frati P. A national survey of Italian physicians' attitudes towards end-of-life decisions following the death Eluana Englaro. *Intensive Care Med.* 2011;37:542-549.
4. McHugh JT. Principles in regard to withholding or withdrawing artificially assisted nutrition/hydration. *Issues Law Med.* 1990;6:89-93.
5. Parere ufficiale della Societa' Italiana di Anestesia Analgesia, Rianimazione e Terapia Intensiva (SIAARTI) in materia di fine vita, stati vegetativi, nutrizione a idratazione. Memoria per la commissione Igiene e sanità della camera dei deputati relativa alla audizione di mercoled ì 7 ottobre 2009.

Early identification of the potential organ donor: fundamental role of intensive care or conflict of interest?

Bell MDD (The General Infirmary at Leeds, UK)
Intensive Care Med 36:1451-1453, 2010

Background.—Organ donations from persons considered brain dead has been accepted based on objectivity in the testing procedure and the acknowledgement that the patient will not respond to further treatment. Brain and/or brainstem death has been nearly universally accepted as a platform for such donations. However, the demand for transplanted organs has far exceeded the supply, placing pressure on critical care practitioners to convert potential donors into actual donors. Among the solutions to the problem are "marginal donors," "elective ventilation," and non-heart-beating organ donation (NHBD). The ethical and legal defensibility of these options remains in question, and some recruitment strategies reveal conflict of interest issues. With this all in mind, de Groot and colleagues from multiple disciplines, primarily based on the Netherlands, propose the concept of "imminent brain death."

The Proposition.—The intention is to increase the conversion rate from potential to actual donor, which responds to criticisms by transplantation services that intensivists do not do enough to maximize donor numbers. The proposed mechanism is an objective assessment to identify early in the process those patients who may qualify as beating-heart donors. Intensivists should see this as a way to minimize protracted futile care and, because it is objective, avoid concerns that decisions are made for utilitarian purposes. Therefore the proposal would seemingly benefit all parties.

Analysis.—Questions arise concerning the objectivity and applicability of the proposal. The Glasgow Coma Scale (GCS) is rarely used when the patient first arrives to determine if active intervention is advisable because of the heterogeneity of brain injury. The focus is on avoiding secondary cerebral injury, so analgesia, sedation, and muscle paralysis are often begun to maximize gas exchange and stabilize the patient's condition while monitoring it to determine the extent of the primary injury. Therapy is escalated to address deranged functions rather than focusing on rationalizing whether active care should be continued or not. It is also difficult to determine how to validate clinical tests of brainstem function, since any cessation of therapy to conduct an evaluation may hasten the progression to brainstem death. If assessments are made after interventions are discontinued, the patient will have survived long enough to make brain or brainstem death less likely. So the mechanism of brain injury, the timing, and the appropriate point in therapy where clinical assessment can give a valid prognosis remain undetermined. Few patients clearly progress toward brain and/or brainstem death by incontrovertible signs. Most challenge the intensivist to determine whether to continue with active support, stop life-sustaining measures and allow the patient to die and become a NHBD, or stop sedation but continue support and do a clinical assessment after sedation has cleared. With a shift away from using the brainstem death criterion, the challenge is to identify futility as the indicator of when to withdraw active support. Patients vary widely in their response to treatment. Neither objectivity nor consistency has been achieved when considering other criteria for futility in brain-injured patients.

Conclusions.—The primary goal of intensive care is to actively treat potentially reversible disease or injury until the patient is no longer responsive to these efforts. It is not to provide organ donors. Donation must be divorced from treatment by using an objective measure to determine futility and ensure there is no conflict of interest.

► In this editorial, Bell surveys the work of de Groot and colleagues in their attempt to develop comprehensive criteria for imminent brain death in potential organ donors in the intensive care unit (ICU) and asks the reader to consider its ethical implications. Bell asks the reader to differentiate between "imminent" brain death and "inevitable" brain death; certainly some proportion of patients with seemingly irreversible brain injury may recover reasonably with aggressive neurosurgery. The authors raise an ethical question: how much risk of misclassification can the intensivist community accept in the early identification of organ donors? Does this entail a conflict of interest?

de Groot, however, is not the first to try to create criteria for early identification of potential organ donors; he builds upon work by the Organ Procurement and Transplantation Network (OPTN) on "imminent neurological death." de Groot tries to improve upon these criteria by adding Glasgow Coma Scale (GCS) to the criteria for imminent brain death: "A mechanically ventilated, deeply comatose patient, admitted to an ICU, with irreversible catastrophic brain damage of known origin (e.g. TBI, SAH, ICH). A condition of imminent brain death requires either a GCS of 3 and the progressive absence of at least three out of six brainstem reflexes, or a FOUR score of EMBR."[1] Adding the GCS to the traditional criteria is fraught with complications, according to Bell.

Other studies have attempted to objectively identify "imminent brain death." In the anesthesiology literature, heart rate variability (HRV) may precede irreversible and catastrophic neurologic injury.[2] Another study in the pediatric critical care literature suggests retrograde flow as shown by transcranial Doppler may herald imminent brain death.[3] These and replicated studies may serve as important adjuncts to the prediction of early brain death.

Bell criticizes this definition's reliance on the GCS, arguing that the intensivist community generally does not use it to decide whether to provide intensive care. Bell argues that many patients in the ICU—by virtue of the therapy they receive—have deranged GCS scores that are unreliable for decision making. The author seems to prefer more objective criteria—such as computed tomography perfusion, angiography, and perhaps Doppler—than the subjective criteria that make up the basis of "imminent brain death." Relying on subjective criteria, Bell argues, creates a potential conflict of interest whereby ICUs serve to identify and prepare organ donors rather than to treat reversible injury and disease. Indeed, relying solely on such "soft" criteria for the irreversibly and traumatically injured patient may undermine the public's perception of medical ethical care in the ICU.

"Primum, non nocere," our medical ethics tell us, which has been translated into the principle of nonmalficence. It is possible that an aggressive approach such as identifying "imminent brain death" may violate some of the tenets of ethical care for our patients. The article by Bell reminds us that our efforts to modify the criteria for brain death should not be motivated by organ procurement but rather by the fiduciary responsibility to the patient.

W. Rafelson, MBA
V. Rajput, MD

References

1. de Groot YJ, Jansen NE, Bakker J, et al. Imminent brain death: point of departure for potential heart-beating organ donor recognition. *Intensive Care Med.* 2010;36: 1488-1494.
2. Rapenne T, Moreau D, Lenfant F, Boggio V, Cottin Y, Freysz M. Could heart rate variability analysis become an early predictor of imminent brain death? A pilot study. *Anesth Analg.* 2000;91:329-336.
3. Bode H, Eden A. Transcranial Doppler sonography in children. *J Child Neurol.* 1989;4:S68-S76.

12 Pharmacology/ Sedation-Analgesia

Recombinant Factor XIII Mitigates Hemorrhagic Shock-Induced Organ Dysfunction

Zaets SB, Xu D-Z, Lu Q, et al (Novo Nordisk, Inc., Princeton, NJ; Univ of Medicine and Dentistry of New Jersey – New Jersey Med School, Newark)

J Surg Res 166:e135-e142, 2011

Background.—Plasma factor XIII (FXIII) is responsible for stabilization of fibrin clot at the final stage of blood coagulation. Since FXIII has also been shown to modulate inflammation, endothelial permeability, as well as diminish multiple organ dysfunction (MOD) after gut ischemia-reperfusion injury, we hypothesized that FXIII would reduce MOD caused by trauma-hemorrhagic shock (THS).

Materials and Methods.—Rats were subjected to a 90 min THS or trauma sham shock (TSS) and treated with either recombinant human FXIII A_2 subunit (rFXIII) or placebo immediately after resuscitation with shed blood or at the end of the TSS period. Lung permeability, lung and gut myeloperoxidase (MPO) activity, gut histology, neutrophil respiratory burst, microvascular blood flow in the liver and muscles, and cytokine levels were measured 3 h after the THS or TSS. FXIII levels were measured before THS or TSS and after the 3-h post-shock period.

Results.—THS-induced lung permeability as well as lung and gut MPO activity was significantly lower in rFXIII-treated than in placebo-treated animals. Similarly, rFXIII-treated rats had lower neutrophil respiratory burst activity and less ileal mucosal injury. rFXIII-treated rats also had a higher liver microvascular blood flow compared with the placebo group. Cytokine response was more favorable in rFXIII-treated animals. Trauma-hemorrhagic shock did not cause a drop in FXIII activity during the study period.

Conclusions.—Administration of rFXIII diminishes THS-induced MOD in rats, presumably by preservation of the gut barrier function, limitation of polymorphonuclear leukocyte (PMN) activation, and modulation of the cytokine response.

▶ This is elegant preclinical work by 1 of 2 laboratories investigating the role of intestinal lymph as a trigger for multiorgan dysfunction.[1,2] A variety of assays are performed suggesting that recombinant factor XIII (rFXIII), in supraphysiologic doses, may increase endothelial stability, reduce cellular injury, and moderate proinflammatory cytokine production.

The model used is widely reported. A laparotomy incision and simultaneous withdrawal of blood to target blood pressure are performed in study animals. Clearly, this model does not replicate severe injury, but it does combine surgical trauma and hemorrhage.

With dosing based on previous experience with rFXIII, the authors demonstrate intermediate improvement in the physiologic and inflammatory parameters studied. In particular, improved ileal histology is seen with rFXIII administration. I would also be interested in pulmonary histology because the lung is examined using myeloperoxidase and Evans-blue dye permeability techniques.

In all, this is an early preclinical study suggesting further investigation of another plasma factor as a means to modify organ dysfunction after injury.

D. J. Dries, MSE, MD

References

1. Deitch EA, Forsythe R, Anjaria D, et al. The role of lymph factors in lung injury, bone marrow suppression and endothelial cell dysfunction in a primate model of trauma-hemorrhagic shock. *Shock*. 2004;22:221-228.
2. Zallen G, Moore EE, Johnson JL, et al. Posthemorrhagic shock mesenteric lymph primes circulating neutrophils and provokes lung injury. *J Surg Res*. 1999;83: 83-88.

Inflammatory Response in Multiple Organs in a Mouse Model of Acute Alcohol Intoxication and Burn Injury

Li X, Akhtar S, Kovacs EJ, et al (Loyola Univ Chicago Med Ctr, Maywood, IL)
J Burn Care Res 32:489-497, 2011

This study characterized the inflammatory response after burn injury and determined whether ethanol (EtOH) intoxication at the time of burn injury influences this response. To accomplish this, male mice were gavaged with EtOH (2.9 g/kg) 4 hours before 12 to 15% TBSA sham or burn injury. Mice were killed on day 1 after injury; blood, small intestine, lung, and liver were collected to measure interleukin (IL)-6, IL-10, IL-18, and Monocyte chemotactic protein-1 (MCP-1) levels. In addition, neutrophil infiltration, myeloperoxidase activity, and edema formation were also measured in the small intestine, lung, and liver. There was no difference in the inflammatory markers in the small intestine, lung, and liver in mice receiving either sham or burn injury alone except IL-6 that was increased in all four tissue compartments after burn injury alone. However, when compared with EtOH or burn injury alone, EtOH combined with burn injury resulted in a significant increase in cytokines, neutrophil infiltration, myeloperoxidase activity, and edema in the small intestine, liver, and lung tissue. Furthermore, a significant increase in IL-6 and MCP-1 was observed in circulation after EtOH intoxication and burn injury compared with either EtOH intoxication or burn injury alone; no other cytokines were detected in circulation. These findings suggest that acute EtOH intoxication exacerbates the inflammatory response after burn injury.

▶ The authors present a murine model involving acute alcohol intoxication followed by burn injury 4 hours later. They investigate short-term inflammatory effects in circulation, small intestine, lung, and liver. The pathway from uncontrolled cytokine levels of interleukin (IL)-6 and IL-18 to neutrophil recruitment to the site of infection and excess neutrophil accumulation in the tissues must certainly be a straight line through multiple organ dysfunction and death in the burn-injured patient.

Although this is a not a human study, the relevance is clear, and exciting. For the first time, alcohol ingestion followed 4 hours later by a small burn injury (12%-15% total body surface area) was directly associated with edema formation. Because edema is one of the biggest challenges in managing burn patients, from airway problems, prolonged ventilator management, impaired gastrointestinal tract functioning, possible compartment syndromes, and worsening of the burn injury, this is a rousing finding. I hope the authors will continue this work in human subjects (although prospective, randomized studies will not be possible, for obvious reasons). Once we know that the pathway is fairly linear in humans, we can investigate ways to dampen increased neutrophil infiltration in the organs studied here (and most probably others as well). Burn-care practitioners should keep these findings in mind as they care for their patients, even with smaller burn injuries.

B. A. Latenser, MD, FACS

Enoxaparin and Antifactor Xa Levels in Acute Burn Patients

Lin H, Faraklas I, Cochran A, et al (Univ of Utah Health Ctr, Salt Lake City)

J Burn Care Res 32:1-5, 2011

Altered pharmacokinetics in critically ill patients have been shown to result in inadequate enoxaparin dosing for venous thromboembolism (VTE) prophylaxis. In the burn unit, routine monitoring of antifactor Xa levels was implemented to ensure adequate VTE prophylaxis. The purpose of this study was to examine the appropriateness of enoxaparin dosing for VTE prophylaxis in this specialized patient population. The authors reviewed patients with acute burn injury from June 1, 2009, to October 20, 2009, who had enoxaparin therapy monitored with antifactor Xa levels. Data collection occurred prospectively. Thirty-eight patients received enoxaparin subcutaneously for prophylaxis of VTE and had antifactor Xa levels measured. Thirty (79%) patients had initial antifactor Xa levels less than 0.2 U/ml. Enoxaparin dosages were subsequently increased as needed to achieve antifactor Xa levels of 0.2 to 0.4 U/ml. Eight of 38 patients never achieved goal antifactor Xa level before enoxaparin was discontinued. The median final dose required to achieve an antifactor Xa level within therapeutic range was 50 mg every 12 hours (range 30–70 mg). In linear regression, final enoxaparin dose correlated with TBSA. Two patients had clinically significant thromboembolic events. There were no documented episodes of significant hemorrhage, thrombocytopenia, or heparin-associated allergy. The low antifactor Xa levels observed in this study demonstrate that standard dosing of enoxaparin for VTE prophylaxis is inadequate for patients with acute burns. In these patients, both a higher initial enoxaparin dose and routine monitoring of antifactor Xa levels are recommended.

▶ This study is the first to examine venous thromboembolic disease/events (VTE) in burn patients from an antifactor Xa perspective. The burn patient population seems to be a high-risk population, with VTE rates dependent on how hard you look. The authors theorize that if VTE prophylaxis is targeted toward normal antifactor Xa levels, there will be fewer VTEs. Interestingly, 79% of patients had initial subtherapeutic antifactor Xa levels, and 8 of 38 patients never achieved goal levels of antifactor Xa.

Some of my concerns with the study include the timing to stop enoxaparin (is ambulating 3 times a day up and down the hallway adequate in this patient population with increased VTE risk?). Nothing in the burn patient responds this quickly to interventions, so why do the authors study VTE prophylaxis on such a short-term interventional basis? With this small study size, there was 1 deep vein thrombosis (DVT) and 1 pulmonary embolism (PE). Is this rate acceptable in patients with an average burn size of 14% total body surface area? Another concern is that we do not know the VTE requirements as patients healed during the study and the burn wound surface area became smaller. Finally, this study is very small and may simply be underpowered to detect a clinically significant finding.

Lin et al found that a higher initial enoxaparin dose is required than that required for a standard surgical patient. Additionally, the enoxaparin dose was held on the morning of surgery, and sometimes the evening of surgery as well. Time of immobility on the operating room table is the exact time when a patient is at high risk for VTE development. I do not recommend holding the enoxaparin dosing for burn/wound procedures or operative interventions, even the day of surgery.

Enoxaparin dosing correlated with burn size, not patient weight, yet current standard enoxaparin dosing for nonburn patients with a body mass index greater than 30 is weight based. Although this study is not designed or powered to answer the question of VTE prophylaxis and patient size, it is an important question that remains to be answered. This is a great first study examining our practice patterns based on antifactor Xa levels. A larger multi-institutional study that can address the appropriate dosing scheme for enoxaparin should be undertaken. All patients will have to be screened for DVT at regular intervals for subclinical DVT/PE.

B. A. Latenser, MD, FACS

The Effect of Ketamine Administration on Nocturnal Sleep Architecture

Gottschlich MM, Mayes T, Khoury J, et al (Shriners Hosps for Children, Cincinnati, OH; Cincinnati Children's Hosp Med Ctr, OH; et al)

J Burn Care Res 32:535-540, 2011

Substantial evidence exists in the acute, rehabilitative and outpatient settings demonstrating the presence of significant sleep pattern disturbances after burn injury. Although the etiology is multifactorial and includes environmental, injury, and treatment mediators, previous clinical studies have not analyzed the critically important relationship of various medications to sleep architecture. The purpose of this investigation was to describe the after-effect of ketamine on sleep patterns in seriously ill burn patients. Forty pediatric patients with a mean TBSA burn of 50.1 ± 2.9% (range, 22–89%) and full-thickness injury of 43.2 ± 3.6% (range, 24–89%) were enrolled in this sleep study. Twenty-three of the 40 patients received ketamine on the day of polysomnography testing. Standard polysomnographic sleep variables were measured from 10:00 PM until 7:00 AM. Chi-square test and *t*-test were used for comparison of descriptive variables between the ketamine and nonketamine groups. A logarithmic transformation was used for analysis when necessary. Ketamine administration was associated with reduced rapid eye movement (REM) sleep when compared with patients who did not receive ketamine on the day of the sleep study ($P < 0.04$). Both ketamine and nonketamine groups were clearly REM deficient when compared with nonburn norms. There was no relationship between ketamine use and effect on nocturnal total sleep time, number of awakenings, or percent of time awake or in stage 1, 2, or 3 + 4 sleep. In conclusion, ketamine was associated with altered sleep architecture as evidenced by a reduction in REM sleep. This finding does not seem to be clinically significant when considering the magnitude of overall REM sleep pattern disturbance observed in both the ketamine and nonketamine groups compared with nonburn norms. Further research is required to identify potential mechanisms of disturbed sleep so that appropriate interventions can be developed.

▶ This prospective, randomized trial examined the after effects of ketamine administration in pediatric patients with very large thermal injuries (average burn size 50% total body surface area). Rapid eye movement (REM) sleep was compared in patients given ketamine with patients who did not receive ketamine on the day of study. Technicians performing the polysomnography and physicians were blinded to the experimental conditions. Although both groups of patients were REM sleep deficient compared with nonburned patients, the ketamine group had statistically significantly reduced REM sleep compared with the nonketamine group. Ketamine did not affect the total sleep time, number of awakenings, or percentage of time awake. The question must be asked: what is the clinical significance of these findings? Most people wake up 1 or 2 times every night, but these burn patients awakened an average of 24 times per night, with or without ketamine. They had more sleep during the day, which was not studied. The authors conclude that the ketamine effect on REM sleep is not significant because the patients spend so little time in REM sleep; therefore, the effect on overall sleep is not significant. This conclusion may understate the effect of ketamine on sleep disturbances in pediatric burn patients with large burns. However, the utility of ketamine in pediatric as well as adult burn patients for procedural sedation, augmentation of narcotics, and use during general anesthetic continues to grow as practitioners become aware of the benefits. I would encourage burn care practitioners not familiar with this therapy to incorporate it into their practice.

B. A. Latenser, MD, FACS

A Blinded, Randomized Controlled Trial to Evaluate Ketamine/Propofol Versus Ketamine Alone for Procedural Sedation in Children

Shah A, Mosdossy G, McLeod S, et al (The Univ of Western Ontario, London, Ontario, Canada)

Ann Emerg Med 57:425-433, 2011

Study Objective.—The primary objective is to compare total sedation time when ketamine/propofol is used compared with ketamine alone for pediatric procedural sedation and analgesia. Secondary objectives include time to recovery, adverse events, efficacy, and satisfaction scores.

Methods.—Children (aged 2 to 17 years) requiring procedural sedation and analgesia for management of an isolated orthopedic extremity injury were randomized to receive either ketamine/propofol or ketamine. Physicians, nurses, research assistants, and patients were blinded. Ketamine/propofol patients received an initial intravenous bolus dose of ketamine 0.5 mg/kg and propofol 0.5 mg/kg, followed by propofol 0.5 mg/kg and saline solution placebo every 2 minutes, titrated to deep sedation. Ketamine patients received an initial intravenous bolus dose of ketamine 1.0 mg/kg and Intralipid placebo, followed by ketamine 0.25 mg/kg and Intralipid placebo every 2 minutes, as required.

Results.—One hundred thirty-six patients (67 ketamine/propofol, 69 ketamine) completed the trial. Median total sedation time was shorter ($P=0.04$) with ketamine/propofol (13 minutes) than with ketamine (16 minutes) alone (Δ −3 minutes; 95% confidence interval [CI] −5 to −2 minutes). Median recovery time was faster with ketamine/propofol (10 minutes) than with ketamine (12 minutes) alone (Δ −2 minutes; 95% CI −4 to −1 minute). There was less vomiting in the ketamine/propofol (2%) group compared with the ketamine (12%) group (Δ −10%; 95% CI −18% to −2%). All satisfaction scores were higher ($P<0.05$) with ketamine/propofol.

Conclusion.—When compared with ketamine alone for pediatric orthopedic reductions, the combination of ketamine and propofol produced

slightly faster recoveries while also demonstrating less vomiting, higher satisfaction scores, and similar efficacy and airway complications.

▶ Procedural sedation is commonly performed in the emergency department. Every physician tries to achieve a level of sedation that allows the procedure to be completed successfully while minimizing complications and maximizing efficacy of patient throughput. This was a well designed prospective randomized trial comparing ketamine alone to a combination of ketamine and propofol (ketofol) for orthopedic procedures in a pediatric population. Ketofol was better in all aspects: shorter sedation by 3 minutes, quicker recovery by 2 minutes, less vomiting by 10%, and better satisfaction scores among patients, nurses, and physicians. There were similar small numbers of respiratory depression/apnea/desaturation among both groups with no serious adverse outcomes. This article is an important piece of a growing body of evidence to support the use of ketofol (at an initial dose of 0.5 mg/kg ketamine and 0.5 mg/kg propofol) for procedural sedation in the emergency department. We have instituted it as an option for physicians, with pharmacy premixing ketofol to avoid the extra time it would take for the nurse to complete this step.

M. D. Zwank, MD

Article Index

Chapter 1: Airways/Lungs

Chapter 2: Cardiovascular

Chapter 3: Hemodynamics and Monitoring

Chapter 4: Burns

Chapter 5: Infectious Disease

Chapter 6: Postoperative Management

Chapter 7: Sepsis/Septic Shock

Chapter 8: Metabolism/Gastrointestinal/Nutrition/Hematology-Oncology

Chapter 9: Trauma and Overdose

Chapter 10: Neurologic: Traumatic and Non-traumatic

Chapter 11: Ethics/Socioeconomic/Administrative Issues

Chapter 12: Pharmacology/Sedation-Analgesia

Author Index

U

V

W

X

Y

Z

Printed and bound by CPI Group (UK) Ltd, Croydon, CR0 4YY
08/05/2025
01864678-0019